Exploring School Counseling
Professional Practices and Perspectives

Tamara E. Davis
Marymount University

Lahaska Press
Houghton Mifflin Company
BOSTON   NEW YORK

Publisher: Barry Fetterolf
Development Editor: Mary Falcon
Editorial Assistant: Lisa Minter
Senior Project Editor: Tracy Patruno
Manufacturing Coordinator: Priscilla Bailey
Marketing Manager: Brenda L. Bravener-Greville

Cover image: © Stephanie Carter/Photodisc Green

Lahaska Press, a unique collaboration between the Houghton Mifflin College Division and Lawrence Erlbaum Associates, is dedicated to publishing books and offering services for the academic and professional counseling communities. The partnership of Lahaska Press was formed in late 1999. The name "Lahaska" is a Native American Lenape word meaning "source of many writings." The small eastern Pennsylvania town of Lahaska, named by the Lenape, is the home of the Lahaska Press editorial offices.

Printed in the U.S.A.

Library of Congress Control Number: 2002109427

ISBN: 0-618-19145-3

23456789-QWF-09 08 07 06 05

CONTENTS

iii

10   The Professional School Counselor as Leader   215

11   The School Counselor as Responsive Leader: School Violence Prevention and Crisis Intervention   235

12 The School Counselor and Advocacy: Taking a Stand   258

13 The School Counselor and Results-Based Accountability   275

PREFACE

This book offers a unique perspective to graduate students in school counselor training programs. The role of school counselors is constantly being transformed, and it is critical to have an understanding, both personally and professionally, of the many roles and responsibilities that school counselors assume in schools. As you develop your personal and professional philosophy about school counseling, it will be helpful to explore and reflect on the practices and perspectives of experts in the field. School counselors are in a unique position to provide support for students as they develop personally, socially, emotionally, and academically throughout their school careers.

Throughout this book, you will read about the practices and perspectives of school counselors, counselor educators, and researchers in the field of school counseling. Included in the text, in elements entitled "My Story," are my own experiences as a school counselor, and it might be helpful to explore what brought me to school counseling in order to get a sense of my perspective on school counseling programs and practices.

I never intended to become a school counselor. Throughout my life, I wanted to be an elementary school teacher and then an elementary school administrator. I pursued a master's degree in school counseling because I knew that a graduate degree would help me get hired as a school teacher, and school counseling seemed to be an interesting blend of education and psychology. What a surprise when I realized that school counseling was a better fit for me! After being a teacher for three years, I found that I was most concerned about the social and emotional well-being of my students. This realization prompted me to move into a job as a school counselor. I knew that I had found my niche. It seemed that it was my calling to work with students on the issues and situations that were their reality. I believe in the goals of education, yet it seemed that students were often so distracted by their life circumstances that they could not focus on becoming effective learners. Helping them work through their difficulties was the most rewarding thing I will probably ever do. So, even though school counseling was not my intended career, it has been the one that has taught me the most about people and about myself. Having the opportunity as a counselor educator to teach others to become effective school counselors actually combines the best of both worlds. However, not a day goes by that I don't miss the day-to-day interactions with students in schools. I remedy this by focusing on school counselors-in-training, with the hope that providing appropriate training for them will result in positive school counseling programs and services for the students, schools, and communities they will serve.

Acknowledgements

I would like to thank many people who were integral to the development and completion of this book. First, the professional school counselors who contributed their practices and perspectives throughout the book added tremendous insight and depth to the chapters. These outstanding practitioners are Renee Orlosky, an elementary school counselor in Fairfax County Public Schools in Virginia; Beth Graney, a middle school counselor and guidance director in Prince William County Schools, Virginia; and Esther Pincus, a high school counselor also in Fairfax County Public Schools. These professionals are truly exemplary in the work they do with students every day. I am awed and amazed by their contributions to students. Second, the contributing professionals for chapters 10, 12, and 13 provided useful information on the transformed roles of school counselors as we move into an exciting time for the profession. Chapter 10, a chapter on the school counselor's leadership role, is contributed by a group of counselor educators that have been heavily involved in recent initiatives that seek to transform the role of school counselors. These counselor educators are Dr. Paul L. Phillips, State University of West Georgia; Dr. Susan Sears, Ohio State University; and Dr. Brent M. Snow and Dr. C. Marie Jackson, State University of West Georgia. Chapter 12 contains a contribution on the topic of school counselors and advocacy from Dr. C. Marie Jackson, State University of West Georgia. Chapter 13 includes a practical approach toward data and accountability that is based on the ASCA National Model and was contributed by Dr. Pamelia Brott, Virginia Polytechnic Institute and State University. The knowledge and insight of these counselor educators contributed immeasurably to the book.

My gratitude goes to the many counselor educators who reviewed the text and gave encouragement, support, and suggestions for improvement during the revisions of the book. The manuscript reviewers included:

Laurie Carlson, Colorado State University

Roberto Clemente, University of Northern Iowa

Teddi Cunningham, Valdosta State University

Claire Cole Curcio, Virginia Polytechnic Institute and State University

M. Sylvia Fernandez, Barry University

Thomas F. Holcombe, Murray State University

C. Marie Jackson, State University of West Georgia

Francis Martin, South Dakota State University

Amy Milson, Iowa State University

Jean Peterson, Purdue University

A. Renee Staton, James Madison University

Thanks as well to my graduate students in school counseling, who, over the last two years, added great insight and material to help develop the examples and cases in the book. The sharing of their "stories" as they progressed through practicum and internships facilitated the development of the manuscript. In terms of book preparation, special acknowledgement goes to Lari Bishop and Michele Chancellor, production managers at Leyh Publishing, who made the final process manageable and enjoyable. I would also like to thank Barry Fetterolf, publisher of Lahaska Press, and Mary Falcon, my editor, who were willing to take a chance on a new author and provided invaluable insight, expertise, and encouragement all along the way.

Most importantly, I would like to thank my mother, Nell Davis, who always understood when I didn't have time to talk on the phone because it was a "writing day," and who always taught me to "bloom where planted," wherever that may be. In that same vein, I thank my husband and best friend, Kenny Kratzer, who understood that I often had to be glued to the computer, reading research, or making changes to the book rather than sharing time with him. He epitomizes the best in counselors, and I dedicate this book to his patience and perseverance as well as his infinite, unconditional love and support.

I hope that this book is the beginning of a meaningful career for you as a school counselor and that students are inspired by your dedication to them and to the field of school counseling.

Exploring School Counseling

CHAPTER **1**

Choosing School Counseling as a Career: A New Chapter in Your Story

*I*f you are reading this book, you are probably seriously contemplating either beginning or making a transition to a career as a school counselor. You may already be in a school counseling graduate program and are preparing for your practicum or internship. You may be a teacher coming into school counseling as a career change, or a mental health counselor seeking to change your specialty. Perhaps you are exploring new career possibilities. Regardless of your path, it is important to reflect on the life experiences that have influenced your decision to consider school counseling as a career.

Each person's life is an unfolding story, with new chapters beginning throughout. In one chapter of your life, you may have encountered a school counselor. Did you have a positive experience with a school counselor and now want to have the same impact on students? Did you have a negative experience with a school counselor and now feel the need to provide a better experience for students? Did your child receive help from a middle school counselor when being bullied? As a parent or student, did a high school counselor help you find college scholarships? If you are a teacher, do you understand the vital role of school counselors because of a negative or positive experience with school counseling colleagues? If you are in a school counseling training program, your peers' stories may be similar to or different from yours, but the desire to become a school counselor is a common bond among you.

FEATURE 1.1

Comments of Graduate Students in School Counseling

- "I feel kids need someone on their side to listen, understand, and fight for their voices to be heard. I want to be that person."
- "Since the shootings at Columbine High School, I have become very concerned with the culture our kids are being raised in, and I want to be part of the solution."
- "I want to be in a position to be an advocate for students. I think counselors have such a wide spectrum of responsibilities that enable them to help students in a variety of ways."
- "In my student teaching, I realized that the most meaningful and enjoyable parts of my day were the interactions with the children— building relationships and helping them overcome any obstacles, social or educational, they encountered."
- "I'd also like to change the stereotype that school counselors seem to have—that they don't help kids. It's simply not true."
- "I hope to be able to help students and families achieve their fullest potential through the services I provide."

Many school counselors-in-training arrive at this decision-making crossroad for a variety of reasons.

Feature 1.1 displays the comments of graduate students in their first year of a graduate program in school counseling. These statements came from people who were in your situation not long ago; perhaps you can relate to their reasons for wanting to become school counselors. You are probably pursuing this career because you have realized that a school counselor is in an ideal position to positively influence the lives of students. You are pursuing this goal with great commitment and are challenged to learn more about this career. Welcome—you are exactly where you need to be!

Meet the Professional School Counselors

Throughout this book, you will read the comments and perspectives of three currently practicing school counselors who, combined, have almost 50 years of experience working with students. It seems essential that, as school counselors-in-training, you consider the knowledge of veterans who have been in the field for many years. Their comments are interspersed throughout each chapter, and they are identified as Renee (ES) [elementary school], Beth (MS) [middle school], and Esther (HS) [high school].

Renee Orlosky (ES)

Renee has a Master of Arts in Counselor Education from Wake Forest University. She was an elementary school counselor in Manassas City Public Schools in Virginia for nine years and has been an elementary school counselor in Fairfax County Public Schools since 1999. Known for her creative counseling skills, Renee has presented at local, state, and national conferences and has served as a supervisor for field experiences, practicum, and internship students from local universities.

Personal Reflection

RENEE (ES)

Why I Chose to Become a School Counselor

I was a Psychology major working on my undergraduate degree. I had never even thought of going into education as a career path. I took an education psychology class that required that we spend a certain number of hours in a local school. I was sent to a local elementary school. After a few weeks, I was hooked. I decided to find a way to use my psychology background and to work in a school. School counseling was a natural fit. I like the variety of what I do each day. I also enjoy working with so many different kids. It helps to be around kids who are well adjusted *and* those experiencing some sort of diffi-culty. You wouldn't have exposure to so many different kids in other counseling specialty areas.

Beth Graney (MS)

Prior to becoming a counselor, Beth was a teacher who taught grades 6 through 12 for twelve years in the Midwest. Beth has been a counselor for 15 years and was the elementary and secondary school counselor for a rural school system for two years. In Virginia, Beth has also been a mental health counselor and is a Licensed Professional Counselor. Beth was named the Virginia Middle School Counselor of the Year in 1992 and again in 1998. She is currently a middle school guidance director in Prince William County Public Schools and has a private practice working primarily with women and adolescents.

Personal Reflection

BETH (MS)

Why I Chose to Become a School Counselor

As a counselor in a kindergarten through 12th grade setting, I worked as an ele-mentary school counselor and then moved into high school counseling, including college prep; but mostly I've been at the middle school level. I think it's the job that fits my personality best. It's what I've been drawn to all my life. As the middle child, I was always the counselor and mediator in the family. Then when I went to college, I was a Resident Assistant. I've always been drawn to jobs where I was working with people. First I wanted to be a nurse because I liked the medical aspect. I think I was confused about what part of the body I wanted to work with, but I eventually decided on the head. I did like teaching, but I found that many times I was just as interested in the social and emotional factors as I was in the academic.

Esther Pincus (HS)

Esther began her work in education in Virginia more than thirty years ago. She taught German in middle school and moved to high school in the early 1980s as a counselor and career specialist. In 2003, she celebrated 20 years as a high school counselor in Fairfax County Public Schools. In addition, Esther has been very active in the Virginia Association for Specialists in Group Work, serving as president from 1998 to 2000, and she remains active on the Board of Directors. Known for her outstanding service to students, faculty, parents, and community, Esther received an American Counseling Association Professional Development Award in 2000. She serves as a role model for school counselors-in-training from local colleges and universities.

Personal Reflection

ESTHER (HS)

Why I Chose to Become a School Counselor

My family history has had a profound influence on my values and my personal choice to become a school counselor. Because both my parents were Holocaust survivors, they suffered great losses during World War II. They lost immediate and extended family members, all their property and possessions, and their freedom. As a result, I vowed to uphold the dignity and worth of every human being. When we are negatively influenced, humanity and even civilization as we know it changes drastically. Everyone has the capacity for tremendous good and evil. Counselors who value humanity work toward ensuring that every generation is allowed to experience positive potential. Counselors nourish humanity. Without the caring and support of school counselors, personal dignity and human worth can be lost.

In addition to the comments of Renee, Beth, and Esther, you will also read about my experiences as an elementary and high school counselor during my nine years as a practitioner. These excerpts are entitled "My Story" and will hopefully provide further insight into the profession of school counseling.

While the experiences and perspectives of four school counselors cannot be generalized or encompass the vast and varied experiences of all school counselors, it is important to learn about school counselors who are still passionate and committed to providing effective services. Consider each perspective and practice as one way of thinking or doing things; more importantly, think about how you might perceive, handle, or respond to the same situation. The shared experiences are intended to be a thought-provoking catalyst for your personal and professional development. Some of the perspectives or practices may not follow the school counseling policies in your state; there is great variation between states, within states, and even within school districts. Use the situations as a springboard to talk with counselor educators and peers about the differences and similarities and to integrate new ideas into your own personal and professional philosophy.

At the end of each chapter, and sometimes at the end of a section, there are Reflection and Discussion questions for you to consider both personally and professionally. Some chapters have more opportunities than others for reflection and discussion because of the topics that are covered. It will be helpful to discuss your thoughts and responses to these questions with peers in order to gain other perspectives and ideas about school counseling. It is my hope that the situations and topics presented in this book will guide you into a new understanding of and appreciation for the role of school counselors and will also enable you to embrace the opportunities and challenges that await you.

A Career in School Counseling: Opportunities and Challenges

There are many reasons for wanting to pursue a career as a school counselor, and it is critical to consider the many roles of school counselors prior to entering the profession. The purpose of this book is to explore this topic and try to answer the following questions: What is the role of professional school counselors in the educational mission of schools today? How are students better prepared for life as a result of school counseling programs? An exploration of traditional roles and the transformed roles of 21st century school counselors will demonstrate that this is an exciting time to enter this profession. However, it is important to first explore the opportunities and challenges that a career in school counseling offers. Table 1.1 lists a few of these opportunities and challenges, and the following sections discuss them to help you better understand the school counseling job.

Opportunities as a School Counselor

Perhaps now more than ever, school counselors have opportunities to advocate and demonstrate the important ways that they contribute to student success. Personal motivation for school counselors might be found in the special opportunities to impact the lives of children, including helping today's youth, providing a path and tools for success, being a positive role model, and feeling that you've made a difference.

HELPING TODAY'S YOUTH   Youth today face a variety of challenges. Do you have an understanding of children in schools today? What is your perception of "at-risk" youth? What would you describe as a problem that might be prevalent with students? Are you informed about the issues that affect schools? The issues youth face and the challenges that daily influence their lives are indeed causes for concern. The decision to pursue school counseling in order to help youth deal with these challenges is a worthwhile goal. One reality that draws people to the profession is the feeling that youth have unique needs that require a great deal of support and attention in today's society. Because much of a child's day is spent in school, counselors become the obvious support personnel to address these needs. School counseling research (Borders & Drury, 1992; Whiston & Sexton, 1998) has indicated that school counseling services positively impact students.

When making this career choice, it is important to examine your response to the challenges students face today. How would you respond to a student who tells you she is pregnant? What reaction might you have to a student who threatens to harm himself or herself, or others? What about situations that are less urgent but are also detrimental to educational achievement, such as a student who is being bullied or having friendship issues? Or a student who is gay or lesbian and wants to come out to his or her peers? While the latter problems

TABLE 1.1
Opportunities and Challenges of the School Counseling Profession

Opportunities	Challenges
Helping today's youth	Personal time and schedule demands
Providing a path and tools for success	Noncounseling duties related to role confusion
Being a positive role model	Taking work home: separating personal and professional life
Feeling that you've made a difference	Getting a job: timing and preparation

may not demand immediate action, they are nonetheless important to the students with the problems. Some situations are difficult to handle; some are more clear-cut. The degree of risk and the extent of support may vary, but school counselors provide essential services to assure that our youth have the best chance possible to become effective learners and productive members of society. Whether it is connecting a student to the appropriate resources or counseling a student on developing resiliency and coping skills, you have a unique opportunity to help young people in schools.

Professional Perspective

BETH (MS)

The reward of being a school counselor is the kids . . . working with kids. Even after all these years, I still have days when I just think, "Wow! Kids are great." It's just so much fun working with them and they have such a delightful way of seeing life. Students spend a significant portion of their time in school, and to know that somebody is there to help you is a big and important thing in a student's life.

Lapan, Gysbers, and Sun (1997) found that schools that implemented a comprehensive school counseling program had the following outcomes: (a) higher student academic achievement, (b) greater student access to career and college information, and (c) a more positive school climate, including increased feelings of belonging and safety (pp. 299–300). Clearly, the assistance provided by school counselors and the implementation of effective and comprehensive school counseling programs is a catalyst for increased success in student development.

PROVIDING A PATH AND TOOLS FOR SUCCESS   The business of school counselors is helping students become effective lifelong learners. The development of National Standards for School Counseling (Campbell & Dahir, 1997) has helped focus the role of school counselors and has provided a path and guide for the goals of successful counseling programs. The focus on the academic, personal/social, and career development of students is related to the overall success of their academic experience. School counselors help students develop skills in all areas, including study skills, social skills, and life skills.

The developmental nature and scope of a comprehensive school counseling program cannot be overstated. School counselor training programs naturally include coursework in human development, with an emphasis on child and adolescent development. Being knowledgeable about the developmental characteristics and stages of children as they grow is an important consideration when planning and implementing school counseling programs. "The developmental program is proactive and preventive, helping students acquire the knowledge, skills, self-awareness, and attitudes necessary for successful mastery of normal developmental tasks" (Borders & Drury, 1992, p. 488).

Skill development may not be an obvious task of school counselors, but it is a large part of the overall school counseling program. The appeal of this opportunity is to help students develop skills that will benefit them in school and in life. One exciting aspect is the variety of methods school counselors can employ to develop these skills: classroom guidance with an entire class of students, group counseling with a small number of students, or individual counseling that focuses on specific tasks and behaviors. Whether in a classroom doing career interest inventories on the computer or working one-on-one to improve test-taking skills, the school counselor provides significant skill development activities.

Professional Perspective

ESTHER (HS)

Counselors contribute to the development of students in several ways:

1. *Counselors promote and observe positive growth.* As a counselor, you get to see student progress and even tremendous change over the course of a few years. Counselors serve as student mentors during a time of critical decision-making, thereby encouraging and fostering personal and academic growth.

2. *Counselors help students broaden their personal perspective.* By shedding light on various options, providing career direction, and expanding educational horizons, counselors help students recognize their academic and career potential.

3. *Counselors assist students in successfully addressing emotional and developmental concerns.* Students grow in self-confidence and develop a mature perspective; they become problem-solvers and look for resources and options.

BEING A POSITIVE ROLE MODEL   School counselors are in a pivotal position to positively influence students, teachers, administrators, parents, and community members. Many situations and interactions necessitate the presence of a person who can effectively respond in a way that is objective, positive, and beneficial for everyone involved. While not all school counselors are model counselors, it is possible and even necessary to change the image that many in our society have of school counselors. As a school counselor-in-training, you can change the negative image that some have of school counselors by demonstrating leadership, action, and accountability.

As a school counselor-in-training, everything you do or say reflects on the profession of school counseling. Within this field, you will find tremendous support among your peers and a wonderful atmosphere of collegiality in most circumstances. Given recent national and international events, there is greater support at the state and federal levels for programs for students. This reflects a positive transition that has exciting implications for school counseling as a profession.

FEELING THAT YOU HAVE MADE A DIFFERENCE It seems a bit cliché to say that you want to be a school counselor so that you and others can feel good, but it is an important part of the equation. You should find great fulfillment in knowing that a young person has benefited from interacting with you. This feeling is called the "Ah-HA" moment. It is the moment when a student comes by or drops you a note just to say, "Thanks, you really helped." It is overhearing students repeating something they learned in a classroom guidance lesson, transferring and using that information in an everyday situation. It is watching the student you feared might not graduate walk across the stage and get a high school diploma, knowing that, in some way, you helped make that happen.

Another key moment in the professional lives of counselors is what may be called the "counselable" moment. You may have heard of the teachable moment—the opportunity to teach a student something that will be relevant and meaningful. Similarly, the counselable moment is the opportunity to reinforce a skill or provide an example so that a student can find personal meaning in that moment. For example, if a student comes to the school counselor and is disheartened because of a difficulty that seems insurmountable, the school counselor can help the student identify innate qualities and characteristics that might help overcome the obstacle. Sometimes students simply need someone to shed light on or clarify a situation in order to realize that they have the capacity to address issues on their own; sometimes they just need a little hope.

Professional Perspective

ESTHER (HS)

Counselors instill hope. Students who face life with the knowledge that eventually things have to get better can cope with even the most difficult circumstances. Students develop resilience and draw on reserves of which they may not have been aware.

It would be misleading to insinuate that the profession of school counseling is always positive and never challenging. The reality is that sometimes the job can be overwhelming and somewhat frustrating. It is important to consider these challenges prior to entering the field in order to develop effective coping strategies for dealing with the adversity that sometimes arises.

Challenges as a School Counselor

Exploring some of the challenges of a career in school counseling will offer a realistic perspective on the job. While the challenges presented here are not present in every school counseling job, school counselors in the field often cite them as concerns.

PERSONAL TIME AND SCHEDULE DEMANDS   School counseling is a career that demands much personal, professional, and emotional energy, and one must be committed to the goals, roles, and mission of school counseling in order to be effective. Because of the time constraints and schedule demands, it is important to consider the potential impact of becoming a school counselor on the other roles in one's personal life. It is not unusual for someone to decide on a career in education because the schedule seems to fit well with other family and personal roles. Women, and often men, have traditionally chosen teaching because it is a career that is conducive to the dual-career professional—educator and parent. It is absolutely feasible to be a parent and a school counselor; many people do it, and do it well, every day. However, the unpredictability of a school counselor's work schedule, coupled with the demands of life outside of work, can be a huge stressor, which may ultimately lead to burnout. Consider this example:

> *You are a parent of three who has chosen school counseling as your profession. Your children (ages 7, 10, and 13) all attend school in your school district. The starting time of the middle school your 13-year-old attends is a little earlier than the starting time of the elementary school your 7-year-old and 10-year-old attend. This works perfectly in your schedule because the 13-year-old rides the bus and you can drop off your other two children on your way to work. Great! However, after-school scheduling becomes an issue. Invariably, two to three days each week you have either a parent conference or a committee meeting after school. Your middle school child has music lessons across town at 4:00 p.m., and though your contract hours end at 3:45 p.m., a parent has called you for consultation after school and your principal is waiting to follow-up with you about a social services referral you made earlier in the day. In the meantime, your two children who attend the elementary school are waiting for you to pick them up. So, all three children are waiting for you, the principal is waiting for you, social services is on hold, and you are on the phone.*

Avoidable? Perhaps. Possible? Absolutely! The school counselor's day often begins earlier and extends later than the scheduled workday. Because of the unpredictability of the school counselor's day, activities such as returning phone calls or e-mails and consulting with parents, teachers, and administrators may occur outside of school hours. This is not to say that school counselors cannot walk away when their contract hours have been fulfilled. As in any profession, one may be able to balance the realities of life and family with career in a very effective manner. However, the unpredictability and spontaneity of the school counselor's day may sometimes require time beyond work hours. While some might view this as an imposition, it is also the appeal of the career for many people: the spontaneity of the unknown challenges within the structure of the school setting. Being aware of this necessary flexibility is integral to choosing a career in school counseling.

In addition, it should be noted that middle and high school counselors often are 11-month or 12-month employees, which means they report back to work up to one month prior to the return of the other school faculty and may also work a period of time past the end of the school year. Depending on your life circumstances, you must take these issues into consideration when deciding if school counseling is a good fit for you. Are there personal or life situations, such as child care arrangements or summer employment, that favor your working a 10-month schedule? The extended schedule may also be viewed as a positive situation in that the school counselor has time to get organized, making the beginning or ending of school go more smoothly. When thinking about your career as a school counselor, also consider the realistic challenges that come with this career in light of your life circumstances. Dealing with these challenges prior to securing a position as a school counselor will alleviate some of the stress and anxiety you might experience if unprepared.

TAKING WORK HOME: SEPARATING PERSONAL AND PROFESSIONAL LIFE   Chapter 14 discusses the types of stressors that often contribute to school counselor burnout and this challenge may be at the top of the list. School counselors tend to be nurturing, caring people who want only the best for others, particularly our students. It is easy to get caught up in the emotional situations that students encounter. It is extremely difficult to know that a child is dealing with or living with circumstances that are (a) out of his or her control and (b) not likely to change. Because school counselors are often privy to private information about students, it is often hard to be detached when students leave the building.

Some students have difficult life situations, such as poverty, neglect, substance abuse, and lack of supervision. These circumstances motivate school counselors to fight for the rights of students, not only as members of the educational system, but also as members of humanity. School counselors are champions for the causes that support the physical, emotional, social, and academic development of students. Taking work home is draining, but it also serves as a reminder that the well-being and healthy development of students is a priority.

My Story

My least favorite part of the school counseling job was making a referral to Child Protective Services. Of course I knew that if I suspected abuse or neglect, I had an ethical and legal obligation to report it to the proper authorities. It wasn't that I didn't want to make the call in order to protect the child, but there were some cases where I wondered if making the call would make the situation worse for the child. I knew that a Department of Social Services worker might visit the house, and I knew that there were measures that would be taken to protect the child. While this should have been reassuring, I often felt unsettled because I didn't know what might happen. It was not unusual for a student to say: "Please don't call . . . I'll just get in more trouble after they leave." There were many long nights after I had made a report when I wondered what was happening and if the child was safe. Dinners often went untouched (sometimes even uncooked) when I could not get the worrisome images out of my head and, more often, out of my heart. Of course, I had talked with the student about what to do if he or she was frightened and who to call when in danger. Somehow, that gave me little comfort as I sat at home with my family. I'm happy to say that nothing catastrophic happened in any case that I reported, but it still made for some very long and emotional evenings. It was comforting to know that I had done what I needed to do in order to protect the best interest of the child and I could only hope that the intervention would have positive results for the child and for the family.

Professional Perspective

RENEE (ES)

You have to learn to separate yourself from the job while still being an involved and caring person who is invested in your students. Sometimes you feel like you don't have the answer, but everyone is counting on you. As long as you do what is in the best interest of the student, then you've been true to your professional and personal responsibilities. It takes some time to learn this . . . and then there are still days when you go home praying that you did the right thing.

NONCOUNSELING DUTIES As a school counselor, there may be duties and activities that do not fall into the category of direct counseling services. It seems that some school counselors have minimal noncounseling responsibilities, while others may spend more time on noncounseling duties than on providing direct services. Many factors influence the amount of and expectation for noncounseling duties. For example, an administrator's perspective of appropriate roles for school counselors, number of other personnel available to do tasks, and the way things have been done historically may influence a school counselor's noncounseling responsibilities.

Professional Perspective

ESTHER (HS)

Paperwork and record keeping take counselors away from direct contact with students. Counselors must keep detailed records and some form of documentation on their student, parent, and administrative contacts. They may also spend countless hours checking on graduation credits, filing test results, report cards, and transcripts.

Noncounseling duties may also include what Gysbers and Henderson (2000) referred to as "fair-share responsibilities," (p. 76) such as bus duty, lunch duty, and hall duty. Test coordination and/or participation in standardized testing are also cited as time-consuming noncounseling duties that many school counselors perform. A discussion of noncounseling duties is included in chapter 4.

In general, school counselors have the opportunity to provide needed counseling services. However, there are days when counseling students falls second to chaperoning a field trip or conducting make-up tests. As members of an education team, counselors often take this in stride. Because counselors typically have flexible schedules, they may be among the first school personnel to be asked to cover classes, proctor tests, or oversee their schools while administrators are out. Consider this situation:

In her first year as an elementary school counselor, Laura was told she would have to teach a one and a half hour reading block for the lower grade students on a daily basis. She had no teaching experience and felt she should not be asked to do this; in addition, she knew that taking 90 minutes from her schedule would interfere with her ability to provide appropriate counseling services. She had two options: (a) teach the reading block as assigned, or (b) let the principal know of her concerns about how this assignment would interfere with her other duties. After much thought, she chose the latter and explained to the administrator that having this responsibility would negatively impact the students since she would not be available to provide needed counseling services during this time. As a first-year counselor, she took a chance on being perceived as defiant and/or not being a "team" player, but the principal accepted her position and respected her right to say no. While this situation worked to the advantage of this counselor (and the students), there are times when counseling services may not be given highest priority.

Dealing with extra duties often comes with the territory of being in an education system. While these duties should not be a deterrent to becoming a school counselor, you should be aware of the noncounseling responsibilities that might be expected. You can hope that the noncounseling responsibilities will be minimal and the emphasis in your school counseling program is on providing direct counseling services. Educating others about the important counseling services you provide is one way to proactively address the time consumed by noncounseling responsibilities.

On the positive side, school counselors can look for opportunities to provide counseling services within noncounseling duties. School counselors can use these duties as a time to check in with students. Having a duty period is one way to get a feel for the pulse of what is going on with students. A brief interaction with a student during bus duty or cafeteria duty might indicate that the school counselor needs to meet with the student that day. As is the case in life, seeing the glass as half full is necessary in order to make the most of a less-than-ideal situation.

GETTING A JOB: TIMING AND PREPARATION   Education is a very cyclical profession in which there are constant occupational shifts. While there may be many openings one year, the next year may be absolutely closed to new personnel. Also, the number of school counselors in a school system is significantly below the number of teachers, so a teacher shortage does not necessarily indicate availability in school counseling positions. Some years there may be a lot of turnover; other years, there may be little. Many factors, such as budgetary issues, student numbers, and geographic location, may influence the number of school counseling positions available in any area. Paying attention to these factors now may be beneficial to you when the time comes to find a position.

Regardless of where you may be in your school counselor training program, it is a good idea to contact school districts to see what the projected need for school counselors will be in the next 3 to 5 years. Chapter 14 provides professional and personal suggestions that will help you prepare for the job search. You can view the challenges presented as unique opportunities to balance your personal life, family life, and career. If you're still reading, you must be ready to begin this exploration of the school counseling profession and the roles that make it such a worthwhile pursuit.

It is important to address how school counseling as a specialty fits into the counseling field in general. While there are similarities between school counseling and other types of counseling, there are also differences that make school counseling unique.

School Counseling: A Unique Specialty in Counseling

Often, a student will earn a graduate degree in one type of counseling and then take extra courses and do an internship to receive certification in school counseling in order to be more marketable in the workforce. This is reasonable and practical. It is important for school counselors to remember that their first responsibility is to be counselors. Most school counseling training programs are counseling programs that include a course or two and/or practicum and internship in the school counseling area. Training as a counselor is critical to the success of counseling in schools, but it is also important to understand the distinction between counseling fields, such as the differences between community or agency counseling and school counseling.

The most obvious difference is simply one of semantics. In school counseling, the individuals we work with are students. In mental health settings, the individuals that receive services are clients. This seemingly small difference in semantics also infers a contextual difference. School counselors work with students in a psychoeducational context and use counseling as a means of helping individuals become better students in the school setting. Schools are not therapeutic by nature and school counselors do not provide therapy. This is not to say that school counselors do not need to intervene to make sure that students receive appropriate counseling services. In fact, school counselors play a critical role in linking students to appropriate mental health services (Wittmer, 2000).

In schools, counseling services are usually prevention- or intervention-based, short-term, and provided within the overall framework of the academic program. Mental health counseling, on the other hand, is considered therapeutic, may be long-term, and is provided to meet the specific needs of the client in a variety of settings. This distinction is very important for persons who plan to move from one area of counseling to another.

Another significant difference between the two types of counseling is the relative governing agency. Mental health counselors function under the American Counseling Association Code of Ethics and Standards of Practice (ACA, 1995), as well as the regulations of the agencies in which they work. School counselors abide by the ethics and standards of the American Counseling Association (ACA), the American School Counselor Association [ASCA] (1998), and the rules and regulations of schools and school systems.

While the ASCA (1998) Ethical Standards for School Counselors are somewhat comparable to ACA's (1995) Code of Ethics and Standards of Practice, there are notable differences that individuals should be aware of if they choose to become school counselors. For example, the ACA ethical code and standards indicate that clients must give consent in order for legal records to be reviewed by anyone. But most school policies allow school faculty and parents access to the confidential records of students, regardless of whether or not the student gives consent, unless the student is 18 years old. Thus, in mental health counseling, the client has more control over the sharing of confidential information than does a student in a school setting. This will be addressed in greater depth in chapter 2.

Ultimately, the school counselor functions within the parameters set forth by the school or school board. While school counselors are governed by the ethics of ASCA and ACA, an additional governing body may affect counseling practices. For example, a school board may have very specific guidelines for dealing with teenage pregnancy or family life education, or a school may have strict rules about scheduling. As an employee of the school district, the school counselor is expected to abide by the policies of the school board. In contrast, counselors in the community and/or private sector often have greater freedom to utilize techniques they feel are effective; the counselor and client determine whether or not a particular treatment option is appropriate.

Professional Perspective

ESTHER (HS)

A school runs on rules and regulations. Often, even the most simple schedule change is thwarted by policy, caps in numbers, teacher preference, guidelines, or prerequisites. Counselors help students navigate the sea of red tape, while constantly looking for the best student-centered solution in an arena of complex problems.

Finally, another difference between mental health counseling and school counseling is the goal of counseling. While the function of counseling is the same in both settings, the goals may be very different. The school environment may dictate and will certainly influence how counseling services are provided. School counselors must help students with issues and concerns with the goal of creating more effective learners; the school counselor contributes to the overall educational process by utilizing counseling services to help students be successful in school. Conversely, a mental health counselor may be able to conduct counseling sessions with a variety of goals, none of which are related to academic performance. For example, goals may be behavioral, social, or family-focused, depending on the needs of the client. The primary goal is to help the client become a healthy, functioning person. Again, it is important to understand this difference and to determine if you can work comfortably within the educational system of schools. It is not unusual for counselors-in-training to change their minds about the settings in which they want to work. This typically occurs after a field or "shadow" experience when students get to spend a day at each level—elementary, middle, and high school. It is an eye-opening experience for students and helps them determine if school counseling is a career they want to pursue. It should not be considered negative if a counselor-in-training decides that school counseling is not a good fit; in fact, it is beneficial when a person comes to this realization before becoming invested and entrenched in a graduate school counseling preparation program. In most cases, the field experience reinforces students' aspirations and motivates them to pursue the goal of becoming a school counselor. Examining your personal motivations and the realities of counseling in different environments will help you determine whether or not working within those environments is desirable.

As counselors-in-training, you must understand that, first and foremost, you will be a counselor. What differentiates school counselors from other types of counselors is the setting in which they choose to practice. Making the decision to change settings or pursue school counseling may require changes in perspective and perhaps changes in practice.

Now that you're here and ready to take on this new challenge, we need to take a quick look at the role of the school counselor from a historical perspective. There is a wise adage that says, "How can we possibly know where we're going if we don't know where we've been?"

A Brief History of School Counseling

There are several books that provide extensive and thorough coverage of the historical trends and activities that have influenced and altered the role of the school counselor (Baker, 2000; Gysbers & Henderson, 2000; Schmidt, 2003). In particular, Baker provided a timeline that highlights the evolution of school counseling throughout the 20th century. For the purposes of this text, we will examine history as it relates specifically to the roles of the school counselor.

The one constant throughout the history and development of the school counselor role is that counseling responds to the trends and needs of society. For example, due to incidents of school violence in the last decade, such as the shootings at Columbine High School in Littleton, Colorado, in 1999, community members and school personnel are recognizing that we cannot afford to focus solely on the academic needs of students. Indeed, schools and communities can no longer deny the value of prevention- and intervention-based programs that help recognize and address the social and emotional needs of students. Therefore, school counselors should advocate for themselves as professionals who are trained to deal with these issues. A historical review reveals distinct time periods in which the roles of school counselors have responded directly to the needs of schools and communities.

1908–1940: Working and War

In school counseling history, Frank Parsons is considered to be the "Father of Counseling." He emerged as a leader around 1908, when the clear emphasis for counselors in education systems was to help students get jobs. They did not perform counseling as it is known today, but served more in a guidance function. The primary role of school systems in general was to train students to be productive workers. Often, teachers were the primary source of guidance, although some schools in metropolitan areas hired personnel specifically to help young people find jobs. Thus emerged school guidance personnel. Their role was based on societal needs—the need for trained, productive workers.

As the United States experienced the First World War and then the Great Depression, the role of guidance personnel in schools shifted slightly. The emphasis was not only on employment, but also on group-administered intelligence tests as a means of classifying young men for service in the armed forces. Using tests as a way to measure or classify individuals became very popular with guidance personnel who were trying to place students in jobs or in the military. The emphasis for school counselors was totally on properly placing youths so that they could contribute most effectively to their country.

Between World War I and World War II, guidance personnel continued to focus on helping identify students for certain vocations or armed service. As World War I ended, compulsory attendance and remediation became additional areas of concern for schools, and school guidance personnel were sometimes given the task of addressing the needs of students in these areas. With the advent of state certification for guidance counselors in 1924, there was some expansion in the role of school guidance personnel (Baker, 2000). While there was no clear definition of the roles of school guidance personnel throughout the 1930s and into the 1940s, the number of trained guidance counselors increased as more students attended and completed school, and more students were seeking gainful employment or educational opportunities after high school.

1940–1960: Increasing Support and Federal Funding

From 1940 into the 1960s, there was an increase in public support of counseling in society and schools. Public interest in the work of Sigmund Freud and key literary works by Carl Rogers in 1942 established a different public perspective of counseling. The emphasis on providing counseling services to students added a new dimension to the school guidance person's role. It was the first time the role included a component of counseling that addressed feelings. Rogers's book *On Becoming a Person: A Therapist's View of Psychotherapy* (1961) redefined society's perception of counseling. His theory of client-centered or person-centered counseling placed greater emphasis on the individual and developing a climate for a positive counselor–client relationship. While the vocational guidance component was ever present, the affective role of counseling became prominent (Baker, 2000).

Public support of counseling was reflected in federal legislation that had direct implications for school counselors. In 1946, Congress passed the George Barden Act, which focused on developing and implementing guidance and counseling activities in schools. The importance of this act, according to Schmidt (2003) was that "for the first time in history, schools counselors and state and local supervisors received resource, leadership, and financial support from the government" (p. 11).

The passage of the National Defense Educational Act of 1958 (NDEA) also had a dramatic impact on school counseling. After the launch of Sputnik, the American people became concerned about the ability of the country to be a leader in the industrial and technical world market. This fear launched a national effort to ensure that the United States regained its dominance as a world power. Through greater funding for academic programs and support services, more school counselor positions were created to improve the academic and vocational preparation of students who would need to function more efficiently in a competitive society. The combination of increased public support for addressing the emotional needs of students and increased funding for academic and vocation programs expanded the school counselor's role.

1960–1990: Role Refinement and Accountability

The 1960s saw continued support for school counselors in both their guidance and counseling functions. The publication of Gilbert Wrenn's *The Counselor in a Changing World* (1962) provided impetus and support for role refinement for school counselors. In the counseling field in general, more theories, such as Albert Ellis' Rational Emotive Therapy (now Rational Emotive Behavior Therapy) and cognitive and behavioral theories, were gaining prominence. This widespread acknowledgement of the presence and need for counseling in society permeated the schools as well. While the 1960s was a time of social unrest, it seemed that school counselors were secure in their roles. A testimony to the perceived importance of school counselors was an amendment to the NDEA in 1964 that provided funding for elementary school guidance counselors (Baker, 2000).

The 1970s saw a decline in the number of school counselors due to dropping enrollment numbers. Most school districts attempted to maintain a reasonable counselor-to-student ratio. While there was a decline in the quantity of school counselors, it seemed that quality was maintained. School counselors still played an active role in the personal/social, academic, and vocational development of students. The passing of the *Education Act for All Handicapped Children of 1975,* while influential, did not spell out specific guidelines for the school counselor, but certainly affected counseling services and roles. This new role emerged to meet the changing needs of a more diverse society and increasing demands for effective educational and support services for all students.

In 1983, a report entitled "A Nation at Risk" raised the public consciousness once more, focusing attention on the condition of America's schools. The report emphasized the declining performance of America's students and the need for more effective schooling. This report did not affect counselors in terms of direct mandates, but the attack on the demise of public schools resulted in a public outcry for better academic preparation and support for students. As a result, school counselors became more accountable for their services and had to produce measurable results that indicated the effectiveness of their programs. The focus on accountability forever altered the role of the school counselor. For the first time, counselors were being asked to prove their worth and their contribution to the educational process. Society wanted to know what school counselors were doing and how well they were doing it.

The 1990s: Role Proliferation and National Standards

The 1990s and current trends have propelled school counselors into myriad roles. The increased emphasis on diversity, gender equity, inclusion for special needs students, school violence prevention programs, and greater accountability has created a smorgasbord of roles and responsibilities for school counselors. For some, the road has had its twists and turns. For example, in 1990 Virginia state legislature mandated a student to counselor ratio in every elementary school of 500 to 1. When the political climate changed in 1996, the legislature overturned the mandate and gave local school districts the option of hiring elementary school counselors or reading specialists, with the goal of improving performance on the reading portion of standardized tests. Whether the act was intentional or not, the message was that elementary school counselors were disposable or optional. This action confused those who did not understand the role of school counseling at the elementary level. The decision to make elementary school counselors optional sent an "either/or" message, when the appropriate message should have been that students need both support resources. In the cyclical nature of education, the Virginia state legislature passed a bill in April 2002 that once again mandated school counselors in all elementary schools. This action indicated a greater understanding of the integral role the school counselor plays at all levels in students' educational careers.

The development of the National Standards for School Counseling influenced the profession in a very positive way (Campbell & Dahir, 1997). This monumental document provided a framework and a standardization model for school counseling programs on a national level. The standards not only define and help structure the development of comprehensive school counseling programs, they also provide three specific areas of student development—academic, career, personal/social—that should serve as the focus for effective counseling services. The National Standards include specific objectives in each of the three areas and provide examples of student competencies at each school level that will indicate that each objective has been achieved. Feature 1.2 lists the general objectives for each of the developmental areas.

Current Events in School Counseling

Recently, at least three major events have influenced the school counseling profession in significant ways. These are the *Transforming School Counseling Initiative* (Education Trust, 2003), the *No Child Left Behind Act of 2001* (U.S. Department of Education, 2002), and the *ASCA National Model: A Framework for School Counseling Programs* (American School Counselor Association [ASCA], 2003a).

TRANSFORMING SCHOOL COUNSELING INITIATIVE The Transforming School Counseling Initiative (TSCI), supported by the Education Trust in Washington, D.C. (Education Trust, 2003), began in 1996 with grant support from the DeWitt Wallace–Reader's Digest fund. The primary goal was to rede-

---

FEATURE 1.2
_____

The ASCA National Standards for School Counseling Programs

Academic Development

- Standard A: Students will acquire the attitudes, knowledge, and skills contributing to effective learning in school and across the life span.
- Standard B: Students will complete school with the academic preparation essential to choose from a wide range of substantial post-secondary options, including college.
- Standard C: Students will understand the relationship of academics to the world of work and to life at home and in the community.

Career Development

- Standard A: Students will acquire the skills to investigate the world of work in relation to knowledge of self and to make informed career decisions.
- Standard B: Students will employ strategies to achieve future career success and satisfaction.
- Standard C: Students will understand the relationship between personal qualities, education and training, and the world of work.

Personal/Social Development

- Standard A: Students will acquire the attitudes, knowledge, and interpersonal skills to help them understand and respect self and others.
- Standard B: Students will make decisions, set goals, and take necessary action to achieve goals.
- Standard C: Students will understand safety and survival skills.

Source: Campbell and Dahir, 1997.

---

fine the role of school counselors in the 21st century. The project connected six higher education institutions with kindergarten through 12th grade school districts to provide training and implementation of comprehensive school counseling programs. The major focus of the TSCI was to refine school counselor training programs and current school counseling practices to include the traditional roles (counseling, coordination, classroom guidance, and consultation) within the framework of the new roles—systemic change, advocacy, leadership, teaming and collaboration, and assessment and use of data. Currently, the goal of the Education Trust is to work with higher education institutions and school districts nationwide to alter the way that school counselor roles support the educational mission of schools and to provide for the successful educational experiences and outcomes of all students. Nationwide training efforts and information are available to school counselor training programs and school districts in order to unify the profession and transform the role of school counselors into one of action and advocacy (www.edtrust.org).

The National Standards and Transforming School Counseling Initiative supports professional efforts that unite school counseling programs nationally and possibly internationally. Another benefit of these programs is that they link school counselors to the No Child Left Behind legislation that is currently the impetus for educational reform.

NO CHILD LEFT BEHIND: CLOSING THE GAP   In January 2002, President Bush signed the No Child Left Behind Act of 2001 (United States Department of Education, 2002). The passing of this act and its inclusion in the Elementary and Secondary Education Act (ESEA) indicated the nation's focus on reform in education, particularly on increasing accountability for our nation's schools. The four primary principles of this act are stronger accountability for results, increased flexibility in state and local education spending, emphasis on teaching methods that are proven to be effective, and expanded options for parents in terms of school choice. While school counseling is not specifically mentioned, it is critical that school counselors understand their role in helping schools and students during this era of reform and engage in practices that promote greater student success. School counselors must be active participants in education reform by rethinking our roles and focusing on the integration of school counseling programs and practices with effective educational programs.

In order to join the era of educational reform, Dahir and House (2002) indicated that school counseling programs must focus on

- closing the achievement gap between the majority and the minority,
- identifying what works (the strategies and practices in counseling that result in student success),
- reducing the bureaucracy and increasing flexibility (recognizing the school counselor's role in leadership and advocacy), and
- increasing options for students (providing services and programs that support the academic, personal/social, and career development of students).

It is evident that recent trends in school counseling in terms of standards and initiatives blend naturally with the goals of educational reform. This merger helps solidify the school counselor's position as an essential member of the education team. The most recent effort, the ASCA National Model, integrates all of the components into a comprehensive and effective school counseling program.

THE ASCA NATIONAL MODEL: BRINGING IT ALL TOGETHER   Most recently, the American School Counselor Association (2003a) has introduced the ASCA National Model: A Framework for School Counseling Programs (see

Figure 1.1). The model contains four elements critical to the creation of effective and comprehensive school counseling services. The first element is *foundation*, which emphasizes that school counseling programs must have a philosophy and mission that are developed within the context of the ASCA National Standards. This foundation is the structure on which school counseling services are built. The second element, *delivery system*, includes the methods through which counseling will occur. These include the guidance curriculum, individual planning with students, responsive services (e.g., counseling, consultation, referral, etc.), and system support. The system support component includes the administration and management of counseling services provided.

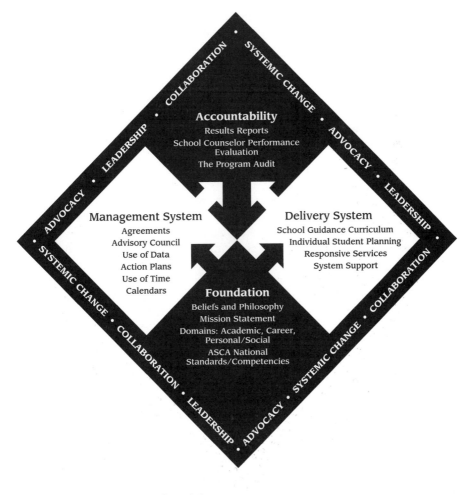

Figure 1.1 ASCA National Model.

Source: From *The ASCA National Model: A Framework for School Counseling Programs* (2003). Reprinted by permission of the American School Counselor Association.

A third element is the *management system* that addresses the overall administration and implementation of the program. The important parts of this element are the use of data for program planning and development, student monitoring, action plans, and the usage of time and calendars. This system focuses on the day-in, day-out management of counseling services, as well as a more global consideration of the counseling program. The final element is *accountability* and includes results reports, counselor performance evaluations, program evaluations, and the development of an advisory council that reviews the reports and evaluations in order to plan and make recommendations regarding the school counseling program.

Forming the framework around the model are key concepts of the Transforming School Counseling Initiative (Education Trust, 2003): collaboration, leadership, advocacy, and systemic change. The National Standards (Campbell & Dahir, 1997) are included under the foundation component of the model. Notice how the foundation of the school counseling program is channeled into the delivery and management systems, which then feed into the accountability process. Accountability then funnels back down to and has implications for the foundation of a school counseling program. This illustrates that each component is directly linked to the others. The ASCA model encompasses all of the essential elements of school counseling programs and school counseling services and is a landmark contribution to the profession of school counseling.

Where Do We Go from Here?

These positive trends in school counseling are exciting, but there is still much work to do. In 1998, Sink and MacDonald estimated that more than 50% of the states emphasized comprehensive school counseling programs. The percentage may be greater today, since many states have adopted the National Standards as the governing document for their school counseling programs since 1998. The National Model for School Counseling Programs (ASCA, 2003a) provides greater professionalism for school counselors and a framework for developing and implementing effective counseling programs. The current trends will forever alter the role of school counselors in a positive way. Gysbers and Henderson (2001) believe this positive trend will continue because of

> (1) Widespread adoption of the Comprehensive Guidance and Counseling Program Model; (2) Excellence and inclusivity goals (to include developmental assistance for all students); (3) Integration of the guidance program and total school mission; (4) Increased human resources for counseling; (5) The advancement of the science and art of counseling; (6) Accountability for resource use; (7) Program and staff leadership. (pp. 254–256)

This brief look at the historical trends that have affected school counseling practices sets the stage for exploring where school counseling is today, as well as potential trends for the future.

Overview of the Book

This book is not intended to cover all of the principles, philosophies, and research related to school counseling. While based on research and trends in school counseling, the book does not provide exhaustive coverage of this material. Instead, it is intended to provide opportunities for thought-provoking consideration and dialogue about current practices and perspectives in school counseling.

In this first chapter, an overview of the opportunities and challenges of a job as a school counselor has been presented. The differences between school counseling and mental health counseling were revealed. A brief historical review indicated that current trends and events in school counseling have catapulted school counselors into exciting new roles that will have positive results for students and reflect positively on the profession of school counseling. This chapter, which is the foundation for what is to follow, is also meant to help readers reflect on and explore the journeys they have made to reach the decision to explore school counseling as a career.

Chapter 2 focuses on the school counselor's role as ethical practitioner. One of the most important roles of the school counselor is to promote and engage in ethically sound counseling practices. Having a clear understanding of ethics and the dilemmas that may be presented in school environments is critical in one's career. An in-depth discussion of the ASCA Ethical Standards reveals that school counselors may find themselves in "gray" areas when it comes to making ethical decisions and deciding how to respond to students and school situations. Tips for ethical decision-making and strategies for being more comfortable when ethical dilemmas arise are offered.

Chapters 3 and 4 focus on the traditional roles of school counselors according to ASCA (1999c): counseling, classroom guidance, consultation, and coordination. Examples and practical experiences from our three veteran counselors provide practical insight and professional perspectives for consideration. The chapters also discuss the various ways in which these roles are demonstrated at the elementary, middle, and high school levels. Critical discussions in chapter 4 include an exploration of the school counselor's role in noncounseling duties, such as testing.

Chapter 5 is a key chapter in this book because it emphasizes what should be the priority role for school counselors—supporting students. This chapter considers the development areas of the National Standards (academic, personal/social, career) and examines how school counselors foster student development in each area. It is especially helpful to hear from our veteran school counselors, who share professional perspectives and practices about their work with students.

Chapter 6 continues the discussion of working with students and explores the important role that school counselors play in working with diverse populations and students with special needs. As our schools become more racially integrated, school personnel will need to respond to the needs of non–English-speaking students and families. School counselors may be at the forefront of connecting schools and families struggling to understand each other. Further, school counselors are involved with students and families who are served by special education programs; it is a necessary role that provides support for students with different needs. Finally, a discussion of working with sexual minority youth is included, as school counselors will need to address the unique needs of this student population.

Chapters 7 and 8 provide an opportunity to consider the school counselor as a member of the education team. Working with teachers, administrators, and other school personnel has important implications for promoting collaborative relationships that will ultimately benefit students. Chapter 7 begins with a discussion of the debate about the efficacy of school counselors with and without teaching experience. The debate is still ongoing and there are considerations, both positive and negative, on each side. The remainder of the chapter explores the school counselor's collaborative working relationship with teachers as well as the need to maintain effective communication and provide support for teachers in their work with students and parents.

Chapter 8 discusses specific interactions between school counselors and administrators, as well as other school personnel. Strategies for gaining administrative support are offered, since school administration practices may strongly influence school counseling programs and services. Working cooperatively with other school personnel is also paramount in order to comprehensively meet the needs of students.

Chapter 9 discusses the school counselor's role in collaborating with parents, families, and communities. Although the consultative and collaborative role of school counselors is discussed throughout the book, this chapter explores a relatively new phenomenon in school counseling: family counseling in schools. Recent counseling practices emphasize working with families in order to help students be more successful in school. Strategies for increasing parent participation and support for counseling programs and services are also discussed.

Chapter 10 moves the reader into considering the transformed roles of school counselors. The school counselor's leadership role is the focus of this chapter, which was contributed by counselor educators at the State University of West Georgia, a partner school in the Tranforming School Counselor Initiative. This overview of school counselor leadership provides essential information about leadership roles and responsibilities of the 21st century school counselor. The "Leadership Development Profile" is offered as a tool to assess your personal leadership attributes.

Chapter 11 serves as a specific example of how school counselors serve as leaders in educational programs. School counselors should be leaders in developing and implementing programs that promote peace and safety in schools. This chapter focuses specifically on the school counselor as an active leader in school violence prevention and intervention, which is a current focus for many schools and school counseling programs.

Chapter 12 includes a professional contribution by Dr. Marie Jackson of the State University of West Georgia, a knowledgeable resource in the area of school counseling and advocacy. An increasingly critical piece of school counselor transformation is the need for personal and professional advocacy across the school counseling program. From local school board meetings to national symposiums, school counselors must advocate for the important services and programs that they provide in order to maximize the success of students in schools. Examples of advocacy are given and school counselors-in-training are challenged to begin advocacy in their preparation programs.

Chapter 13 focuses on school counselor accountability. This chapter, contributed largely by Dr. Pam Brott of Virginia Tech, editor of *Professional School Counseling*, offers practical suggestions and examples to help school counselors develop useful ways to utilize and report data to support the efficacy of school counseling programs. Accountability and results-based evaluation are going to be the norm in education systems, and school counselors must be prepared to rise to the challenges of the age of accountability. The chapter also discusses school counselor performance evaluation and offers information to help prepare school counselors for the ways in which their performance may be evaluated or assessed. The chapter's focus on data and evaluation are timely in this educational era of accountability.

Chapter 14 brings everything full circle and ends up where we began: personal and professional considerations about school counseling and whether or not it is a "fit" for you. The need for professional development and developing a professional identity is emphasized, and strategies for developing a professional portfolio are offered. While developing a professional identity is crucial, it is superceded only by the need to personally take care of oneself. Personal and professional demands can take a toll on school counselors, which sometimes leads to burnout. Prevention strategies and words of wisdom from our veteran counselors are offered.

In the following chapters, you will explore the many roles and practices of school counselors at the elementary, middle, and high school levels. You will learn from school counseling research and the real-life experiences of practicing counselors at each level and at various points in their careers as they share professional practices and perspectives. Most importantly, you will have the opportunity to examine your own motivation and commitment to becoming an effective school counselor. As you read these chapters, it is my hope that you begin to develop your own chapters as well.

CONCLUSION

As we continue to explore school counseling, we must recognize that as society continues to grow and change, the profession must continue to be responsive to the needs of society. With the growing national concerns about school violence, higher test scores, and building collaborative relationships, the school counselor is an obvious person to ensure that students are successful in their academic careers by attending to the personal, social, and emotional needs that might interfere in the learning process.

Looking at the progress in the field of school counseling, it is exciting to see the new directions and paths that are available to us as a profession. As professional school counselors move forward to a promising and successful future, there will always be a need to consider and explore practices and perspectives in order to maximize the educational potential of students and provide effective counseling services to foster student success in school and in life.

REFLECTION AND DISCUSSION

1. What is your motivation for becoming a school counselor? What experiences or events brought you to this decision? Discuss this with your peers.
2. What did you learn in this chapter that either reinforced your decision or made you question your decision to become a school counselor?
3. What societal forces do you see at work that may influence school counseling in the next decade?

CHAPTER 2

The School Counselor as Ethical Practitioner: Doing the Right Thing

*N*o other element of the school counselor's role is more important and more challenging than the ethical responsibilities that are inherent to the profession. While the American Counseling Association's (1995) Code of Ethics and Standards of Practice and the American School Counselor Association's (1998) Ethical Standards provide support and guidelines for the boundaries of school counseling practices, making ethical decisions and "doing the right thing" are difficult and stressful. But behaving ethically is the essence of what school counselors do. More so than other school personnel, a school counselor is in a position to advocate for students both legally and ethically. Although all school personnel are considered "mandated reporters," a school counselor is typically (a) the person to whom people report concerns and/or (b) the person who makes the contact to Child Protective Services (also referred to as the Department of Social Services).

This chapter will discuss the importance of being aware of one's worldview when dealing with ethical issues. We will examine each section of the American School Counselor Association Ethical Standards. It should be noted that school counselors are also guided by the ethical code and standards of the American Counseling Association; for the purposes of this discussion, focus will be primarily on ASCA standards. Each of the standards discussed in this chapter is from the most recent revision of the ASCA Ethical Standards (1998), and a copy of the standards is included in the Appendix at the end of the book for your reference. Also, there are references to ASCA Position Statements throughout the chapter and the book; these documents can be accessed through the American School Counselor Association Web site at www.schoolcounselor.org.

In most counseling books, ethical and legal issues are considered simultaneously (Corey, Corey, & Callanan, 2002; Remley & Herlihy, 2001; Remley, Hermann, & Huey, 2003). This discussion will focus on ethical responses in school counseling, but will also cover legal aspects when appropriate. Finally, a model for ethical decision making will be provided.

The Philosophy of Ethics: A Snapshot

Ethics, whether personal or professional, are infused throughout our daily lives, and most decisions that we make are influenced, at least in part, by our ethical worldviews. Looking at the larger picture helps provide a framework in which the ethical principles of school counseling can be contemplated. However, before dealing with specific ethical situations and decisions, it is important to consider personal values and how they play into our thoughts, feelings, and ultimately our behavior.

Becoming Aware of Your Worldview

It would be naive to believe that we do not bring our own values and judgments into life situations. A personal worldview is made up of internal and external entities. The internal components might be the values, opinions, and morals that are intrinsic to who we are. External factors might include how we were raised, socialization, and life experiences that influence our views of the world in which we live. This worldview will affect what we believe to be right or wrong and our responses to ethical dilemmas.

As school counselors, our worldviews must be open and tolerant. We need to believe in working for the needs of the individual and the greater good of society. While worldviews are unique and personal, there are some basic tenets that seem desirable in the worldviews of school counselors:

1. Students ultimately want to achieve.
2. Every child has the potential to be successful; accessing that potential is the challenge.
3. Every child deserves a chance to be successful.
4. Ultimately, the student is empowered with the choice of being successful or not, depending on ability and capacity for success.
5. It is the student's actions that are fallible, not the individual.
6. School counselors facilitate growth and change; they do not impose it.
7. We should not assume anything.

It is vital to understand the magnitude of the influence school counselors can have on students. Our worldviews can affect how we interact with students, as well as our ethical responsiveness.

It is not unusual to hear school counselors say, "Well, I just went with my gut feeling about the situation and it turned out fine." Frequently, these instinctual actions are appropriate; however, there are safeguards school counselors can use to support their decisions and actions in situations with ethical implications. We will now look at the ethical codes that govern the behavior of school counselors and provide the protocol for action when necessary.

Ethical Standards for School Counselors

The Ethical Standards for School Counselors proposed by the American School Counselor Association (ASCA) were last revised in June 1998. The passage of the 1998 standards decreased the number of ethical inquiries from prior years and seemed to provide greater clarity on issues of concern for school counselors (Dansby-Giles et al., 1999). ASCA updated and added ethical standards related to current events in schools. For example, the ethical standards cover the use of technology for record keeping by acknowledging the need for confidentiality when maintaining those records. Other alterations and additions have responded to the present circumstances of school counselors. Remley, Hermann, and Huey (2003) offered a comprehensive overview of the ethical and legal issues in school counseling.

The ASCA Ethical Standards begin with a preamble that addresses the global rights and responsibilities of school counselors: "The school counselor assists in the growth and development of each individual and uses his or her highly specialized skills to protect the interests of the counselee within the structure of the school system." The preamble uses the words *personal* and *professional* to indicate that these standards address the responsibilities of the individual as well as the professional—the responsibility school counselors have to their constituents and the profession in general. The word *responsibility* implies an obligation and dedication to the school counseling profession and the community it serves. Let's examine each responsibility individually.

Responsibilities to Students

The first section of the standards is devoted to school counselors' responsibility to the students with whom they work. It is appropriate that the first group addressed in the ethical code is students. All decisions and practices must focus on the best interest of each student. As student advocates, school counselors must also understand the extent of those responsibilities. Consider this example:

> *Joe is a high school counselor in a rural area. The community he lives and works in is very politically and religiously conservative, and the school system has a strict policy about talking to students about alternative lifestyles. Joe is to promote healthy and "normal" relationships (in the school system's view, heterosexuality), and school personnel are not to impose their opinions or values on the students. Joe is working with a student who seems to be struggling with her sexuality and has implied that she believes she is a lesbian. Joe believes he should help the student with her awareness of her own sexual orientation. He thinks it would be valuable for this student to participate in a support group for gay and lesbian students, because he knows of other students who struggle with the same issues. Joe also knows of community organizations that provide information for youth who are struggling with their sexuality. As Joe starts to bring this up to the student, he wonders if he might be reprimanded for sug-gesting that the student explore this possibility. He also wonders if he is advo-cating a particular lifestyle, which is an ethical violation. What should Joe do?*

Ethically, Joe has to do some soul searching. In Ethical Standard A.1, the man-date is to treat each student with respect as a unique individual. Joe is responding appropriately by demonstrating concern for the student and sup-porting her in this difficult stage of her life. However, the same section also states that professional school counselors are to "Refrain from consciously encouraging the counselee's acceptance of values, lifestyles, plans, decisions, and beliefs that represent the counselor's personal orientation" (Ethical Standard A.1.c). Although Joe wants to help the student in this struggle, making a suggestion or trying to influence a student's values or lifestyle is an ethical violation. It is spelled out very clearly in the standards that school counselors should not impose their values or beliefs on the students in their care. Can Joe provide support for this student? Absolutely. While Joe is not advocating a homosexual lifestyle, he must be cautious when working with the student. Even when a problem is not as controversial as sexual orientation, school counselors must be cognizant of how their own beliefs, values, and lifestyles could permeate their counseling practices. It is appropriate for Joe to help the student sort through feelings and insecurities about this issue. Guiding students to their own solutions or conclusions is very different from encouraging or influencing them based on one's personal life experience or beliefs. The objectivity that is necessary to make these important ethical decisions is not always innate. However, becoming familiar with the ethical standards could prevent problems for Joe in his role as a school counselor.

But what should Joe do? First, he must consider the school community in which he works. There does not appear to be great tolerance for alternative lifestyles, to the extent that the school board has instituted policy against promoting any lifestyle other than heterosexuality. Where does the school district draw the line? If students wanted to start a support group or approached Joe or other counselors about the need for a group, is it possible that Joe might approach the administration about providing group counseling on this topic? It would be wise for Joe to talk to colleagues, the guidance director, or the administration about the possibility of beginning this support group. These persons might have a better feel for the pulse of the school district and the likelihood of the idea being accepted.

CONFIDENTIALITY

> A student has the right to privacy and confidentiality. ASCA recognizes that a counseling relationship requires an atmosphere of trust and confidence between the student and the counselor. Confidentiality ensures that disclosures will not be divulged to others except when authorized by the student or when there is a clear and present danger to the student or others. (ASCA, 2002a, p. 1)

At first glance, the parameters of confidentiality seem fairly concrete. The Ethical Standards are very clear about when school counselors must break confidentiality: when there is clear and present danger to the student and/or other persons or when ordered by the courts to release information. According to Dansby-Giles et al. (1999), there were 50 ethical inquiries of the ASCA Ethical Committee from 1997 through 1999. The majority of those inquiries were related to issues of confidentiality, although concerns also included parental consent for counseling, preparing for court appearances, and student cases that involved duty to warn. Legal aspects of confidentiality include privileged communication, which protects the privacy of counselor–student communication in a court of law. In states that do not have privileged communication, school counselors may be required to break confidentiality if ordered by the court.

One issue that often causes disagreement among school counselors is students engaging in risky behaviors, such as sexual activity. Sexual activity in particular generates intense discussion in graduate courses due to the personal, moral, ethical, and emotional concerns that surround sexual issues and minors. The biggest dilemma is whether to inform parents about the sexual activities of their children or to maintain counselor–student confidentiality. Is sex among young people a threat to them or others? If one considers the likelihood of sexually transmitted diseases and pregnancy, then sexual activity is probably a threat. If sex is consensual and protection is used, does that minimize the danger and mean that confidentiality should be maintained? Maybe. What if the counselor has a strong moral and ethical belief that premarital sex is wrong? Condoning the behavior and doing nothing goes against personal ethics and values. Trying to coerce students by proclaiming that premarital sex is wrong is an ethical violation because the counselor is imposing personal views and beliefs. If the school counselor does not maintain confidentiality, the student may not seek help from the counselor again. Finally, do the parents have a right to know? School counselors usually support the rights of the parents to raise their children and guide them in the decisions that they make regarding personal behavior. Sometimes, the school counselor's ethical dilemma is made easier because a school district has a policy that states that if school employees become aware of student sexual activity, they are to report the activity to the parents. While this might seem to alleviate the difficulty of decision making, it also compromises the counselor's ethical responsibility to keep information confidential. This dilemma is never an easy one, and rarely is there agreement even among school counselors on issues of confidentiality.

A survey by Davis and Mickelson (1994) indicated that there was less than 50% agreement among school counselors who were presented with dilemmas involving confidentiality and parental rights. Most counselors will agree, however, that ethical issues involving confidentiality are often the most ambiguous and difficult to address.

Isaacs and Stone (1999) conducted a study with 627 school counselors in Florida, posing 22 scenarios that related to confidentiality. The participants were asked to respond to the scenarios and decide if the counselor in each should breach confidentiality. The results provided interesting information on the issue of confidentiality.

> Our findings suggest that school counselors protect younger students to a greater degree by warning others or including families in children's issues. Middle and secondary school counselors seem to be considering the privacy rights of older students more frequently. Thus, school counselors believe that regardless of professional ethics and rules, the age of the child is the most significant variable in dealing with dilemmas related to confidentiality. (p. 265)

This finding makes the assumption that chronological age may be a deciding factor in questions of confidentiality, but what about emotional maturity or developmental factors? Obviously, there is much to consider when dealing with situations involving confidentiality and the rights of students and parents.

One of the most difficult aspects of confidentiality is making sure that students understand its limits. It is good practice to teach students about confidentiality as early as possible so that they understand the school counselor's ethical responsibility to maintain it and the circumstances under which information must be shared.

Professional Perspective and Practice

BETH (MS)

I think a tough ethical situation is when you want students to have confidence in you and feel that they can talk with you freely, but at the same time, you have to be responsible to state, federal, and local guidelines on what you have to report. One way that I handle the issue upfront is when I go into classrooms at the beginning of the year to introduce myself, I tell the students exactly what I can keep confidential and what I cannot and the reasons why. This way, if a student does come in and tell me something, I've already put the confidentiality limitations out there. Then the choice of what to tell me is the student's. I also gently remind students that there are things that I can't keep confidential, and then they can decide how much information they want to share.

Student confidentiality is obviously much more complex than simply keeping counseling sessions private. As ethical practitioners, school counselors have an ethical responsibility to maintain student privacy and confidentiality to the extent possible.

Confidentiality of Records　The privacy of student records was discussed briefly in chapter 1. School records are handled somewhat differently than client records in other types of counseling settings. The confidentiality of records also has a legal component. The *Family Educational Rights and Privacy Act of 1974* (P.L. 93-380), also known as the Buckley Amendment, gives parents of minor students the right to review student school records. The passage of this act resulted in greater concern about what was placed in students' records, as well as who had permission to review them. In some schools, the school counselor serves as the gatekeeper of student records and must review the records regularly to ensure that the information contained within is appropriate and legal. It should be mentioned that if parents or guardians disagree with any of the contents of their child's record, they may provide a written objection to the content and the letter must be added to the student's folder.

Sometimes external agencies submit requests to see a student's attendance record or academic record in order to determine if some event or situation has negatively affected the student's progress. Ethical Standard A.2.e specifically addresses this issue. While most school systems have strict policies about who has access to student records, in addition to the federal guidelines, it is sometimes hard to monitor who is and is not seeing the records. ASCA (2002a) states, "It should be each school's policy to guarantee adequate working space for secretaries so that students and school personnel will not come into contact with confidential information, even inadvertently" (p. 2). The ethical standard referring to confidentiality of records includes records kept on computers. Many school systems have moved to technological maintenance of records. Using computers to store confidential information creates new challenges to confidentiality. While most confidential documents are protected by passwords or are accessible only to a select few persons, other people may figure out alternative ways to enter the system and access the information. Also, what if the system loses information or crashes and information cannot be retrieved? On the positive side, technology provides quicker access to information, as well as more advanced tracking of student progress and transition from grade level to grade level. The paper trail can be quite extensive in a student's file, and computer-based data systems provide a concise way to monitor student records. Assuring confidentiality of student records will continue to be a goal as school systems rely more extensively on technological maintenance of records.

Informed Consent The final standard for protecting the confidentiality of students involves informed consent. Informed consent has both ethical and legal implications. Legally, only parents of minor children can give informed consent, although obtaining student assent to services is certainly advantageous to the counseling process. There is some debate about acquiring parent permission for school counseling services, and the rules for obtaining parent permission for counseling services may vary from school district to school district. Glosoff and Pate (2002) reported that "Some school districts or school principals have policies that require counselors to obtain parents' permission before beginning counseling students, and others require counselors to seek permission if they see students for more than a specified number of counseling sessions (e.g., two or three)" (pp. 21–22). It seems reasonable that seeking parental consent and student compliance with counseling would be the best in terms of potential efficacy of counseling services and embracing the notion of building collaborative relationships.

The second half of Ethical Standard A.2.f discusses confidentiality in group counseling. "In a group setting, the counselor sets a high norm of confidentiality and stresses its importance, yet clearly states that confidentiality in group counseling cannot be guaranteed" (Ethical Standard A.2.f). When conducting group counseling, confidentiality is stressed from the beginning of the group process and is reviewed each time the group meets. Because there are multiple members in the group, the chances of breaching confidentiality increase significantly, particularly when students may not fully understand the concept of confidentially.

Students share family issues, relationship issues, and private information with school counselors and expect that these disclosures are protected by confidentiality. The practice of confidentiality, as well as the ethics and rules governing confidential information, must be followed in order to protect the rights and privacy of students.

My Story

As an elementary counselor, I was working with a group of upper elementary students on social skills. The group had met four times, and each time we discussed the rules of confidentiality. I was sure that each person understood the rules. One afternoon, two group members came to me and said that they had heard a third group member telling a group of students (non-group members) what one of the other members had said about a family situation during the group. They reported that she was telling the story as if it were gossip. I thanked the students for sharing and told them we would talk about this in group later. In the meantime, I sent for the student who had breached confidentiality. When I began asking her about the situation, she admitted that she had told the story. She stated that she "forgot" about the rules of confidentiality and that she was sorry that she had done it. I asked her if she was willing to apologize to the group member whose private information she had shared. She agreed and I got the two group members together.

The member whose confidentiality had been breached was very upset but agreed to forgive the other member. After I spoke with the two members together, I asked the person who had breached confidentiality to leave. When I talked to the member whose confidentiality had been broken, I could tell she was hurt and angry. I knew that the damage had been done. When I asked her how she wanted this to be handled in the group, she said she did not want to kick the other member out of the group, but she did not feel like she could trust the group anymore. I asked if she still felt comfortable coming to the group and she responded that she did, but only to do the activities, not to share. When the group met the following week, there was a great deal of animosity toward the member who had broken confidentiality, even though we processed the negative feelings. I knew that group cohesion was not going to be regained because of the distrust that was obvious among group members. The group terminated after two more sessions and I do not think that group goals were achieved. However, I do think there were some important lessons learned. After that group experience, I worked much harder on making sure that group members understood the boundaries of confidentiality, as well as the limitations. It helped to give concrete examples of how confidentiality might be broken, even accidentally.

COUNSELING PLANS School counselors, as part of their ethical responsibilities to students, must involve students in the development of the plan for counseling services. One way to do this globally is to conduct a needs assessment survey of the entire student body. Based on the results of this survey, a school counselor can create a school counseling program. For example, if there has been a series of loss events in the school community, the school counseling program may focus on grief and loss issues. The services provided could include individual, small-group, and large-group counseling, depending on the responses from the survey.

Ethical Code A.3 focuses on the collaborative relationship between the school counselor and the student. A school counselor has the responsibility of facilitating a plan for counseling sessions. The counselee should be an active participant in planning and is responsible for informing the counselor if the plan is either not working or not congruent with the student's needs. Another crucial component of this standard is the need for regular review to determine if the plan is effective. But often, the changes that occur in counseling are either immeasurable or not obvious. If the school counselor cannot see the benefits of the counseling plan, the first and most obvious action would be to talk to the student. How is the student feeling about the sessions? Is the counseling service meeting his or her needs? If so, how? If not, how could it be more effective? Other important resources for gauging the efficacy of counseling services are the teachers who interact with the student or the student's parents. Have they noticed any difference in the child's attitude or behavior in the classroom or at home? Ongoing evaluation is a necessary component of an effective counseling program. Whether it is an evaluation of an entire program or a single interaction with a student, school counselors must constantly consider efficacy and make revisions as necessary.

DUAL RELATIONSHIPS   The issue of dual relationships arises often in discussions about counseling ethics. A school counselor has the paramount task of maintaining a boundary between the role as school counselor and other roles in his or her life. This can become tricky, especially when the school counselor lives in the community in which he or she works. The likelihood of running into parents of students at the grocery store, in church, or at the pool is quite high. How do school counselors balance the school counseling role, a role in the community, and the ethical standards that govern school counselor behavior? There are a few instances when dual relationships could occur:

- when a school counselor is the counselor assigned to a family member, close friend, or close friend's child;
- when a school counselor is a coach of a school team or the sponsor of a club or activity other than those that are counseling-related; and
- when a school counselor is the assigned counselor to children in the neighborhood in which the counselor lives.

It is very important that school counselors are not assigned to counsel relatives if at all possible. At the secondary level, this is usually handled by simply transferring the student to another counselor. If you are an elementary counselor, perhaps the only one in the building, this is a much greater challenge. This situation, however, is covered in the second part of the standard, which states: "If a dual relationship is unavoidable, the counselor is responsible for taking action to eliminate or reduce the potential for harm" (Ethical Standard A.4). If there is a situation in which objectivity cannot be maintained, consult with a colleague or see if there is another professional available to see the student (e.g., school psychologist, school social worker, etc.). Another option would be to refer the student to outside counseling, depending on the nature of the presenting problem.

When school counselors are coaches or sponsors of teams (academic or sports), the role boundaries can become blurred. Often, students are closer to their coaches than any other adult in the school building, so most people would think it ideal for the two roles to be combined. But counselors must be cautious when they are involved with students on so many levels. Can objectivity as a counselor be maintained when coupled with a supervisory role? Counselors must answer this question on a case-by-case basis. Being aware of the level of objectivity is key in this situation. If for any reason the counselor feels his or her objectivity is being affected, he or she needs to refer the student to another counselor.

Does this mean that if you are a school counselor, you should not coach a team or sponsor a club? No. However, a school counselor must be cognizant of conflicting roles and how they impact the ability to be an effective counselor.

APPROPRIATE REFERRALS Making referrals to outside resources is a major component of the school counselor's job. As ethically responsible practitioners, school counselors must ". . . [have] knowledge of available resources and make proper plans for transitions with minimal interruption of services" (Ethical Standard A.5). The counselor must therefore develop a list of potential counseling resources and make it available to parents/guardians so that they can make decisions about appropriate outside counseling.

To stay informed about available resources, school counselors should develop relationships with counselors and other mental health professionals in the community. Finding an appropriate professional for a student's needs requires that the school counselor have some familiarity with counseling professionals and their specialties. The school counselor must also determine to what degree the outside counseling will affect the counseling services provided in school. If the student is going to be in outside therapy, it might be best to decrease or eliminate counseling sessions in school. The school counselor could provide support through group counseling or by simply checking in with the student. It is important for the school counselor and the outside therapist to consult with each other, first making sure that they both have written parental consent to do so.

GROUP WORK The ASCA Ethical Standards do not go into great detail about the ethics of group counseling. They address the need for pre-group screening and adherence to group goals. In addition, they emphasize protecting the members from physical and psychological harm in the group sessions. It should be noted that the Association for Specialists in Group Work (1998) developed *Best Practice Guidelines* that specifically address ethical standards in group counseling.

DANGER TO SELF OR OTHERS   A school counselor is a *mandated reporter*, which requires the counselor to report suspicions about a student being a danger to self or others to the appropriate authorities. Ethical standard A.7 addresses this legal responsibility. The legal terms "duty to warn" and "due care" used in the standards resulted from the famous *Tarasoff v. California Board of Regents* case, in which proper authorities were not notified about a clients' threats to kill a college student, and the client carried out the threat. School counselors must take threats to harm self or others very seriously and respond by notifying appropriate authorities. The ethical guidelines are clear when there is "clear and imminent danger to the counselee or others" (Ethical Standard A.7). However, this guideline is not always as concrete as one might think. Consider this situation:

> *Robert comes into his middle school counselor's office, throws his backpack on the floor, and plops down into a chair. Ms. Jackson can see he is angry, practically in tears, and ready to explode. She and Robert have developed a good rapport since school started, and she has met with him about school issues as well as personal/social issues. She has never seen him so upset. When she asks what happened, Robert screams: "I cannot take his constant teasing anymore; I'm going to kill him. It's either him or me, and it isn't going to be me!" Ms. Jackson tries to calm him down, but his anger seems only to become quiet rage. She convinces him to stay with her in the office and talk about the student who is bothering him. Robert does not want to reveal the student's name and Ms. Jackson is not exactly sure who he is talking about. It will be difficult for her to figure out, since Robert has been teased by several groups of students. As she continues to explore his thoughts and feelings with him, Robert obviously begins to relax. However, he maintains his desire to hurt the other student. "I've just had it, Ms. Jackson. If I don't shut him up today, this will go on forever. He is just getting what he deserves."*

Ms. Jackson has an ethical dilemma. How serious are Robert's threats? How can she find out who the other student is without breaching confidentiality with Robert? What about her relationship with Robert? Ms. Jackson knows she is going to have to let appropriate authorities know about the threat Robert has made. She also knows she is going to have to tell Robert that she is telling other people, including his parents. Will that destroy the relationship they have developed? What if she can't find out who the student is and Robert attacks him? It is her ethical responsibility to protect the student and inform his parents. How can she when she doesn't know who the student is? And what about the issue that was the catalyst for the entire situation? If Robert is being bullied, isn't he in danger as well? How does Ms. Jackson begin to investigate? Again, it is wise to consult with other counseling professionals before making a decision. Discussing the case with a counseling director or director of guidance prior to making any decisions is also important. In some schools, especially if there are no other counseling professionals onsite, it would be appropriate to inform an administrator of the volatile situation and seek his or her input. Most secondary schools have school resource offices or police personnel that could be helpful in investigating and monitoring these types of situations. Therefore, there is some comfort in the realization that maybe this is a decision that does not have to be made alone.

Informing the counselee of the plan of action is probably the hardest part of fulfilling this standard. The first step may be to remind the student of ethical responsibilities and the limits of confidentiality. Students need to understand the seriousness of their statements when they threaten to harm themselves or others.

In cases of abuse, reporting involves informing Child Protective Services or the Department of Social Services in the school district. There are strict state and federal guidelines that provide protocols for reporting cases of abuse, as well as local school district regulations regarding these reports. The ASCA *Position Statement: Child Abuse* (ASCA, 2003b) commits school counselors to direct involvement in suspected cases of abuse or neglect. Not only are school counselors to report suspected abuse, they are also responsible for providing support services afterward. The ethical responsibility to report is only one role that school counselors must perform when involved in child abuse cases. The other roles are prevention of abuse and neglect if possible and intervention when necessary.

STUDENT RECORDS   We discussed some aspects of student records in the section on confidentiality, but there are other ethical issues to be addressed, particularly for counseling records. There are at least two different perspectives on maintaining and securing counseling records. Some professionals feel that school counselors should maintain detailed student counseling records, similar to case conceptualization where the presenting problem is defined and a written counseling plan is developed. Because of the risk of having records subpoenaed, depending on the laws of privileged communication in the state, others advocate maintaining minimal notes on student progress in counseling. Regardless of the viewpoint, it is an ethical responsibility to make sure the student records are secure, follow legal guidelines for maintenance, and ensure confidentiality. A good rule of thumb is never record anything that you would not want others to read or hear in a court of law.

EVALUATION, ASSESSMENT, AND INTERPRETATION   A school counselor's role in testing and assessment may vary from school to school. The school counselor may be in charge of or involved in standardized testing and assessment. Typically, school counselors are not trained to administer specialized tests, such as psychological instruments or intelligence tests. School psychologists and/or educational diagnosticians typically perform these assessments. Counselor education programs usually require a course in testing and assessment so that counselors are informed about different types of assessment, understand what certain tests measure, and are able to interpret results.

According to Ethical Standard A.9, it is the professional school counselor's responsibility to understand the nature and purpose of testing that occurs in the school setting. Probably the most important aspect of this knowledge is the ability to interpret test results and help the counselee and the parent/guardian understand them. School counselors are often called upon to talk to parents about the results of testing in order to minimize the anxiety that sometimes comes from having one's child tested. Whether the testing is for special needs, gifted services, or general knowledge, all parties involved have the right to know what the results mean. The limitations of the test, level of significance, and meaningfulness of results are all components that should be explained to the counselee and his or her parents, depending on the age of the counselee.

When explaining test results to parents, it is necessary to break things down to the most basic level. It is probably easiest to interpret percentile rank, if it is available, because most people are familiar with the 100-point scale. For example, if a student scores in the 82nd percentile, one might say: "Imagine that there are 100 students your child's age standing in a line. Your child would be number 82 in line; that is, she did as well or better than the first 81 students." If the test is one that is not on a 100-point scale, for example, an IQ test, it is best to talk in terms of ranges. Most people understand above average, average, and below average. If the school counselor does not understand a test or does not feel confident interpreting the results, it is an ethical responsibility to consult with school personnel who can aid in that process. Part of our responsibility to students involves making sure they understand the reason for the testing, as well as having the results explained in a way that is meaningful.

School counselors sometimes conduct informal testing, such as career assessments using computers. This will be discussed in the next section.

COMPUTER TECHNOLOGY   The first section of Ethical Standard A.10 discusses using computers as counseling tools. They indicate three steps to follow when using computers as a medium for counseling: (1) The computer program should meet the individual needs of students; (2) the students should understand how to use the computer program; and (3) the counselor(s) should follow-up with students to answer any questions. One example of computer-assisted counseling is online career assessment. There are several of these types of computer programs, one of which is Bridges (www.bridges.com). Secondary school counselors might have the entire class come into the computer lab and go through the step-by-step process to assess interest in and aptitudes for certain career fields. But having students complete the career exploration task is not enough. School counselors have an ethical responsibility to discuss the results with each student following the computer activity.

The second part of Ethical Standard A.10 addresses communicating with counselees via the Internet. The National Board of Certified Counselors has developed a set of standards for Internet counseling (www.nbcc.org/ethics/ webethics.htm). You should review the cautions and guidelines provided on the NBCC Web site if you are considering conducting any type of counseling online.

PEER HELPER PROGRAM   The ethical standards for Peer Helper Programs reiterate the responsibilities of school counselors when working with programs in a supervisory or training capacity. These responsibilities will be discussed at length in the discussion of peer mediation programs in chapter 11, but the ethical emphasis is on serving both the students and the trainees. Looking out for the welfare of the participants is another important component of maintaining an effective peer helper program.

This section on "Responsibilities to Students" has covered many areas related to a school counselor's ethical responsibilities to students. Within the standards are some important guidelines that may challenge your personal and professional ethics and values. Take some time to consider how you will comply with the guidelines without compromising your personal position.

Responsibilities to Parents

It is imperative that school counselors collaborate with parents on student issues in order to provide a holistic approach to helping the student reach his or her full potential. As school counselors walk the tightrope between responsibilities to students and responsibilities to other involved parties, it becomes evident that the ethical role of school counselors may be fragmented and may vary with each individual situation. The one constant that cannot be denied is the necessity of a collaborative relationship between school counselors and the parents and guardians of students.

PARENT RIGHTS AND RESPONSIBILITIES   The first standard addressing the school counselor's ethical responsibilities to parents speaks volumes about the significant relationship between parents and school counselors. The most important part of the statement refers to the responsible school counselor who "endeavors to establish, as appropriate, a collaborative relationship with parents to facilitate the counselee's maximum development" (Ethical Standard B.1.a). Collaboration should create an effective working relationship between home and school that benefits the student as much as possible. Further, collaboration with parents and/or guardians seems much more likely to result in healthy progress for the student, regardless of the nature of the presenting problem.

When school counselors are developing relationships with parents, they need to be aware of the issues of cultural and social diversity, which is mentioned in the third section of the Ethical Standard. Having developed a personal world-view based only on one's own experiences may lead to intolerance of cultural differences or ignorance of how cultures differ. Consider the following example:

> *Erica is a kindergartener in your building. She and her family have recently moved here from Mexico. In the first week of school, Erica is late each day. The second week, she is absent two days, and late the other three. When the mother brings her in to school, the school secretary informs her that she is late and needs to be here on time. Because Erica is late, she has missed key instruction in learning the alphabet. The teacher approaches you about Erica's tardiness and absences. As a school counselor, how might you respond?*

It is important that someone from the school connect with Erica's family immediately. From the outside, it may seem that Erica's family is not invested in or does not value her education. Erica's tardiness, however, may be a result of cultural customs. Also, Erica may be a first generation school attendee, or her parents may have limited education or little knowledge of English, so notes or phone calls to her parents may not be understood. Cultural sensitivity often involves education about the rules and laws of our country. An effective way to approach this situation is to team up with the English as a Second Language teacher and approach the family together. The family needs to understand the laws of mandatory school attendance in this country and the consequences of truancy. Communication should always be respectful of cultural traditions, yet informational in terms of helping parents from different cultures understand the laws and customs of the United States. Chapter 6 will discuss the need to be culturally responsible in school counseling practices.

PARENTS AND CONFIDENTIALITY   As mentioned in the discussion of confidentiality, the boundary between responsibilities to students and responsibilities to parents can be obscure. Isaacs and Stone (1999) cited competing perspectives of school counseling researchers, one side advocating that parents have access to all information about students and the other side arguing that such disclosure is a breach of confidentiality and should not be counseling practice unless it is school board policy. One cannot deny that parents are entitled to know what is going on with their children. The problem is when parents ask that counselors share information about the student that does not need to be or have to be shared, or when the sharing of the information is not what is best for the student. Glosoff and Pate (2002) wrote, "In these cases, we suggest that counselors attempt to educate parents about the counseling process and how disclosing against the child's wishes may result in negative consequences" (p. 27).

The school counselor–parent relationship is vital to the successful implementation of a comprehensive school counseling program. The importance of this relationship is noted in ASCA's *Position Statement: Parent Consent* (ASCA,

---

My Story

As a practicing school counselor, one way that I made sure I was not violating confidentiality was by asking a student what he or she wanted me to say to his or her parents. We would decide how much information the student felt comfortable sharing and what would stay confidential. This worked well for two reasons: (a) The student was informed that I might talk to his or her parents and knew the nature of that conversation, and (b) the parents usually appreciated the information I shared with them. On occasion, a parent might say, "What did she say specifically?" I would remind the parent of my ethical obligation to maintain confidentiality, but I would also offer some suggestions based on the general nature of my sessions with the student.

1999a). School counselors protect the relationship by explaining the confidential nature of the counselor–student relationship to parents. The counselor should inform them in writing (e.g., brochures, newsletters, personalized letters) and provide opportunities to discuss the issue in person via a "Counselor's Coffee" or an evening parent program to explain school counseling services. Parents who do not understand the boundaries of the confidential relationship may have difficulty accepting that they are not privy to what their children say during sessions. Therefore, establishing the parameters early on is the best way to avoid conflict over this issue.

Another ethical responsibility of the professional school counselor is to provide parents with "accurate, comprehensive, and relevant information in an objective and caring manner . . ." (Ethical Standard B.2.b). School counselors develop skills in speaking in generalities about information that students share in counseling sessions. Instead of saying, "Tommy said that he is really angry with his dad because he has grounded him from using his car," the ethically professional response might be, "Tommy has some strong feelings about things that have been happening. What do you think he might be feeling?"

The final section of Ethical Standard B.2 discusses honoring the wishes of parents/guardians regarding sharing information about their children. In addition to the ethical responsibility of receiving written permission to talk with others about a child, the school counselor must make sure that the parents feel comfortable with information about their child being shared with anyone. For example, if a student is being presented to the Special Needs Team or Child Study Team for review, the school counselor should consult with the parent(s) and the student before sharing any of that information with the team members. Honoring the wishes of parents and guardians is an essential part of building a collaborative relationship that will, in turn, provide for more comprehensive services for students.

Responsibilities to Colleagues and Professionals

PROFESSIONAL RELATIONSHIPS   Two chapters of this book will cover in detail the importance of building collaborative relationships with faculty, staff, and administration in your school building. Ethical Standard C.1.a indicates that the professional school counselor's working relationship with school personnel is a necessary component for providing "optimal counseling services." The second part of this standard emphasizes the need for school counselors to let school personnel know the boundaries and extent of their counseling roles and responsibilities. Confusion about the school counselor's role and ethical responsibilities comes about, in part, because those who interact with the school counselor do not have a clear understanding of what school counselors do. It is a professional and ethical responsibility to provide insight into the practices of school counselors.

A second statement in this standard focuses on treating colleagues with "professional respect, courtesy, and fairness" (Ethical Standard C.1.b), which seem to be obviously desirable habits for school counselors. However, within the context of the school setting, it is not uncommon to find that one's viewpoint or opinion about something differs from a colleague or administrator's opinion. This situation provides a great opportunity to practice effective empathy and respectful listening. It is certainly appropriate to agree to disagree with someone's opinions or actions, but it is also helpful to do so in a respectful manner. It is this type of professional behavior that will ensure ethical behavior.

The third section of Ethical Standard C.1 offers guidelines for the optimal utilization of referral sources and organizations in the profession. This concurs with standard A.5 and reiterates the ethical responsibility of school counselors to have knowledge of appropriate referral sources through the development of professional relationships with colleagues in the community.

SHARING INFORMATION WITH OTHER PROFESSIONALS   The ethical standard for sharing information with other professionals supports the earlier standards regarding confidentiality and consultation with others. Maintaining student confidentiality can become quite troublesome for counselors when school personnel ask for information about students. For example, a teacher may believe that by learning about the issues or concerns of a student, he or she can better help the child in the classroom. This interaction, though well-intentioned, puts the school counselor in an awkward position.

Professional Practice

RENEE (ES)

If a parent or teacher refers a student to the counselor, he or she often wants to know what is causing the observed problems. Obviously, if someone is in danger, I let the child know that I am required to share what I have been told.

I always remind children of this requirement at the beginning of the school year and again if their conversations with me appear to be heading in that direction. Often I will say, "Do you think it would be helpful for your teacher or parents to know what is going on, so that they understand why you are having difficulty right now?" The student almost always agrees. Then we talk about who should talk to the parent or teacher. Sometimes the student will want to talk to the involved parties alone, and sometimes he or she asks me to speak to the parents and teachers alone or with him or her.

School personnel are often unaware of the ethical codes that govern school counseling practices. Certainly, school counselors want to be viewed as team players, but they are often privy to student information that might be misconstrued or taken out of context. It is a good idea to consider how you, as a school counselor, will deal with school personnel who ask specific questions about counseling sessions with students. Refer to the "My Story" box for further discussion of this issue and Figure 2.1 for an example of how to communicate effectively and ethically with teachers about student issues.

My Story

One of the most difficult things I encountered as a beginning school counselor was communicating with teachers about students I had counseled. A teacher would send a student to see me, I would have a session with the student, and then I would see the teacher later and he or she would ask: "So, what did Susie have to say? What's going on with her?" I would find myself stammering and looking for a way to generally describe the session without breaching the confidentiality of the student. Over time, I learned a couple of effective strategies for not alienating my colleagues and providing useful information for the teachers. After I would meet with a student, I would complete a form like the sample shown in Figure 2.1.

When I started providing this kind of feedback, I decreased the need for teachers to ask me for specific information about their students. I didn't have to look at them and say, "Oh, I can't tell you, it's confidential," creating a barrier between us. I was able to make helpful suggestions for working with particular students in class. I gave enough general information for them to understand that a particular student was under some kind of stress and provided strategies that might help the teachers work more effectively with the student. I also let students know that I was going to inform their teachers of certain issues in order to create more support for them in class. Many times, the student and I would complete the form together so the student would know exactly what I was going to share with teachers and be comfortable with it.

Dear _____: Date: _____
I met with _____ from your class today. Based on the content of
our session, I would suggest these classroom considerations when working with
him or her.
1. _____
2. _____
3. _____

An example:
After meeting with Susie today, I would recommend the following classroom
considerations when working with her:
1. Extended time for working on assignments, as she may be a little distracted.
2. Close monitoring in social situations and encouraging her to participate with others.
3. Positive reinforcement upon completion of a task.

Figure 2.1   Sample counselor communication with teacher.

Another difficult situation is when school administrators request student
information that is confidential. Consider the following situation:

> *Mr. Adams, a middle school administrator, approached the school counselor at*
> *the beginning of the year and wanted to know about the counseling plan for*
> *next year. The school counselor provided information about the themes of*
> *classroom guidance, the groups that would be offered, and general informa-*
> *tion about special activities, such as the Career Fair. Mr. Adams then asked the*
> *counselor for a list of students who were seen individually last year for per-*
> *sonal/social counseling, especially if it pertained to behavior. The adminis-*
> *trator wanted to try to intervene with these students and keep the list handy in*
> *the event a student came to the office for a behavioral problem. Mr. Adams*
> *believed his request was reasonable, as he wanted to be better informed about*
> *the students and their needs.*

This dilemma could be very unnerving because it involves ethical responsibilities to the student and the request of a supervisor. What should the school
counselor do? The first requests are reasonable and it is a good idea to keep
the administration informed about the counseling program, plans, and services
that will be offered. The problem arises when the principal asks for specific
names of students who are being seen for counseling services. ASCA's Ethical
Standard A.2.b states that counselors should keep information confidential
unless the child or others are in danger. Further, the position statement of
ASCA regarding the professional school counselor and confidentiality (ASCA,
2002a) clearly states that, unless there is certain danger to a student or others,
confidentiality must be maintained. Therefore, if the principal comes to you
and says, "John Smith is in my office and says he wants to kill himself. Has he
been in any counseling services in the past year?" it would be ethically responsible to share information about interaction with John. The school counselor

should also offer to get involved with the case and help with the decisions that will be made about how to handle John's statements. However, in the current situation, the principal is requesting the list of names simply because he wants to know and possibly use the information in administrative situations. The first step might be to clarify the administrator's need to know: Why is this information useful or necessary to the principal? Will it alter how he approaches the student? Does he plan to use the information for data purposes? Clearly, releasing the names of the students violates the ethical standard of confidentiality, so unless there is an ethically supported reason for giving him this information, the professional school counselor would not. So, how does the school counselor inform Mr. Adams that he or she cannot comply with his request?

In the example given, the school counselor should inform the principal that he or she will certainly provide the information he has requested about the counseling plans for the year. In terms of his request for student names, it would be helpful to make him aware of the ethical codes that prevent this. Rather than defiantly stating, "I can't do that," it is important to explain the rationale behind the code. For example, "As much as I am willing to share information that would be helpful for the student, I am bound by my professional code of ethics to maintain the confidentiality of the student unless there is clear and imminent danger to the student or others. Might I suggest that you ask students sent to your office if they have participated in counseling services? Then they can tell you what they want you to know about the counseling services they have received, and I have not broken their trust or my ethical obligation."

The standards ethically support the sharing of information as long as the data is "accurate, objective, concise, and meaningful" and is used "to adequately evaluate, counsel, and assist the counselee" (Ethical Standard C.2.b). Professional school counselors must decide what information should be shared to benefit the child while also protecting the ethical codes of confidentiality. For example, subjective information, such as the content of counseling sessions or feelings expressed during a counseling group, should not be shared. It is easy to get involved in conversations with colleagues about cases and fall into the trap of giving more information than is necessary. Learning to limit the sharing of personal information regarding students is a skill that is necessary for ethical school counseling.

Ethical Standard C.2.c is an important one. If a school counselor learns that a student is being seen by a mental health professional outside the school and is also participating in counseling services in school, the school counselor should seek written consent from the student and the student's parent/guardian if the student is younger than age 18 to share information with the outside professional. When a student is receiving counseling services outside of the school setting, it is often helpful for the school counselor and the outside therapist to consult regarding the process and progress in each arena so that counseling services and objectives are not being duplicated. Any time a student's case is being discussed, school counselors must make sure the confidentiality of the student is being maintained and that proper consent has been given. Consider the following example:

> *Mr. Lincoln is a middle school counselor who has been working with a student who has an eating disorder. The student was in denial for some time, and Mr. Lincoln worked closely with the student and her family to get the student to agree to professional intervention. The parents hospitalized the student for 3 weeks in order to address the physical immediacy of the disorder and the student participated in individual and group counseling experiences while hospitalized. When the student returned to school, Mr. Lincoln met with the parents to find out what types of services the student had received while in the hospital. In this meeting, he learned that the student was continuing to receive individual therapy from a specialist on eating disorders. The student was attending sessions twice per week and as needed in between. The parents requested that Mr. Lincoln continue to provide counseling services for their daughter while she was in school, which he agreed to do. Mr. Lincoln then requested that the parents sign a form allowing the school and the external counselor to release information so that they would not create confusion for the student. Based on that conversation and the agreement between the two professionals, Mr. Lincoln could determine the depth of services he needed to provide at school.*

Mr. Lincoln certainly demonstrated ethically responsible behavior in this scenario. In addition, Mr. Lincoln probably should let the parents know that the underlying issues that result in eating disorders are probably beyond the level of training that he received in his school counseling training. (This ethical responsibility is noted in Section E of the Standards.) When a student is in counseling outside of school and also has counseling with the school counselor, he or she can sometimes burn out on the counseling experience. Over-counseling or overemphasis on counseling could be detrimental to the student's progress, both in school and in counseling.

Responsibilities to the School and Community

RESPONSIBILITIES TO THE SCHOOL Because school counselors are employees of a school system, they have an ethical responsibility to help support the best interests of the school. The professional school counselor "supports and protects the educational program against any infringement not in the best interest of the counselees" (Ethical Standard D.1.a). If the school counselor sees that some part of the educational program is psychologically, socially, or emotionally harmful, it is essential for the school counselor to inform the appropriate school officials. Standard D.1.b obliges the school counselor to serve as an informant when a condition or situation could result in damage or detriment to the school program, property, or mission. For example, if a school counselor learns that a group of students plans to pull the fire alarm during final exams, he or she must let an administrator know. In this type of situation, a school counselor might encourage the students to tell the administration themselves. The school counselor should offer to go with the children to tell the administrator and applaud the students for their honesty.

Another key responsibility that school counselors have to their schools is to only accept employment in positions for which they have the proper education, training, and credentials (Ethical Standard D.1.d). The flip side of this responsibility is that administrators *should* hire only those individuals who are competent and qualified for school counseling positions. However, when there is a shortage of qualified candidates, school administrators may feel they must fill positions with persons who may be less than qualified for the position. The American School Counselor Association is clear about the level of expertise that is necessary to work effectively with students: "In situations in which noncredentialed personnel are performing school-counseling–related activities, these services must be limited to the scope of the role of the service provider, based on training and capabilities" (ASCA, 2000b, pp. 1–2).

The final section of this Ethical Standard, D.1.e, includes a comprehensive description of the professional school counselor's responsibilities to the overall academic program in a school. It highlights the school counselor's involvement in (a) the development of curricula that are appropriate for the school, (b) the creation of an environment that promotes student learning, and (c) the planning and implementation of programs and procedures that are developmentally appropriate and congruent with student needs. Further, the school counselor is also responsible for the ongoing, systematic evaluation of counseling services and programs in order to collect data and use the results for planning effective counseling services. Chapter 13 will cover the issues of evaluation and accountability in detail.

RESPONSIBILITY TO THE COMMUNITY   Though brief, the ethical standard addressing the professional school counselor's responsibility to the community emphasizes the collaborative relationship between agencies, organizations, and individuals in the community. The school counselor is often in a position to serve as liaison between the school and the community. This relationship is vital to promoting good public relations and support for school projects and activities that necessitate community involvement. The second half of the statement provides another warning against dual relationships. School counselors should not use their connections with the community for any personal, professional, or monetary gain.

Responsibilities to Self

While much time is spent focusing on how school counselors are responsible to everyone else, the Ethical Standards also mandate that school counselors should take care of and protect themselves. The school counselor's ethical responsibility to develop professionally and contribute to the profession of school counseling represents a continuous process that spans one's career.

PROFESSIONAL COMPETENCE The first three standards in this section address the professional school counselor's ability to recognize his or her competence and to make sure that professional development and personal functioning are always at a level that is conducive to serving the counseling needs of the students. The concept of nonmalfeasance (avoiding doing harm) is not unique to codes of ethics, but school counselors must remember that we often work with people who are vulnerable, emotional, and sometimes even irrational. The last section advocates for the continuous professional development and personal growth of school counselors throughout their careers. Securing a job is the first goal of counselors-in-training upon leaving their graduate programs, but continuing to develop professional competence is an ethical responsibility and the best way to stay informed about changes in school counseling. Being informed about new practices is an absolute necessity for and professional responsibility of effective school counselors. There will be more in-depth discussion about the development of professional competence in chapter 14.

MULTICULTURAL SKILLS The ethical standard for multicultural skills is also brief, but describes a great responsibility of the school counselor. The standard describes the importance of school counselors being culturally knowledgeable and aware of the diverse needs of students from various cultures and the need for school counselors to constantly revisit their own thoughts, feelings, and beliefs about diversity. Ongoing evaluation of one's personal worldview and how it affects counseling practices is a major practice of culturally responsive counseling. Chapter 6 provides an extensive discussion of multiculturalism and diversity and the implications for school counselors.

Responsibilities to the Profession

PROFESSIONALISM The ethical code governing professionalism holds school counselors to very high standards. Ethical Standards F.1 and F.2 provide specific guidelines that govern school counseling behavior.

First, school counselors should know the protocol for reporting an ethical violation by joining and maintaining memberships in professional school counseling organizations (Ethical Standard F.1.a). These organizations can provide specific guidelines for handling challenging situations. Further, the American School Counselor Association provides the opportunity for its members to purchase professional liability insurance. Thus, professional membership benefits the school counselor by identifying a process for filing an ethical violation, as well as offering protection in the event of a claim filed against the school counselor.

Ethical Standard F.1.b speaks to professional conduct and advocates leading by example. This refers back to one of the school counselor's opportunities discussed in chapter 1—to be a positive role model. School counselors are human and will certainly demonstrate human emotions and frustration.

My Story

When I disagreed with something or if a situation came up and I knew there was a discrepancy between how I wanted to handle it and how the school policy said I should handle it, I consulted with my colleagues and administrators to see how I should proceed. My job was valuable to me and I did not want to lose it, but I had to come to some sort of compromise between my personal feelings, my professional responsibilities, and the policy. Sometimes, the policy dictated how I was to respond as an employee of the school district; at other times, I found that there was some flexibility in how the situation was handled and I was happy with the compromise.

However, losing one's temper or acting inappropriately will damage the image of the effective counselor who helps others deal with their emotions. Further, when the time comes to make an ethical decision, the professional school counselor will demonstrate sound moral principles and follow the standards of the profession. Dansby-Giles (2002) identified these moral principles as

- autonomy—promoting self-determination;
- beneficence—promoting good for others;
- nonmalfeasance—avoiding doing harm;
- justness—providing equal treatment to all people; and
- fidelity—keeping promises (p. 23).

The third part of the standard (F.1.c) describes the ethical mandate for school counselors to conduct research and report results that are useful for educational and psychological purposes. This is an area that seems to challenge our profession. One of the pitfalls of school counseling practice is that it is difficult to measure success. The reality is that counseling is a qualitative field with subjective overtones and often immeasurable outcomes. Trying to quantify that a student feels better is a tough task. Evaluation of the participants in a group or a counseling services needs assessment survey of parents are simple ways to gather data for a school counseling program and promote effective planning for future counseling practices. We will devote much more time to the discussion of use of data and accountability in chapter 13.

Ethical Standard F.1.d asserts that school counselors are responsible for adhering to not only the ethical standards of school counseling, but also the standards pertaining to counseling that are published by federal, state, and local governments. In addition, school counselors must also follow the standards of local school boards, which are governed by local laws. This may be the most difficult, as school board policies may not always concur with personal ethics or one's worldview.

The next standard (F.1.e) requires that school counselors make a distinction between personal statements and actions and professional statements and actions. It is not easy to separate who we are from what we do, especially in the school counseling profession. People primarily pursue this career because of the way they feel about young people and the desire to help them. This standard emphasizes the need for objectivity and separate personal and professional viewpoints or practices. School counselors are certainly entitled to opinions about politics, social action issues, and controversial subjects. The ethical conflict arises when those viewpoints are expressed and are perceived as being representative of the school, school district, or school counseling profession. Learning to identify appropriate arenas in which to share those opinions is ethically responsible behavior.

Ethical standard F.1.f prevents school counselors from recruiting clients for other types of interaction outside of the school counseling setting. For example, some school counselors are also licensed to have private practices, and it would seem that the school is a likely and even desirable place to find clients. Ethical issues, such as dual relationships, come to the forefront in this situation and clearly prohibit this action. The ethical code also prevents school counselors from using their position to "seek and receive unjustified personal gains, unfair advantage, sexual favors, or unearned goods or services" (Ethical Standard F.1.f). Sometimes, ethical standards are simply good common sense. It should almost go without saying that one cannot use a professional position to take advantage of others or as a trade-off for a good or service. The rationale for established ethical standards is that at some point in time, these issues came up and had to be addressed. It is better to provide clarity and understanding up front than to face the repercussions of unethical and irreparable actions.

CONTRIBUTIONS TO THE PROFESSION   Some might interpret Ethical Standard F.2 as indicating that professionals must publish articles or books about school counseling practices in order to contribute to the field. While these are certainly professional options, contributing to the profession also includes networking with colleagues and sharing ideas and expertise. Attending and presenting at conferences is the best way to network, share ideas, gain support, and feel rejuvenated about the profession. Conferences are a great way to learn about new ways of doing things and to hear the experiences of other counselors. Professional interaction leads to greater skill development and professional competence. There is also reciprocity in this process; typically when contributing to the profession, you also come away with new ideas and skills that you can implement in your own program.

Maintenance of Standards

Section G of the Ethical Standards refers to the manner in which professional school counselors should respond to potential or actual ethical violations. The first paragraph entitles school counselors to take action to rectify any situations that are deemed unethical or are an infringement of the ethical standards. The steps provided in Ethical Standards G.1 through G.5 define a clear protocol for how to handle ethically challenging situations:

1. Consult with colleagues to see if they concur that the situation is a violation of professional ethics.

2. Approach the colleague or person about your ethical concerns related to the situation and try to resolve the issue.

3. If no resolution is reached, follow the chain of command in reporting ethical concerns, starting locally and moving more globally. Refer first to the guidance director or school district person responsible for school counseling personnel and programs, then contact the state level school counseling or counseling organization. Finally, the American School Counselor Association has an Ethics Committee that deals solely with issues or concerns regarding ethical standards and violations. This committee, as described in Ethical Standard G.5, has the responsibility to recommend changes in code and also has a responsibility to receive, process, and respond to ethical requests of its membership. Another good reason for membership in professional organizations is support for situations and concerns that arise.

Resources

The final section of the Ethical Standards for School Counselors is a reference list of all sources utilized for developing and supporting the statements in the standards. There have been three revisions to the ethical standards, and the Ethics Committee continuously reviews the need for changes to any information contained in the ethical standards. These resources are research support for the standards, as well as supplements that address specific categories of the document. It would be worthwhile to examine these resources, as they provide the framework for current standards and practices in school counseling.

A Model for Ethical Decision Making

School counselors must take their ethical responsibilities very seriously, and one way to act responsibly is to participate in continuing education workshops and training sessions on ethical and legal issues in counseling, particularly in school counseling. A study by Hermann (2002) found that school counselors who had participated in ongoing legal and ethical training opportunities felt they were better able to deal with ethical and legal issues that emerged in their schools.

Ethical decisions are not always black and white. However, the ethical standards are an important support system when ethical decisions have to be made. There are general guidelines to consider when an ethical situation arises. First and foremost, make sure that your decision is in the best interest of the child, regardless of the consequences that might result in terms of your relationship with the child. For example, when reporting suspected abuse, the parents may become upset with the school system and withdraw consent to have the student continue with counseling services. It may be necessary to explain to the student that this might happen, but that he or she will continue to have support as much as possible at school. It is also important to identify other adult resources in the school building (teachers, school social worker, school psychologist, administrators) that could help the student.

Second, review the ethical guidelines and the impetus behind the need for ethical consideration. Is the issue moral, ethical, legal, or some combination of the three? In this review, it is important to consult with colleagues, and it may also be appropriate to consult with a professional organization in order to make a decision about how to proceed.

Finally, the best decision is an informed and well-thought decision. Ambiguity sometimes clouds obvious and clear-cut solutions to ethical decisions. It is good practice to have a copy of the ASCA Ethical Standards (1998) accessible so that they are readily available as a reference in the event of an ethical dilemma. In addition, close adherence to the ethical codes helps solidify the school counselor's position and responsibilities in many situations that arise in schools. It is often comforting to know there are guidelines for ethical behavior and following the standards demonstrates professionalism in the school counseling field.

Professional Perspective

ESTHER (HS)

ADVICE: Team with a seasoned counselor to share ethical and other dilemmas. Look for a broader perspective and share in the wisdom of experience.

CONCLUSION

This chapter has been devoted to the role of the school counselor as ethical practitioner. Though not always easy, the ethical issues and situations that exist in schools must be dealt with professionally and ethically. School counselors should address areas that are "gray," such as confidentiality in certain situations, by following ethical standards, state and local laws, and school board policy. It is always good to consult with colleagues or professional organizations about situations in which the ethical decision is not clear. Chances are that others have experienced similar challenges, and being aware of prior actions and protocol may alleviate the difficulty of ethical decision making.

The professional school counselor is ethically aware and prepared to deal with difficult situations and behaves in a manner that reflects positively on the profession. It is critical, as a school counselor–in-training, that you devote considerable time to becoming knowledgeable about ethical practices in order to become an ethically sound practitioner.

REFLECTION AND DISCUSSION

1. Consider your personal values and belief system about controversial issues that might arise in schools (e.g., sexual orientation, parental rights to information, etc.). What issues do you think might challenge you in terms of your ethical response?

2. Outline your plan or protocol for handling an ethically challenging situation. What would you do first? What next? How would you follow-up?

3. In addition to ethical responsibilities, there are legal aspects to some of the issues that school counselors face. What is the best way for you, as a school counselor in training, to be informed about these issues? What are specific actions you can take in order to prepare yourself to be an ethically sound practitioner?

4. Why do you think the role of the professional school counselor as ethical practitioner is important? What priority should it have in terms of other school counselor roles?

CHAPTER 3

Counseling and Classroom Guidance

*A*ccording to the American School Counselor Association (1999c), a school counselor's duties can be categorized into one of four roles: counseling, classroom guidance, consultation, and coordination. Recent emphasis has been on the importance of a fifth "C," collaboration, which serves as an umbrella under which the other roles operate. The *Transforming School Counseling Initiative* (Education Trust, 2003) identified the collaborative role of school counselors as encompassing all that school counselors do.

When considering the role and function of school counselors, it is important to consider how counseling services are provided. The American School Counselor Association (1999c) has identified the traditional roles of school counselors as classroom guidance, counseling (to include individual and small-group services), consultation, and coordination. Gysbers and Henderson (2000) categorized the roles to encompass many of the other services school counselors provide: guidance curriculum, individual planning, responsive services, and system support. These roles are included in the delivery systems component of the ASCA National Model for School Counseling Programs (ASCA, 2003a). The *Transforming School Counseling Initiative* (Education Trust, 2003) expands on the traditional roles by including leadership, advocacy, teaming and collaboration, and the use of data for systemic change.

While this book will move from traditional roles into the transformed roles of school counselors, it is crucial to explore all of the roles that school counseling services comprise. Because each role assumes several tasks, this chapter will focus solely on the first two Cs—counseling and classroom guidance—which are direct services for students.

Counseling

The American School Counselor Association (1999c) has defined the counseling function as ". . . a confidential relationship which the counselor conducts with students individually and in small groups to help them resolve or cope constructively with their problems and developmental concerns" (p. 1). In discussing the counseling function, consideration is given to both *individual counseling* and *group counseling*.

Individual Counseling

Probably the most distinctive role of a school counselor is the opportunity to spend time with individual students working on academic, personal/social, or career problems. The picture that comes to mind when discussing individual counseling sessions is the counselor and student engaged in an intense conversation behind closed doors for extensive periods of time. While this may occur, individual counseling sessions can take many forms: private sessions in the counseling office, one-on-one sessions outside a classroom, checking in during common periods (i.e., lunch, before school, changing classes), or a conversation at a school-sponsored event. Though these more public interactions risk an absence of confidentiality, the school counselor can get a good sense of the pulse of the school or the personal state of the individual from these brief interactions.

Professional Perspective

ESTHER (HS)

Individual counseling at the high school level takes place in both a planned and spontaneous fashion. Students come in with a variety of problems and can also be in a state of crisis. The counselor is both proactive and immediate in individual counseling. Follow-up is critical.

One common misconception is that the school counselor is a therapist. While some might use the terms *counselor* and *therapist* interchangeably, there is a distinction to be made, especially as it applies to school counselors. The training that occurs in school counseling preparation programs typically prepares students for counseling as it relates to the school setting. In mental health counseling or community counseling programs, there is much greater emphasis on diagnosis and treatment by applying the Diagnostic and Statistical Manual of Mental Disorders, Text Revision (DSM-IV-TR) (American Psychiatric Association, 2000). School counselors do not make diagnoses, and the treatment plans they develop are appropriately referred to as counseling plans. Explaining this difference is an important distinction when helping others understand the parameters of the school counseling role.

The primary goal of individual counseling is to help students, one-on-one, explore issues or situations that are affecting their ability to function inside and outside of school. Many individual sessions are unscheduled and occur in casual encounters. A student may walk by, see that the school counselor is available, and come into the office to talk. Table 3.1 lists issues that might be addressed through individual counseling with students.

Sometimes, sessions that seem short-term or simple become complex. For example, a student comes in because he or she has lashed out at a classmate. You discover the reason for the behavior is that a parent physically disciplined the student last night; upon further investigation, you find a bruise on the student's arm. This requires a referral to Child Protective Services and all of the counseling services that come with this referral. It is important to never assume that a case or situation is going to be easy.

In some situations, long-term sessions will be necessary. Students who are really struggling with a situation at home or at school might need more extensive support. It is important that the school counselor's role as an individual counselor is clearly defined and given priority. Sometimes it seems that

TABLE 3.1
Examples of Issues That Might Be Addressed Through Individual Counseling

Elementary	Middle School	High School
Friendship issues	Academic difficulty	Classes or class schedule
Difficulties with teachers	Relationship issues	College and career planning
Difficulties at home	Crisis situations	Attendance or truancy issues
Behavioral or academic difficulty	Transition to high school	Relationship problems
Crisis situations (fighting, sudden loss, etc.)	Issues with parents	Issues with parents
Emotional issues, such as moving, divorce, death of a loved one, etc.	Difficulty with school faculty or administration	Difficulty with school faculty or administration
	Academic scheduling	
	Career planning	

individual counseling sessions are at the bottom of the priority list and occur only if there is time to see students. Again, counseling is a primary role for school counselors. Communicating this to administrators and teachers is critical. There is nothing more frustrating or disheartening to a student than to feel that the counselor—the person who is supposed to be the student advocate—either does not have time for or does not give high priority to individual sessions

My Story

I used to refer to unplanned sessions as "walk-bys" because as students would walk by my open door, they would often stop, backpedal, and come into the office. As a school counselor, I implemented an open-door policy to encourage students to come in. Sometimes this would result in what I called "frequent flyers" because there were always a few who came by weekly, if not daily, just to check in. It was the opportunity to talk about something specific or just vent that seemed to help them manage their academic and personal lives. Another phrase coined by one of my school counseling interns captures the essence of the brief interactions—"two-minute touch base." This refers to checking in with students in the hallway, in the cafeteria, before school, after school, or between classes in order to monitor how they are doing. While it is not a complete counseling session, the "touch base" approach may be appropriate for some students, especially those in need of follow-up.

with students, especially when they are scheduled. An effective way to manage this is to make sure that school personnel understand that, unless there is an emergency situation, individual sessions take priority.

INDIVIDUAL COUNSELING SKILLS Most school counseling training programs include a course that teaches specific skills and techniques for counseling students. One of the questions that beginning counselors often ask is, "How will I know what to do?" The first response to this question is: *Meet the student where the student is.*

When a student enters the counseling office for individual counseling, it is important to know how he or she got there: Did the student come on his or her own or did someone else refer him or her? A quick assessment might note the obvious: How upset is the student? What is his or her body language? What kind of comments is he or she making? Does the student seem receptive to counseling? The answers to these questions may determine a great deal about how counseling should proceed. Once the student seems comfortable in the counseling session, more in-depth questions might be appropriate. These might include

- "Tell me more about what has brought you here today."
- "How have things been going for you lately?"
- "I can see that you feel strongly about this. Tell me more about what you're feeling."
- "What would you like to share with me about this issue?"
- "How would you like me to help you?"

These questions or statements are good icebreakers for initiating counseling sessions with students. Of course, counselors can use specific theoretical techniques to work with students, such as behavioral contracting, art, and play therapy. Recently, there has been a trend toward solution-focused brief counseling in schools. Brief interventions should be explored as a useful method for working with students within the time constraints of the school day.

SOLUTION-FOCUSED BRIEF COUNSELING Although solution-focused brief counseling (SFBC) is considered a relatively recent phenomenon, its roots actually began in the 1950s at the Mental Research Institute in Palo Alto, California. In the 1960s, Fisch and colleagues based their work on a model that narrowed the treatment focus to problem solving (Capuzzi & Gross, 2003). A team of therapists developed the tenets and principles for what is currently referred to as solution-focused brief counseling. The Brief Family Therapy Center was opened in the early 1980s in Milwaukee, Wisconsin. Early proponents of SFBC (de Shazer, 1985; de Shazer et al., 1986; O'Hanlon & Weiner-Davis, 1989) advocated for the new short-term approach to counseling based on the assertion that "solution-focused counseling departs from the problem-solving strategies, in which most counselors have been trained, by identifying what individuals are already doing well and building on those things. The approach focuses on beliefs about change, beliefs about complaints, and creating solutions" (LaFountain, Garner, & Eliason, 1996, p. 256). O'Hanlon and Weiner-Davis (1989) also emphasized the overriding elements of optimism and hope that permeate the concepts of solution-focused counseling. Birdsall and Miller (2002) concisely described the utility of SFBC in school settings: "School counselors are ready for an approach to working with students, their families, and school staff that takes less of a time commitment and is more effective at the same time" (p. 1).

Part of the appeal of brief counseling approaches is the simplicity and action-oriented philosophy that directly focuses on goals and solutions. In recent years, Metcalf (1995) and Sklare (1997) have written entire books that provide specific applications of solution-focused concepts and techniques in schools. These are useful resources for a professional counseling library; the books provide extensive coverage of solution-focused brief counseling and describe numerous strategies for implementing solution-focused counseling services. Many workshops and conference sessions focus on brief counseling, and the trend continues to dominate much of the literature on theoretical approaches to school counseling.

Key Concepts and Principles   Originally, the delivery of brief counseling services was based on the Brief Counseling Model (Bruce, 1995; Bruce & Hopper, 1997). The steps in this model are:

1. The counselor and student build a working alliance while also identifying the presenting problem.

2. The counselor and student discuss the solutions and consequences of previously attempted solutions. It is during this time that the counselor identifies student strengths or capabilities that might be used in the solution to the problem.

3. The counselor and student participate in goal setting and consider all the possible solutions to the problem. Goals are to be immediate and measurable.

4. The student implements the intervention and reports the results back to the counselor. Success or failure in achieving goals should be discussed, and alterations to the goals or changes in the implementation may need to occur until the problem is resolved.

More recently, Thompson (2002) presented an SFBC model that focused specifically on the stages to be followed when using SFBC in the school counseling setting. She suggested that once a new positive behavior has been acquired, it is important to identify how things have changed and how the student might respond differently should a challenging situation occur. Capitalizing on strengths and learning to respond in more productive ways when crises arise are two important solution-focused practices. SFBC is a positive, no-nonsense approach to counseling students in schools, and it makes sense that this approach would appeal to school counselors, whose time is limited and whose caseloads are often overwhelming. Students may also respond positively to the direct, solution-focused approach to their problems and the hope that their issues can be resolved.

Techniques   The techniques of solution-focused brief counseling also appeal to counselors because they are user-friendly, direct, and help students progress toward meaningful goals. The techniques include:

- *The miracle question*—"Suppose that tonight, while you are sleeping, a miracle happens and when you wake up, your problem has gone away. What does that look like for you? What is different now that the problem is solved?" Having the students describe their lives without certain problems is the first step in helping them resolve issues so that they can create their reality without the problem.

- *Scaling*—"On a scale of 1 to 10, with 1 being the worst and 10 being that the problem is solved, where do you think your problem is right now?" Scaling can also be used to gauge emotion and cognition. "On a scale of 1 to 5, with 1 being the most anxious and 5 being totally relaxed, how are you feeling right now?" This gives the counselor some sense of the severity of the student's situation and will help with goal setting and progress toward a resolution.

- *Looking for exceptions*—The counselor listens for times or circumstances when the student has responded in a way that will help resolve the problem. For example, if a student comes to counseling because he or she is anxious about a new or unfamiliar situation, the counselor can help the student remember other times when he or she has successfully entered new situations and identify the strengths that helped him or her feel positive in the new situations.

- *Coping questions* (Birdsall & Miller, 2002)—The counselor focuses on the student's coping resources by asking, "How have you managed this so far?" The student then realizes his or her coping mechanisms and capacity for adaptation, which helps motivate him or her toward problem resolution.

Research on Brief Counseling and SFBC in Schools   Research on the efficacy of brief counseling with students has important implications for future practice in schools. Littrell, Malia, and Vanderwood (1995) conducted a study in which 61 high school students were counseled using one of three types of counseling approaches: (a) a problem-focused brief counseling approach that did not include a task, (b) a problem-focused brief counseling approach with a task, and (c) a solution-focused brief approach with a task. The results indicated that "brief counseling provided a vehicle for students to reduce their concerns about problem situations, move closer to their goals,

and diminish uncomfortable feelings about their problems" (p. 456). There was no significant difference between the three brief approaches, whether the approach was problem-focused or solution-focused; the factor that seemed to be most critical was the brevity of the sessions, not whether the focus was on the problem or on the solution. In a study with younger students, Bruce and Hopper (1997) found that the Brief Counseling Model was as effective if not better than traditional counseling methods in individual counseling sessions.

A more comprehensive study by LaFountain, Garner, and Eliason (1996) explored the use of solution-focused techniques in small-group counseling with elementary, middle, and high school students. The results indicated that the students who received solution-focused counseling experienced the following: higher levels of self-esteem in areas other than academic progress, higher self-perception scores, and a greater ability to cope than the control group that did not receive solution-focused counseling.

To examine the efficacy of SFBC from the counselor's perspective, Mostert, Johnson, and Mostert (1997) conducted a one-year study of solution-focused brief counseling with five counselors. The counselors were trained in SFBC and asked to utilize the methods and techniques of SFBC in their counseling programs with students and parents. Results indicated that the counselors felt SFBC was helpful in promoting collaborative relationships with all members of the school community. Further, the counselors felt SFBC was a useful and effective way to work with students and parents.

Because SFBC in school counseling is relatively new, research is just beginning to measure its impact on school counseling. Research has indicated that SFBC has been used successfully with adolescents with ADHD (Dielman & Franklin, 1998), with students with learning disabilities (Thompson & Littrell, 1998), and with the school avoidance behavior of seventh graders (Schopen, 1997). Gingerich and Wabeke's review of literature (2001) suggested that SFBC has been effective when involving parents in a student intervention and in counseling work with parenting groups. While there is certainly room for expansion, it appears that SFBC has been used successfully in a variety of school settings and populations.

Advantages and Disadvantages of SFBC While solution-focused brief counseling seems to be an ideal fit for the school counselor, it is important to be cautious before fully embracing its philosophy. School counselors must make sure that they do not become so focused on the solution that they overlook more serious problems that might require long-term intervention (Birdsall & Miller, 2002; Littrell, Malia, & Vanderwood, 1995). Brief counseling may be a perfect choice for dealing with some problems, but may not be effective if student problems are more intense or require long-term intervention. Issues such as child abuse, eating disorders, and clinical depression cannot be resolved quickly. School counselors must be able to identify when SFBC may not be the appropriate course for counseling.

Another incorrect assumption is that solution-focused techniques are easy because they are concrete and concise. "For example, considerable counseling skills are required to help students set small and meaningful goals. In addition, assigning tasks to help students move in the direction of their goals also requires skill and sensitivity on the part of counselors" (Littrell, Malia, & Vanderwood, 1995, p. 457). As with any counseling technique, education and practice are necessary in order for counselors to gain experience and expertise in providing appropriate services. A less obvious pitfall of SFBC is the training or educating of other school personnel in the principles and techniques of SFBC (Birdsall & Miller, 2002). Because of the time needed to make others aware of the solution-focused counseling approach, time will be taken from other school counseling activities.

Much literature and research has supported SFBC as advantageous for school counselors for several reasons. The advantages that emerged from the Littrell, Malia, and Vanderwood (1995) study included efficiency in terms of managing large groups of students and positive student responses to the brief, goal-directed focus of sessions. Murphy (1994) cited other advantages, including an increased sense of cooperation with parents and teachers, which influences the overall school environment.

Solution-focused models are compatible with the problem-solving approaches in education in general. In fact, all members of the education community have received the concept of a *solution-focused school* positively; educators are answering the challenge to shift perspectives in order to view the overall school mission in a more positive light (Davis & Osborn, 1999). "This means not dwelling on the problems we are faced with each day, but instead focusing on the overwhelming abundance of positive, exceptional occurrences taking place in our schools everyday" (Davis & Osborn, p. 42). Solution-focused school counseling contributes to a positive atmosphere by focusing on what is already working and creating solutions based on these strengths. This compatibility between school counseling practices and the overall school mission contributes to the opinion that solution-focused brief counseling may be the method of choice for many school counselors.

Another appealing characteristic of solution-focused brief counseling methods is that they integrate well with other counseling theories. Watts and Pietrzak (2000) identified the similarities of SFBC and Adlerian therapy in terms of perspective, the counselor–client relationship, and the process of change. Further, SFBC and behavior therapy may be integrated if the counseling goals developed are related to behavior change. Behavior modification strategies may fit into brief counseling methodology if that is the student's goal. Finally, Glasser's Choice Theory complements solution-focused counseling therapy because it is also brief and focused on goal setting. Counselors-in-training do not need to adhere to only one theoretical philosophy; however, it is important to have a professional and practical understanding of an identified theoretical orientation prior to beginning school counseling practicum and internships. The theoretical orientation of a school counselor will influence counseling practices, so it is critical that counselors-in-training develop a professional counseling philosophy with a strong theoretical foundation. Thus, a solution-focused counseling approach should be considered, along with the various other theoretical paradigms that have proven to be effective in school counseling practices.

RESPONDING TO STUDENT NEEDS   The techniques described in the previous sections assume the counselee has come to the counseling session ready to talk. This may not always be the case. Consider the following story:

> *A first-grade teacher comes to the school counselor about a student in her class named Molly. Molly has not spoken a word to the teacher in the first four weeks of school. The teacher has observed Molly talking to other students, but never above a whisper. Despite the teacher's efforts to get Molly to talk, Molly simply drops her head and does not respond to the teacher. The teacher has met with the mother of the child who says this has not been a problem before. Molly is not new to the school and seems to have normal peer and adult relationships outside of school. The teacher is asking for help.*

Since the behavior of concern is lack of communication, the school counselor should not expect that Molly will easily disclose her concerns. Instead, he or she may need to employ a variety of techniques in order to see if Molly will communicate in other ways. For students who are nonverbal or who do not seem to want to talk about the problem right away, school counselors may need to be creative in building the rapport that is necessary to gain the student's trust. Art therapy techniques such as drawing or writing are often used to get students to express emotions. Playing games or going for walks may be other options for getting students to open up. The concept of meeting the student where the student is means that school counselors may have to use different techniques and ideas in order to relate to and connect with students. Whether using a puppet or going out to shoot baskets, school counselors must have a repertoire of techniques to use when working individually with students. When working with older students, discussing other interests in their lives, such as music or relationships, may be an effective strategy for building rapport and fostering communication. Chapter 5 presents further discussion about assessing student issues and developing counseling plans to address student needs.

RESEARCH ON INDIVIDUAL COUNSELING IN SCHOOLS   In a survey of 80 practicing counselors in two southeastern states, Burnham and Jackson (2000) found that the percentage of time devoted to individual counseling ranged from 2% to 75%. More than half devoted up to 25% of their time and one-fourth spent 50% of their time performing individual counseling. On the surface, these results are pleasing; however Burnham and Jackson are cautious about the implications of their findings:

> We believe the counselors relied too heavily on individual counseling for numerous reasons. The counselors most likely found individual counseling

convenient, easy to schedule, and a comfortable way to work with students. We also recognize that traditionally, the focus of counselor education training programs has been on individual counseling skills; thus, many counselors feel most prepared to function in this mode. This is a dilemma since current counselor education programs emphasize individual counseling as the least efficient way to reach all students. (p. 46)

This study implies that while individual counseling is a primary task for school counselors, it should not dominate a school counselor's time. Individual counseling, in combination with the other counseling roles, should be part of a balanced school counseling program.

The significance of individual counseling as part of the counseling role cannot be overstated. Students often have the answers to their own problems before they enter a school counselor's office, and school counselors may serve as sounding boards to confirm their plans of action. In other cases, students may need more direction or guidance when working through problems. It is often after the fact that school counselors realize the impact they have had on students, but it is the individual counseling process that provides support for students to develop the important life skills of problem-solving and decision-making.

Group Counseling

Group counseling is probably the most efficient way to provide direct counseling services in the school counseling program. *Group counseling* refers to small groups of no more than eight members who meet, usually once per week, to discuss a specific topic. *Group guidance* (also known as *classroom guidance*) will be discussed in the next section.

Professional Practice

ESTHER (HS)

I am responsible for organizing and promoting group counseling at our high school. I publish a *Groups Guide,* which details 22 student enrichment seminars (counseling groups) for students to choose from. One copy is given to every student in our school, and to every parent at grade level meetings during the school year. Students are self-referred for our counseling groups. Referrals also come from teachers, parents, and administrators. I tally and organize the student requests and get the lists to the counselors in our department who conduct these specialized groups (myself included). Our counseling department evaluates the offerings yearly, and new group materials are created to serve student needs. Counselors work in pairs and involve the school social worker, school psychologist, career center specialist, and school nurse as group leaders.

It has been my experience that group counseling occurs more frequently at the elementary level than at the secondary level, although there are exceptions. Ripley and Goodnough (2001) offered strategies that would help high school counselors plan and implement group counseling at the secondary level. These strategies included developing awareness about group counseling and how it supports the curriculum, giving students greater access to group services, and planning and preparing to offer group counseling services.

Counselors-in-training typically learn about the group process through a course specifically on group counseling. Implementing groups in schools begins with seeking referrals for group membership. Typically, teachers and parents make referrals, although students, especially older students, may self-refer or sign up for groups themselves. Once a group has been selected, members will progress through a series of sessions, typically weekly, that address student needs. The goal of group counseling is to help the individual members, as well as the group as a whole, move toward certain goals. Goals are related to the overall purpose of the group and the individual needs of the group participants.

The pros and cons of group counseling become quickly evident when a school counselor implements small group counseling services. Table 3.2 lists the potential benefits and challenges of group counseling in the school arena.

BENEFITS   As indicated in Table 3.2, group counseling can be beneficial because a wide range of student needs can be addressed. Group topics might be remedial (e.g., study skills, retention), supportive (e.g., changing families, children of alcoholics), developmental (e.g., peer relationships, identity development), or preventive (e.g., anger management, conflict resolution). Table 3.3 provides a list of possible group topics for kindergarten through 12th grade school counseling programs. While not exhaustive, the list represents the range of topics that are appropriate in a small group counseling forum. Conducting a needs assessment of students, teachers, and parents will provide valuable input when deciding about topics for small group counseling.

In addition to addressing topics to meet students' needs, groups also provide a *safe environment* in which students can express their thoughts and feelings and practice new behaviors prior to trying them out in the world. The thought of being ridiculed is sometimes overwhelming to children, regardless of age, and the group setting provides a safe haven for students to get comfortable with themselves, as well as any new behaviors that might emerge as a result of group counseling. Students who might have difficulty expressing themselves or experiencing life on a larger scale might feel more secure and confident about expressing themselves in a small group. Perhaps the most obvious benefit of group counseling is that more students can be served in a group than in individual counseling. ASCA (2002b) posited:

> Many components of a comprehensive school guidance program are best
> delivered by means of group counseling. Small- and large-group approaches

TABLE 3.2
Benefits and Challenges of Group Counseling

Benefits	Challenges
Can be remedial, supportive, developmental, and/or preventive	Teacher resistance due to missed classes
Gives students the opportunity to share experiences in a safe setting and understand that they aren't alone	Students might feel ostracized if forced to participate in group sessions
Is a more efficient way to service a greater number of students	Scheduling difficulties: In elementary schools, must schedule around language arts and math blocks; in secondary schools, you must alternate class periods missed, which is hard for students to remember
Greater likelihood of behavior change due to peer role modeling and the ability to rehearse new behaviors in a nonthreatening atmosphere	Large number of referrals (especially at the elementary level); there may be more children referred for a group than can possibly be seen on a weekly basis

are the preferred medium of delivery for developmental guidance and counseling activities, in terms of efficiency as well as effectiveness. (p. 1)

Small group and individual counseling often go hand-in-hand. Many of the issues that emerge during individual counseling sessions may result in an invi-

TABLE 3.3
Possible Topics for Groups (Remedial and Support)

Remedial	Support
Study skills	Changing families
Assertiveness skills	Grief/loss
Building self-concept	New students
Social skills/Friendship skills	Bullying (victims or perpetrators)
Test-taking skills	ADHD
Anger management	Multicultural or diversity issues
Stress management	Substance use or abuse (self or family member)
Behavior management	Teenage pregnancy
Attention issues	Age-related or gender-specific issues
	Students with common medical problems (e.g., eating disorders, physical challenges)
	Adopted or foster children
	Homeless students
	Students who are retained

tation for a student to participate in group counseling. Group counseling may be the final step for students who had been receiving long-term individual counseling. For example, after seeing a student for issues surrounding a parental divorce, the counselor might invite the student to participate in a group on changing families. This seems to be a logical progression of counseling services because the student has been working through the initial stages of grief/loss, and it is probable that the student might benefit from participating in a group with other students with similar issues. Once the student has completed a 6- to 8-week group experience, the student's needs would be evaluated to determine if further counseling is needed. Likewise, it might be that group counseling becomes a catalyst for individual counseling. An example of this might be a high school student who discloses information about drug use or sexual experiences during a group session; this would certainly prompt the need for individual counseling to explore the issues in the student's life. The link between these counseling roles is an important one that allows for more comprehensive coverage of student needs.

It is not surprising that most students are more responsive to information from their peers than information from adults. The result has been the advent of peer mediation and peer counseling/tutoring programs at all school levels. It makes sense that students, especially as they approach adolescence, respond better to input and encouragement from their peers. Thus, one of the benefits of group counseling is that *peer modeling* is a natural part of the group counseling process. Through role play and other means of rehearsal, students can observe and emulate model practices of other students. Further, it is beneficial to have peer role models in a group, particularly groups that are focused on behavior change. School counselors help foster peer interaction and the positive results of peer modeling by providing opportunities for students to observe each other responding to relevant and challenging situations.

CHALLENGES   Perhaps the biggest challenge for school counselors in their role as group counselors is dealing with the issue of students' *missed class time* while participating in group sessions. In many states, recent pressure from state and local agencies regarding testing and time-on-task has made it difficult to recruit members for groups. Almost all states require a competency test or some type of assessment for students to (a) pass core subject area tests, (b) pass from one grade level to the next, or (c) graduate from high school. In addition to the effect on the student, some states also connect accreditation and faculty competence to student performance on these statewide assessment instruments. This phenomenon in schools has also affected the role of the school counselor in the delivery of counseling services. We will explore this in greater detail in chapter 4.

Because of the pressure for improved academic standards and higher test scores on standardized tests, teachers and administrators have had to rethink their priorities in school programs. In many situations, programs that are not directly related to the test subject areas have low priority. Specialists, including the school counselor, often find that their time with students is either cut back or, in some cases, eliminated, except as it relates to the academic program. Even in schools where the counseling program is considered a priority, teachers are hesitant to have students miss class to attend group counseling sessions.

Professional Perspective and Practice

BETH (MS)

When teachers are resistant to let counselors pull students from class, the counselors need to do some grassroots work with the teachers and let them know why this group might be helpful for the child and, in turn, helpful for them. If you can convince them that the time missed from class might result in some change in behavior that will help the student perform better in class, you're more likely to get them to allow students to come to group counseling sessions. I've found that scheduling groups on a six-week schedule, rotating periods each week has worked best in my school. This way, I can tell the teachers right from the get-go that Joey will miss Period 1 this week, Period 2 next week, etc. Then I try to the best of my ability to maintain that schedule.

It is understandable that the pressure for academic success has resulted in hesitancy of school personnel to allow time for activities that are not directly related to the academic progress of students. At the elementary level, even the most supportive teacher may express concern about a student who misses the language arts or math block. In secondary schools, even missing half a class is sometimes antagonistic to the demands of preparing for standardized testing. The school counselor can connect with faculty by acknowledging the priority of the student's time in class. Also, mentioning that the student has personal/social issues that could be detrimental to academic performance helps others understand that counseling is an important service with an ultimate goal of student academic success.

One of the challenging tasks of group counseling, especially at the middle- and high-school levels, is soliciting members for the group. At middle- and high-school levels, peer relationships and peer perception are paramount in the students' lives. The result may be greater resistance to group participation. More than any other factor, peer influence determines the degree of student support for counseling services. Individual or group counseling may be stigmatized in certain schools or among certain groups within a school. This situation varies from school to school. Many middle and high schools have popular counseling groups that cover a wide range of topics relevant to the students. In schools where group counseling may not be the norm, counselors should implement strategies to change the attitude toward counseling services. Though change is hard, the end result could be a greater appreciation for and participation in group counseling services.

My Story

A response that I often used that seemed to reinforce the importance of group counseling while also acknowledging the importance of class time was, "I know how important it is for Jesse to be in class and I will try to schedule the session so that he misses as little time as possible. However, it does seem that Jesse has a lot going on in his life right now and unless we work through some of these issues, he is not going to be at his academic best in order to learn the material he needs to do well in school and on the test. I think if we work together on this, he can do both and be successful. What do you think?"

Professional Practice

ESTHER (HS)

Tips for new counselors: Don't wait to do groups. Work in teams to co-lead groups with other professionals in your department, or bring in outside resource people. Teamwork provides support, generates a wider variety of ideas, and offers different approaches and counseling styles to students. Counselors learn something new each time they conduct a group. This learning comes from the students, co-leaders, or from taking a different direction or approach. Group work is challenging, exciting, and rewarding!

RESEARCH ON GROUP COUNSELING IN SCHOOLS In Burnham and Jackson's (2000) study, 90% of the counselors conducted small group sessions; in addition, they spent 10% to 23% of their time on small group counseling. While this is good news, these results must be interpreted cautiously. We must consider not only the quantity of services, but also the quality of services. Perhaps the most important role of the school counselor in terms of group counseling is to ascertain that it is effective. The characteristics of effective groups include cohesion, trust, and progress. Two problems emerged in the Burnham and Jackson study: (a) Groups often included too many students (groups should have six to eight members) and (b) groups were usually held on an irregular basis (p. 46). The school schedule itself is often inconsistent, so it follows that groups might be postponed or rescheduled and progress might be interrupted. As a school counselor, it is important to provide as much consistency as possible in the opportunities and scheduling of group counseling sessions.

Although there are barriers to conducting group counseling sessions in schools, groups are an effective way to provide prevention and intervention services to students. A meta-analysis by Whiston and Sexton (1998) of outcome-based school counseling research between 1988 and 1995 found that counseling in a group format was an effective intervention for a variety of student issues, including social skills development, family problems, behavioral issues, academic difficulties, and stress management. Reeder, Douzenis, and Bergin (1997) found that small group counseling sessions improved racial attitudes and increased cultural awareness of second grade students. More recently, there has been support for adventure-based group counseling in schools (Glaser & Shoffner, 2001), group work with students experiencing homework difficulty (Rowell & Hong, 2002), group counseling interventions with gifted learning disabled students (McEachern & Bornot, 2001), and group counseling interventions with at-risk adolescent girls (Zinck & Littrell, 2000). These studies give evidence of the efficacy of group counseling as an intervention in schools and as a valuable service provided by school counselors.

Conclusion

The counseling role of school counselors, both individual and small group, is probably one of the most enjoyable services that school counselors perform, since counseling is probably the component of the job that attracts most people. It is essential that school counselors remember that counseling is the crux of the job and should remain a priority.

Professional Perspective

RENEE (ES)

Individual and group counseling is the foundation of everything else I do as a school counselor. When I am counseling a student or group of students, I see myself as a facilitator of change. There may be a behavior, attitude, interpersonal dynamic, or mindset that is getting in the way of a child's learning. My role is to help students (or parents or teachers) develop strategies that will enable them to overcome these obstacles and get on with the job of learning. New counselors should keep in mind that counseling is the most important thing they do. Never lose sight of that and get too caught up in other tasks that will keep you from this role.

REFLECTION AND DISCUSSION

1. The counseling role is the crux of the services school counselors provide for students, parents, and faculty. In what ways could school counselors ensure that counseling remains a priority?

2. Some students are resistant to individual and/or small group counseling. How might you recruit or encourage students to take advantage of these services? What types of outreach could you provide to foster

greater student participation in individual and group counseling services?

3. Individual counseling or group counseling typically requires parental consent for students who are under age 18. If parents contact you to ask about the benefits of individual or group counseling for their children, how would you respond? What specific points would you want to include?

4. Consider the variety of socioeconomic, geographical, and cultural settings you may work in as a school counselor. What implications do these factors have for providing effective counseling services?

Classroom Guidance

The phrase *classroom guidance* is sometimes referred to as *large group guidance* in literature. Gysbers and Henderson (2000) and the National Model for School Counseling Programs (ASCA, 2003a) calls this delivery system "School Guidance Curriculum." For the purposes of this discussion, classroom guidance will refer to counseling in a classroom or other large group setting to provide instruction and discussion on topics that are relevant to the developmental needs of the students. For example, at the elementary level, classroom guidance might focus on themes that relate to student experiences at each grade level. In middle school or junior high, topics might include resisting peer pressure, time management, or sexual harassment, as these are more relevant to the developmental needs of adolescents. At the high-school level, classroom guidance might address college/career planning, preparing for tests (e.g., SAT, ACT), or selecting courses for next year's schedule. Given that school counseling programs should be developmental in nature, the topics covered in classroom guidance should be appropriate for the grade level and age group to which they are being presented.

Professional Practice

RENEE (ES)

I cover a variety of topics in classroom guidance. During the school year, I am likely to include lessons on career education, problem solving, social skills, appreciation of diversity, and awareness of self. Often teachers will approach me and ask me to address particular issues with their classes. I see this as an affirmation that they see the counseling program as supportive and useful.

BETH (MS)

We cover a variety of topics at the middle-school level. The topics could include: decision making, bullying, refusal skills, drug education, career education, and character education. I often will ask the kids or the teachers what topics they think are needed. I try and make the classroom lesson interactive if I can, using role plays or discussion groups. I have even used a talk show format—one of the students is the host, others are the guest panelists, and the class asks questions—somewhat like Oprah. I just try to get them involved using a format that is fun and that they have seen before. We also do high school scheduling in the classroom. I prefer that because I can see more students, yet still respond to their individual needs as they select their classes.

ESTHER (HS)

Classroom guidance at the high-school level focuses on a variety of areas. Every year, counselors do activities focusing on career and college selection. They discuss personal values as they relate to career choice and college majors. Counselors also assist with the college search process. Classroom guidance also includes presentations on test preparation and interpretation of the results of the PSAT and the SAT. Counselors share units on health and safety issues and transitional issues, such as entering high school from middle school, moving from high school to college, and transitioning from school to work.

Benefits

Myrick (2003) suggested that classroom teachers and counselors conduct in-class guidance lessons together so that the teacher can reinforce concepts and observe results during everyday classroom activities. Some curricula use teachers and/or parent volunteers to teach lessons on topics that the counselor typically addresses. While involving the teachers and parents in the presentation of some topics, school counselors should coordinate the presentations, using teachers and parents when appropriate. For example, in some school districts, school counselors are responsible for training students about sexual harassment. Ideally, a partnership exists between parents, teachers, and counselors. If the counselor provides a lesson for or discussion with students about a topic, teachers and parents are provided with enough information to reinforce the concepts and respond comfortably to questions and situations that arise as a result of greater student awareness of new, sensitive, or volatile issues. It is this collaborative relationship that ensures the success of classroom guidance lessons on any topic.

There are basically two ways to reinforce the concepts that are covered in classroom guidance sessions: (a) Ask teachers to participate or observe so they have an awareness of the ideas and topics covered and (b) inform parents that their children participated in a classroom guidance lesson on a chosen topic, and offer some tips on how to help students implement the ideas/strategies outside the school setting. Open communication is necessary to the success of a classroom guidance lesson and fosters positive interaction and support among involved parties.

Professional Perspective

RENEE (ES)

I see classroom guidance as an opportunity to develop a relationship with students and teachers alike. When you can facilitate a learning experience through activities that are meaningful and dynamic, the students will see you as someone who is knowledgeable and who can help them when they have problems. This is also an area where you can demonstrate your ability to connect with the students. This will go a long way in developing your relationship with the teachers in your school.

Challenges

Basically, there are two challenges in conducting classroom guidance: (a) scheduling a time with teachers to conduct classroom guidance lessons and (b) finding time in the midst of other counseling responsibilities to conduct classroom guidance. The best way to handle both challenges is to include classroom guidance as a priority in your program. The primary advantage of classroom guidance is that it gives school counselors access to the most students. For students who never seek counseling services, classroom guidance might be their only exposure to counseling services. It is important for students to see a counselor in a regular class, dealing with developmental or social issues that concern all students, not just those who are perceived as having problems. Having a presence and being visible in the classroom will help students have a greater awareness of the school counselor's role and may increase the likelihood of a student visiting the counselor's office or seeking counseling services.

Research on Classroom Guidance in Schools

Most research supports the use of large group counseling or classroom guidance for a variety of topics. Lee (1993) conducted a classroom guidance program for students in grades 4 through 6 and found that the lessons positively impacted student academic achievement in math. Brown (1999b) concurred that classroom guidance units that focus on improving test-taking skills may foster academic achievement. Classroom guidance lessons have also been effective in addressing concepts such as fairness (Kelly, 1996), and classroom guidance activities have been used to increase empathy and positive interactions between students without disabilities and their peers with special needs (Bruce, Shade, & Cossairt, 1996).

Nicoll (1994) indicated that research regarding classroom guidance has been positive, but has also produced nonsignificant outcomes. He suggested, "the limited research support for the effectiveness of classroom guidance programs is probably more a reflection of inadequate program development and intensity rather than an indication of limited effectiveness" (p. 360). For this reason, Nicoll advocated classroom guidance programs that target the developmental stage of students. For example, lessons on understanding self and others, developing empathy, effective communication skills, cooperation skills, and fostering responsibility should be repeated at each grade level, but should focus on age-appropriate activities in order to make them more applicable to the students' needs. This makes sense within the framework of comprehensive developmental school counseling programs. One might conclude that effective classroom guidance must foster social–emotional growth throughout a student's school career.

Meeting students where they are continues to be a focal point for developing classroom guidance lessons, but it is also important to assess student growth and development as a result of participation in classroom guidance. Planned developmental classroom guidance curricula with measurable outcomes are a positive step toward more effective counseling services for students and greater accountability for school counselors.

REFLECTION AND DISCUSSION

1. Choose a school level in which you would like to provide a classroom guidance unit. What topics might be appropriate? How would you plan to conduct the classroom guidance unit?

2. One area that is sometimes lacking in classroom guidance units is follow-up. What are some specific ways that you could follow-up in order to reinforce concepts that were covered in classroom guidance or to ascertain that students benefited from the lesson(s)?

CONCLUSION

This chapter has explored the direct counseling services that school counselors provide. In the counseling role, school counselors conduct individual and group counseling sessions that are prevention- and intervention-oriented, as issues emerge for students. While individual counseling sessions focus on the specific needs of students, group counseling addresses the common issues of a group of students. Classroom guidance, which is mostly instructional and preventive in nature, can also address current problems or issues that arise throughout a school year. Individual planning and large group activities can help students plan or prepare for challenges in their future. These roles are the primary mode in which school counselors directly interact with the students and determine, to a great extent, the effectiveness of the school counseling program.

REFLECTION AND DISCUSSION

1. Counseling and classroom guidance are considered direct services to students. What do you think is a realistic amount of time that should be devoted to providing these direct services in a week? In a day?

2. Although important, counseling and classroom guidance sometimes get bumped by other roles or duties of the school counselor. What are some ways that you, as the school counselor, might prevent this from happening? How can you keep these essential services a priority?

3. Choose a school level or age group of students with whom you would like to work. What topics do you think might be relevant to their experience at this age or level? How might you address these topics through counseling and/or classroom guidance?

CHAPTER 4

Consultation, Coordination, and Noncounseling Roles

*W*hile counseling and classroom guidance are roles that enable the school counselor to interact with students, consultation and coordination are roles in which the school counselor interacts with all invested players in the educational process—administrators, parents, teachers, central office personnel, support services personnel, community members, external counseling agencies, and other mental health professionals. These important affiliations have a direct effect on the efficacy of a school counseling program because connecting information, input, and services provides a holistic approach that benefits students. This chapter will focus on the consultation and coordination roles of the school counselor. We will also consider noncounseling duties that school counselors may perform, including the school counselor's role in testing and assessment.

Consultation

Kurpius and Fuqua (1993) developed a working definition of consultation: "In general, consultants help consultees to think of their immediate problems as part of the larger system, and not only to understand how problems are solved but also to understand how they were developed, maintained, or avoided" (p. 598). For school counselors, consultation includes myriad interactions, contacts, and relationships with people inside and outside the school community. More than any other, consultation may be the role school counselors perform the most without actually realizing or documenting it. Burnham and Jackson (2000) found that 78 of 80 counselors indicated they spent time consulting, but the time spent ranged from 1% to 80%. One reason given for this wide range is that consultation in school counseling is not well defined. The role is fragmented, and consultation often occurs in a crisis situation, over the phone, or in informal conversations rather than as planned sessions.

Models of Consultation

There are several models of and approaches to consultation in counseling (Brown, Pryzwansky, & Schulte, 2001), and most advocate for collaborative problem solving (Dustin & Ehly, 1992; Keys, Bemak, Carpenter, & King-Sears, 1998). Kurpius and Fuqua (1993) advocated that the consultation relationship is triadic, involving the consultant, the consultee, and the person or situation that needs to be addressed. According to Kurpius and Fuqua, consultation may occur in one of four modalities: provisional, prescriptive, collaborative, or in mediation. Provisional consultation occurs when the counselor provides something to meet the consultee's needs. In prescriptive consultation, the counselor serves as an expert and prescribes a remedy for the consultee's problem. Collaborative consultation involves teamwork between the counselor and consultee to find a viable solution to the problem. Finally, a consultant may serve as a mediator who helps resolve an issue between two disputants (Kurpius & Fuqua). School counselors may use each mode in isolation, or in some combination.

Kahn (2000) suggested that school counselors take a solution-focused approach to consultation in order to emphasize solutions rather than problems, strengths rather than weaknesses. Kahn noted that a possible benefit of solution-focused consultation is that the consultee might transfer learned skills into other life situations and problems.

In general, school counselors provide consultation to at least three groups: school personnel (teachers/staff and administrators), parents/guardians, and community agencies (counselors, agencies, etc.). An exploration of each of these areas will identify ways that consultation can be most effective.

Consultation With School Faculty/Staff/Administration

The most common type of consultation typically occurs when colleagues consult with school counselors about students or their situations and there is some uncertainty about how to respond. Teachers often approach counselors about students who are consistently having difficulty in class. For example, at the elementary level, a concern might be students who are exhibiting problem behaviors that interfere with schoolwork and disrupt the class. At the secondary level, consultation might occur to discuss a student who is lethargic or sleeps in class.

Professional Practice

BETH (MS)

Sometimes consultation occurs in places where others might not consider it consultation, such as the lunchroom or hallway. A great deal of consultation is informal and may be as simple as letting a teacher know that a student's life is pretty tough right now, making the gentle suggestion to consider this when working with the student.

Counselors often handle situations by meeting with the student, calling a parent, or establishing a working alliance with the teacher to help meet the needs of the student. A key component of consultation, regardless of the situation or conditions of the problem, is *taking action as quickly as possible*. Teaching colleagues have indicated that they sometimes feel that their requests for help go unanswered. Often, they are unaware of the demands on a school counselor's time and the number of students for which a counselor is responsible. However, even if requests for help cannot be acted upon immediately, school counselors have an obligation to let staff, faculty, and administrators know that the issues they have identified will be addressed.

Professional school counselors must prioritize situations on a daily basis. For example, a middle school counselor is working with students on next year's schedules when a teacher comes in to report a student who is failing every class.

At the same time, an administrative assistant calls the counselor to report that a student has threatened to commit suicide and wants to leave the building. The school counselor must decide which takes precedence. Obviously, the student threatening suicide must be the priority because it is an acute crisis. Scheduling students can be addressed at another time. Consultation with the teacher must happen sometime in between for two reasons: (a) The failing student needs an intervention quickly in order to salvage grades and get back on track academically, and (b) the teacher has come to the counselor asking for help and needs to feel that help will be forthcoming.

Consultation will not always fall somewhere in the middle. Depending on the nature of the consultation, there will be times when immediate action must be taken to address a problem. For example, a faculty member reports that a student has said she is being sexually abused and isn't sure how the report should be handled. This type of student problem requires immediate action and the teacher should be commended for coming forward. In situations that are not as dire or when the need to respond is not immediate, school counselors should take the time to listen to the consultee and discuss possible options.

Professional Perspective and Practice

RENEE (ES)

The majority of the consultation I do is with teachers. Typically, teachers will seek me out if they observe student behaviors that may interfere with learning. Keep in mind that you cannot fix every problem on your own. People go into school counseling because they want to help others. That can result in a tendency to say, "I'll take care of it" whenever teachers come to them with concerns. However, sometimes it is more helpful to assist teachers by giving them some possible strategies to deal with situations on their own. Ultimately, this may give teachers some skills that will be helpful down the road.

The skills needed for effective consultation parallel those needed for effective counseling. As Gysbers and Henderson (2000) indicated, consultation is not a function in and of itself, but is a function *across* other roles. Consultation is a critical role of school counselors and requests for consultation must be addressed immediately, if only to schedule a time to meet later to discuss the consultee's concern. Once the meeting occurs, the consultation process can be utilized to generate ideas and strategies for maximizing the successful resolution of the teacher's or administrator's concern.

Consultation With Parents

Consultation with parents may occur throughout all of the school counselor's roles. Research has indicated that consultation with parents is important in a variety of circumstances (Dunn & Baker, 2002; Keys, Bemak, & Lockhart, 1998;

McEachern & Bornot, 2001). From a phone call about grades to an intense meeting at school, consultation with parents serves as one of the gauges by which one's program is measured. The following material describes four ways to facilitate effective consultation with parents.

Professional Practice

BETH (MS)

With parents, consultation is a bit more formal. Either they call you or you call them to indicate that there is a need to talk about their child. That interaction is very important, and how you handle it the first time can affect the relationship and their confidence in you if they need your help in the future.

BE AVAILABLE AND ACCESSIBLE   In this age of voice mail and e-mail, parents do not accept that school personnel don't receive or check messages for several days. In fact, many school counselors now feel that e-mail has become an efficient way to provide consultation. In contrast to a lengthy phone call, e-mail allows the sender and recipient to be concise in the statement of the problem and options for possible solutions. However, relying on e-mail as the only mode of communication has some inherent problems. The brevity of e-mail and the inability to give it voice eliminates two important features of consultation: the level of emotion of the parent telling the story and the counselor's interpretation of the story. School counselors must be careful about confidentiality when responding via e-mail or voice mail. Addressing student issues in writing via e-mail or leaving a message via voice mail opens accessibility to private or personal information and is not fail-proof in terms of confidentiality. Therefore, making contact through e-mail or voice mail to set up a time to meet in person may be the best way to protect confidentiality for all parties involved.

A final caution for school counselors is to make sure that, regardless of the medium of information (e-mail, voice mail, in person, or in writing), the whole story is heard. Making a choice or decision with only part of the story would be like trying to find a destination with only a portion of the map. School counselors are trained to be fair and objective listeners and should facilitate communication from all involved parties in order to proceed with the most effective intervention.

RESPOND AS QUICKLY AS POSSIBLE   Unless a parent meets the counselor in the hall or bumps into him or her at the nearest shopping mall, most consultation with parents will result from a request to meet with the school counselor. It is important that the school counselor respond to this request as soon as possible. Even if it is going to be some time before the school counselor's schedule allows a meeting, parents need to be reassured that their request has been acknowledged and some action will be taken. More often than not, parents will usually try to tell the story to the counselor as soon as they have made personal contact. If time allows, the counselor should listen and respond to the parent in a supportive and reassuring manner. Some solutions are generated easily either by the school counselor agreeing to see the student, the parent taking some action outside the school setting, or the counselor determining if other persons, either inside or outside the school setting, might be better equipped to help the parent. Consultation can range from very simple to very complex; some situations may be resolved with a brief response, while others may require more complex intervention. The key is to respond, even if only to say, "It might be a few days before I can give this matter my full attention; but rest assured, we will work together on this situation."

DO NOT GET CAUGHT UP IN FAMILY ISSUES   It is not unusual for school counselors to become familiar with families and their circumstances. While it is advantageous to work collaboratively with families to address student issues, it is also important to be aware of the tendency to get caught in the middle of a dysfunctional family system. One way to know this is happening is to consider the content of conversations with parents. What is the majority of the conversation about? Is it about the student? Is it about the parent or parents and what is going on in their lives? This analysis is necessary to identify the actual problem or issue, and it also helps the school counselor recognize and establish boundaries when deciding how to address the problem.

FOLLOW-UP WITH PARENTS   Once a plan has been established or a question has been answered, it is important for the school counselor to follow-up with the parents to determine if there has been a change in the situation. While some consultation may be as simple as passing along information, it is important to check back with parents to say, "Were you able to find what you needed?" For more complex situations, it is imperative that the school counselor check in with parents to let them know about a student's progress or challenges. When parents receive a phone call from school personnel, the first response is usually, "What did she do?" or "What's wrong?" Imagine their pleasant surprise when they hear a counselor saying, "I just wanted to let you know that I spoke with Johnny's teacher and she has noticed he seems much more involved in class discussions. I think we're on the right track."

Consultation With the Community

Connection is the word that comes to mind when considering how school counselors consult with parties that are external to schools. An important part of effective consultation with community members, businesses, agencies, and other mental health professionals is making a connection with these members of the community early in one's position as a school counselor. "Given the movement toward integration of school and community services and school-community partnerships, collaborative consultation adds a critical dimension to the school counselor's consultative function" (Keys, Bemak, & Lockhart, 1998, p. 385). These partnerships and connections are very valuable to school counselors because often the counselor serves as a liaison between the school and community. For example, teachers, parents, or administrators may need to find a particular resource in the community for a project or to sponsor a school function. If the school counselor has already made connections with various members of the community, it will be easier to secure help.

In addition, the connection between school counselors and community members bodes well for advertising the school counseling program to persons in the community who may not have school-aged children. The community must see that the school counseling program is beneficial and integral to the overall school program to garner support should school counseling programs come under attack for financial or political reasons. School counselors should be leaders in fostering these important relationships.

Counseling-Related Types of Consultation

In counseling-related consultation, school counselors often make referrals to counselors or therapists outside the school setting. Parents frequently ask school counselors about reputable practitioners in the community; it is reassuring when the counselor can offer a list of mental health practitioners who might be appropriate to work with their child. It is easy to hand out a resource guide or a list of mental health resources, but this may be overwhelming to people who are seeking professionals to meet their individual needs. Therefore, it is imperative that school counselors develop a networking relationship with mental health professionals throughout the community in order to provide information for parents who are looking for counselors to address specific needs or issues. While a school counselor should be cautious about recommending a specific counselor, it is helpful for parents to have a list of several counselors to choose from so that they can make an informed decision about which counselor might best meet their child's needs.

There are several ways to learn about mental health facilities and practitioners in one's community. First, local offices and agencies often sponsor meetings where professionals can gather, exchange business cards, and discover licensed counselors and therapists who specialize in particular areas. These experiences are valuable because they provide opportunities to personally connect with community resources. Second, talk to people who have received services from local counselors and therapists to gather specific information about the professionals in your community. A final way to connect with outside counseling professionals is through professional meetings, conferences, and workshops.

Another type of counseling-related consultation is when outside mental health professionals who are involved with students contact the counselor at

---

My Story

I found an effective counselor in our area by going to a workshop on ADHD and learning about a therapist who specialized in treating boys with ADHD. Because ADHD was a relatively new phenomenon at the time, it was wonderful to find someone who could deal specifically with students who had severe ADHD issues. Even better, the therapist's wife was a substance abuse counselor who worked mainly with adolescents and young adults. By attending one workshop, I had managed to find two reputable counselors who treated students of varying ages with specific issues. This was information that I used time and time again in my career as a school counselor.

---

the school. Once written permission is received from students (if age 18) or parents/guardians, the school counselor may share information about students with mental health professionals outside of the school setting (refer to the ethical guidelines for disclosure of information in chapter 2). It is also appropriate for the school counselor to ask the outside counselor, "Based on things that have been addressed in therapy, can you think of any way we can help this student be more successful in school?" This type of collaboration and connection can only benefit students and is an example of effective consultation.

This section has provided examples of consultation and has discussed the three most obvious groups for whom school counselors most often provide consultation. But school counselors consult with multiple groups on a variety of issues. Even though the amount of time spent on consultation varies widely among counselors, this is clearly a counseling service that is imperative when meeting the needs of all constituents in the education community.

Professional Practice

ESTHER (HS)

Counselors consult with parents, teachers, administrators, students, fellow counselors, other helping professionals such as psychologists and social workers, college admissions personnel, vocational academic representatives, proprietary school specialists, athletic and school representatives, ROTC and military representatives, and potential employers. In each case, the counselor coordinates programs, presents information, develops materials, makes suggestions, receives information, makes referrals, or uses the information to assist the student and the family in future planning, problem solving, or decision making.

REFLECTION AND DISCUSSION

1. Consider the tripartite relationship among the members involved in the consultation process. What factors do you think might impede the consultation process? How detrimental is it if one of the components of the triadic relationship will not cooperate or change?

2. Sometimes, consultation requires sharing information about students or families in a way that might threaten confidentiality. How might you ensure that you do not breach confidentiality? What types of information are appropriate to share?

3. Consider the groups with whom a school counselor might consult. Which group do you think might be the most challenging to work with? Which group would be the easiest?

Coordination

While coordination is identified as one of the four major roles of school counselors, school counseling literature does not always cover it as a distinct role. Schmidt (2003) stated that coordination is typically a more indirect counseling service, so broad in its scope that it is often hard to identify. Keys, Bemak, and Lockhart (1998) noted specifically that coordination is a critical role for school counselors in working with at-risk youth. "Program coordination also includes informing school-based community agency professionals of school policies and procedures; supervising such professionals; facilitating communication between agencies, the school and families; and monitoring program implementation and evaluation" (p. 385). The following "Professional Practice" offers examples of coordination activities as described by our veteran counselors at the elementary, middle, and high school levels. Clearly many of the other school counselor roles are embedded in the process of coordination.

Professional Practice

RENEE (ES)

School counselors coordinate many events. One event that I coordinate is the Career Fair, which supports career education. I have approached this event in different ways, depending upon the needs of the school in which I am working. Parent involvement, school policy regarding instructional time, and teacher support may influence how large an event I will plan. I have hosted Career Weeks, during which we had guest speakers and school-wide activities for an entire week. In other schools, I have simply hosted a Career Fair one morning and invited representatives from a variety of career fields to manage booths at which students could learn about jobs. All in all, I think effective coordination requires organization and responsiveness to the needs of the school.

BETH (MS)

The counselors at my school coordinate the peer mediation program and the mentorship program. In mediation, we either train the students or provide for their training. Then we coordinate the actual implementation of the mediations and schedule the students to serve as mediators. We serve as supervisors when the students are mediating, and as consultants if the mediators feel they need us to intervene in a situation.

We also coordinate parent programs and the crisis response plan in the event of a death of a faculty member or student. Another example of coordination is our work with the new students in our building. This is not really a group, but it is an on-going support service for students who are new to our building each year.

ESTHER (HS)

An example of an activity that I coordinate is the College Partnership Program. My role is to coordinate our school's program with those of other schools throughout the school district, and to provide monthly programming. The College Partnership Program is designed to promote college admission for under-represented student populations. I work with minority students in our school to promote their admission to college. I coordinate the assignment of academic mentors to each student, poll students for appropriate topics for monthly programming, schedule parent meetings, organize a graduation program to recognize sessions in the program, monitor student academic progress, recognize "star performers," schedule career speakers, provide information on college trips and student scholarships, and coordinate an annual conference trip for these students.

Coordination implies harmonious interaction of events, ideas, or services. When applied to the school counseling program, there are three distinct phases of the coordination function—*planning, implementation,* and *management.* These phases do not necessarily occur in sequence; in fact, they often occur in varied order or simultaneously.

Planning

The school counselor's role of coordination is critical to the planning phase of any project. The most effective and efficient planning begins globally (program-oriented) and becomes very specific (activity-oriented). Consider, for example, planning a Career Week in March for an entire school. Feature 4.1 presents a sample month-by-month plan for coordinating the event.

The planned schedule in Feature 4.1 assumes that there is only one school counselor working on the Career Week activities. In an elementary school, this

FEATURE 4.1

Month-by-Month Career Week Coordination Plan

August to September

- Make sure that the dates for the Career Week are established and entered into the school's calendar of activities. This should actually occur when the school calendar is being developed, probably in spring of the prior school year.
- Review last year's career activities and the evaluations of participants (teachers, speakers, students). Consider any input and decide how to implement and improve any suggestions that seem appropriate.
- Assess the need for new or additional materials related to careers, and review any materials that may have come in over the summer months.

September (or within the first 2 to 3 weeks of school)

- Advertise the Career Week at parent information sessions or other school events that involve parents, and start to identify and recruit parents who might be interested or willing to help.
- Communicate with teachers about the recruitment of speakers and volunteers, and about any new ideas for planning and implementing Career Week.
- Begin developing classroom guidance lessons that either the counselor(s) or teacher(s) can conduct with students. Keep an eye out for ideas and lessons that might be used.

October

- Develop a format for Career Week. Will the speakers be in one place with students rotating through? Will students stay in class with the speakers rotating? Will each student select a few speakers of interest and only hear from those speakers? The format will be the impetus for much of the planning for Career Week.
- Secure the facilities needed for Career Week. Even if the format has not been determined, it is important to secure the space needed. This is extremely important, as space is often a hot commodity in schools. For example, if the multipurpose room is also the gym, consult with the physical education (P.E.) teacher and discuss the likelihood of using that space during the week. The displacement of the teacher can be handled in a couple of ways: (a) Invite the teacher to bring his or her P.E. classes to speakers during their scheduled class times, or

(b) make sure the P.E. teacher has priority access to outside space in the event that the weather cooperates and P.E. classes can be held outside. Working out these potential problems in advance helps alleviate any issues that might surface when Career Week arrives.

- Continue to recruit guest speakers. Consult with other counselors in the school district to get recommendations for speakers they have used. Start networking with representatives from community businesses and organizations to see if they would be interested in coming to share information about their careers.

November

- Continue searching for and securing speakers for Career Week.
- Enlist volunteers to help implement the week's events.

December

- Continue securing career speakers.
- Meet with a committee composed of teachers, administrators, and parents to discuss ways to make the week a success. Get input from all members regarding ideas for helping the week run smoothly.
- Advertise for career guest speakers in newsletters, flyers, and other types of media. Make sure there is a blurb about the upcoming Career Week and who to contact for more information.
- Reconfirm the space needed to implement the week's activities.

January

- Secure written contracts from people who have verbally committed to be guest speakers.
- Keep teachers informed about the time frame of the week and provide a tentative schedule of events.
- Plan for career counseling lessons in the week(s) prior to Career Week. Make sure the lessons are developmentally appropriate for each grade level.
- Send a letter home with students to invite parents to be guest speakers during Career Week. The letter should have a detachable return slip that parents can send back with contact information and availability.
- Identify students to serve as hosts for the career speakers. Keep them informed about the week's events and how they will be involved.

(Continues)

February

- Conduct or have teachers conduct classroom guidance lessons on careers. Depending on the age group, lessons should focus on career awareness (elementary), career exploration (middle), or career decision making (high school).
- Begin announcing and putting up posters about the Career Week activities.
- Continue securing career speakers and develop a master schedule that indicates when, where, and to whom speakers will be speaking.

One week prior to Career Week

- Make phone contact with all career speakers and confirm the day and time they will be coming; make sure they have directions to the facility.
- Reserve any audiovisual equipment that career speakers might need.
- Confirm space for career speakers and make sure space is ample enough to contain the number of students that will be participating.
- Meet with the student hosts and give them specific schedules (in writing) that indicate exactly where and when they should meet the speakers and how they should transition them from space to space.
- Make final contact with teachers and give them a schedule of the week's activities. In addition to the full week's schedule, let teachers know that they will receive daily communication and that each day's schedule will be in their mailboxes the afternoon before.
- Decide what will happen if a speaker does not show or cancels.
- Announce the Career Week activities and get students excited about participating. Give teachers a list of activities they might want to do in their classrooms related to careers and Career Week.
- Make sure administrators and office staff are given schedules so they will be aware of where students are, where classes are, and where the Career Week activities are taking place.
- Plan a break room where career speakers can relax between sessions.
- Furnish snacks and beverages for the speakers; often, this can be worked out jointly with the school cafeteria.
- Make nametags for each speaker and volunteer.
- Secure tables, chairs, easels, screens, etc. that might be needed throughout the week.
- Inform specialists, custodians, and cafeteria personnel about any changes that might alter their schedules. For example, if a class will

be arriving 15 minutes late for lunch, talk with the cafeteria manager and see if it would preferable for the class to come to lunch as soon as they can or if it might be better to have grade levels switch lunch times for that day.

Day before the beginning of Career Week

- Review all the activities that will be going on the next day.
- Be available for any questions or issues that arise concerning the schedule, location, etc.
- Make sure everyone has the schedule and sticks to it.
- Have a place where career speakers can leave their mailing addresses so that thank you letters can be sent.
- Plan to sit in on a few of the activities to enjoy watching how the students benefit from a well-planned event.
- Get a good night's sleep the night before Career Week begins.

might be true, so it would be helpful to seek out a parent volunteer or a teacher who is willing to share the responsibility of planning. At the middle and high school levels, students may have the opportunity to participate in a Career Fair or Career Night instead of a Career Week. The planning process is still challenging and typically involves all of the counselors in some capacity. Sharing the planning responsibilities is effective because of the opportunity to share ideas, give and receive feedback, and have unconditional support for the week or the night.

The planning component requires a great deal of coordination, as well as organization. One of the characteristic traits of effective school counselors is the ability to juggle many things at one time, or multitask. It is important for school counselors not only to be involved in the planning of upcoming activities or events, but also to maintain the overall goals of the counseling program. While school counselors can be entrenched in the day-to-day demands of their jobs, it is always important for them to consider future plans and activities simultaneously.

Implementation

The second important element of the coordination role is *implementation.* Implementation duties could range from carrying out plans for classroom guidance lessons at the elementary level to facilitating a scholarship program at the high school level. In a forum on program development and management,

Gysbers and Henderson (2002) identified the following key elements for successful program implementation:

- counseling program improvement goals,
- yearly program plan,
- weekly schedules,
- leadership,
- individual job descriptions,
- counselor professional development goals,
- weekly campus staff meetings,
- monthly district staff meetings, and
- established accountability for student results, program standards, counselor performance, and program improvements.

In essence, these elements address both the general school counseling program and the professional growth of the school counselor. In addition, several of the key elements address support systems for the counseling program and the need for ongoing professional development and evaluation. The implementation of counseling services encompasses the vastness of the school counseling program and its goals, as well as the specific tasks and strategies for program success.

Concepts that support effective implementation in a school setting are *predictability* and *consistency.* Predictability refers to school counselors doing what they say they will do. For example, if teachers, parents, and students are expecting a program or activity that is being organized by the school counselor or counseling office, there needs to be a high probability that that event or activity will occur. While certain cancellations are unavoidable, poor planning is not an acceptable excuse. If there are going to be changes, alterations, postponements, or cancellations, you must inform all involved parties as soon as possible and provide reasons. If the reasons are confidential or personal, say exactly that. If not, explain them. Consistency refers to equal distribution and quality of counseling services among all the grades encompassed by a school counseling program. Because comprehensive school counseling programs are developmental, it is appropriate for school counselors to create plans specific to each grade level.

Implementation is the action phase of the coordination process. It provides an opportunity to present school counseling in a positive light, which contributes to the overall success of school programs. The Career Week example in Feature 4.1 ends when the planning is complete and the school counselor is ready to begin implementing those elements of Career Week that were so carefully planned. Implementation activities might include:

- Place a schedule in teachers' mailboxes daily; include any changes or alterations to the master schedule; send e-mail notifications of changes if possible, and announce changes to the faculty as soon as they are known.

- Make sure the facility/space is ready with any equipment the speakers might need. Provide evaluation forms for the teachers as they exit the activities so that they can offer immediate feedback and responses.
- Circulate when activities are underway to make sure that transitions occur on time and smoothly. Establish a signal to indicate to speakers when they are running out of time.
- Ascertain that the student hosts are with their guest speakers and are guiding them from one place to another.
- Inform guest speakers of the refreshment room and always offer water as they are doing their presentations.
- Give the speakers the opportunity to evaluate their experiences with the students. Be sure to find out if they would return in the future.
- At the end of each day, assess how things went and make notes so that when the entire experience is evaluated, there will be a list of changes needed to implement Career Week next year.

Whether a school counselor is conducting classroom guidance, consulting with a parent, or making sure speakers are all in the right rooms with the right groups, organization is key in making sure the implementation process goes smoothly.

Management

It is often the school counselor's role to manage the entire school counseling program, making sure it runs efficiently and effectively. This may include the management of any suggestions for changes, improvements, additions, deletions, or strategies for coordinating counseling services. This is especially true in elementary schools, which often have only one counselor. At the middle and high school levels, guidance directors often manage the overall school counseling program and delegate responsibilities to different counselors. Following are suggestions for effective management of a school counseling program:

- intermittent written and verbal communication with teachers regarding the need for counseling services;
- revision of counseling services as needed to meet the needs of students, faculty, parents, and community;
- adherence to the time line that is established for the school year;
- delegation of responsibilities as needed for the effective implementation of services and events;
- ongoing evaluation of the efficacy of services, as well as plans for follow-up;
- scheduling facilities and rooms in advance for special events or activities; and
- monitoring student, faculty, and parent response to services, programs, and activities provided by the school counselor(s).

In conclusion, coordination is involved in all aspects of the school counseling program and is a role that is integral to the effective delivery of services. Strong organization and management skills are certainly assets in this function of school counseling and, as always, commitment and dedication to providing essential services is the impetus for fulfilling this necessary role.

REFLECTION AND DISCUSSION

1. This section has described several types of activities that fall under the school counselor's coordination role. What professional skills or personal qualities do you think one might need to possess in order to coordinate the school counseling program effectively?

2. The coordination role of school counseling requires the ability to juggle many things, or multitask. What types of experiences might you seek out in your practicum and internship that will help prepare you for this role?

3. Imagine that you have been asked to coordinate a Cultural Appreciation event in your school. Describe a process for how you might plan, implement, and evaluate this event.

Noncounseling Roles and Responsibilities

Conversations with school counselors reveal that many of the duties that counselors perform do not fit neatly into the categories of counseling, classroom guidance, consultation, or coordination. While most duties are related to the school counseling field, others are almost the opposite of the roles that school counselors want to perform. We focused briefly in chapter 1 on the noncounseling roles of school counselors. These activities include the roles, responsibilities, and duties that a school administrator or school policy might deem as part of the school counselor's job.

Burnham and Jackson (2000) indicated that a majority of the counselors they surveyed participated in nonguidance (mainly clerical) activities. These activities included scheduling, enrolling students, and activities involving the upkeep and maintenance of student records. Burnham and Jackson's survey results indicated that percentage of time spent on nonguidance tasks ranged from 1% to 88%, highlighting a disparity in the implementation of school counseling roles. Perhaps more enlightening is the finding that half of the counselors reported handling 5 of the 10 clerical tasks included in the study, specifically student records, scheduling, transcripts, office sitting, and supervising clubs and organizations. The evidence suggests that school counselors still spend an excessive amount of time in noncounseling activities and duties. This has a definite impact on the quantity and quality of services that can be implemented with students.

Gysbers and Henderson (2000) acknowledged that some activities fall into the "fair-share responsibilities" (p. 76) category that includes duties that are naturally a part of a school employee's tasks (i.e., bus duty). However, Gysbers and Henderson warn, "Care must be taken, however, to watch the time given to system support duties because the prime focus for counselors' time is the direct service components of the comprehensive guidance program" (p. 76).

From bus duty to testing coordinator, probably all school counselors can list a number of duties and roles they assume that are unrelated to their counseling roles.

Professional Practice

ESTHER (HS)

Because counselors are considered part of the total school team, they often are called upon to perform noncounseling functions, such as lunch duty, attending faculty advisory meetings, writing letters of recommendation, completing college and scholarship applications, or filing, interpreting, and maintaining student records.

One of the biggest challenges for school counselors is promoting an image as a team player while maintaining the integrity of the school counseling role. Participating in activities that are not job-specific is not unusual in schools. Most teachers and administrators acknowledge that job expectations often go beyond the duties that they were trained to do. School counselors share in this dilemma. The issue is *when asked to do or participate in something that is not directly related to a counseling role and/or function, do we (a) refuse to do it because it is not part of the job description, (b) agree to do it and take time from other counseling responsibilities, or (c) do it and overload ourselves so much that we feel ineffective at everything?* This is a huge question that school counselors must consider. In order to best discuss this issue, let's look at each potential response and determine which might be the most reasonable.

- *Refusing to do it because it is not part of the job description*—While many of the duties and responsibilities assumed by school counselors are not specified in their job descriptions, some school counselor job descriptions include a statement that reads: "Assumes other duties as assigned by the building administrator." The consequences of refusing to participate in activities or perform duties that are assigned by school administration are potentially job-threatening. *Insubordination—* refusing to perform duties as assigned—is grounds for dismissal. Therefore, blatant refusal is not a good idea. While school counselors are often viewed as part of the administrative team or as specialists, teachers hopefully view school counselors as peers and colleagues. The unspoken understanding is that everyone pitches in to do things like bus duty, which no more fits the role of a teacher or administrator than a school counselor. In situations where school counselors are not required to perform duties that teachers perform, resentment may lead to negative feelings toward the school counseling program. The two consequences—being cited for insubordination or negative implications for the school counseling program—are valid reasons not to refuse to perform noncounseling duties.

- *Agreeing to do it but losing time from counseling responsibilities*—While taking on noncounseling responsibilities may result in acceptance as a team player, it may also result in neglecting some of the necessary roles and functions of the school counseling program. For example, school counselors may be asked to cover a class until a substitute arrives. This may involve canceling classroom guidance lessons, meetings with students, and group counseling sessions until the teacher or teacher substitute arrives.

- *Do it and overload the schedule in order to compensate for lost time*—This is probably the response that most counselors ultimately choose. Many feel they have no other choice. School counselors are governed by the ethics of ACA and ASCA, but are also bound to the rules, regulations, and responsibilities of the school system. If an administrator informs the school counselor that he or she will be the testing coordinator for the school, it is difficult to argue or refuse to do it. One goal of school counselors is to be viewed as a necessary part of the overall school program, so school counselors may agree to duties that may not be directly related to counseling in order to support the overall education program. While this helps with the image of school counseling, it often places a huge burden on counselors.

Professional Perspective

BETH (MS)

I think the best way to minimize the noncounseling duties is for your colleagues and administrators to believe your time is too important to be consumed by those other duties. Sometimes, you have to get in there and let them see that you're running groups, counseling individuals, coordinating programs, and that your time is really too valuable to have to assume duties unrelated to counseling. It may take a year or two for people to see what the school counselor is doing. It's also important to advocate for yourself and say, "Well, if I'm doing lunch duty, then I can't do lunch groups," or "I can't be available for students who might need some extra support during their lunch periods because they can't be taken out of academic classes. So, if the school wants me to perform these important duties, then I have to be freed up from other noncounseling duties so that I can provide the needed counseling services."

There probably is no right answer or magical solution to this problem, which plagues school counselors at all levels. It *is* appropriate, however, for school counselors to advocate for the importance of time and opportunities to provide effective counseling services. Many duties, such as sponsoring a club or class, supervising a lunch period, or assuming the role of administrative designee when other administrators are out of the building, offer hidden counseling opportunities. Observing students' interactions with their peers may provide insight into issues that arise in counseling sessions. Dealing with a crisis or behavioral issue when the principal is unavailable may give the school counselor a unique opportunity to intervene before a situation becomes out of control. As a school employee, you will probably assume extra duties, but you should plead your case for avoiding job responsibilities that seriously interfere with the ability to provide effective counseling services. Often, those making requests may not realize the extra duties may detract from the ability to do the school counseling job effectively. However, recognize that noncounseling roles sometimes present opportunities to enhance your effectiveness as a school counselor. Finally, school counselors need to continue to educate others about their counseling roles and the impact of effective implementation of those roles on the overall success of school programs.

One noncounseling role that many school counselors must assume is involvement in testing and assessment. It is important to discuss where school counselors might fit into the testing process. The next section explores the school counselor's role in this area.

The Role of the School Counselor in Assessment

A current trend affecting schools across the country is the implementation of mandatory state testing as a means of assuring academic growth and progress. The standards-based reform movement has been the catalyst for the emphasis on testing students to ascertain that they have developed a certain level of competency in core subject areas. Administrators, teachers, students, parents, and school counselors are feeling the stress of standardized testing demands.

Proponents of student testing see it as a way to establish standards and clear expectations for student performance. Further, testing appears to be the only objective way to hold schools accountable for imparting basic knowledge in core areas. On the other hand, critics of standardized testing or assessment used for promotion or graduation argue that it is simply unfair to measure all students by the same yardstick. Poor or minority students who have limited access to resources might be misplaced into a lower program of study or not promoted or allowed to graduate, in part because they did not have equal access to the education resources that other students were given. These are valid concerns that must be addressed if testing and assessment are to achieve their intended goals.

But what does this mean for the school counselor? The American School Counselor Association's (2002c) position on high-stakes testing focused primarily on the school counselor's role of explaining the tests and reporting results. The role statement does not specify what the school counselor's role should be in terms of participation in the administration of tests.

Professional Perspective

BETH (MS)

I believe that school counselors are trained to interpret test data. I don't believe we are a more reasonable choice to administer tests than any other personnel in the school. I think people have confused test interpretation with test administration. Test administration is not a cost effective use of our services. School counselors are highly skilled, and having them count out test booklets is not a productive use of taxpayers' money.

It should come as no surprise that school counselors' involvement in school testing programs varies from state to state, district to district, and school to school. Within each school district, there is probably great variation in the role of school counselors in testing programs, and school counselor involvement may range from no involvement to serving as testing coordinator.

THE ROLE OF TESTING COORDINATOR   In a school where the school counselor is the testing coordinator, much time will be spent preparing the tests to be administered, training school personnel to administer the tests, arranging for proctors to be present during the testing period, collecting and accurately counting tests, reporting any testing inaccuracies, arranging for make-up testing, and packaging the tests to be sent away to be scored. If testing only occurred once a year in schools, this might not be such a time-demanding job. However, in most schools, there are typically two or three different types of tests administered during the school year. For example, a high school might administer the Preliminary Scholastic Assessment Test (PSAT) in the fall to all juniors, statewide standards testing for all 9th and 12th grade students in the spring, and Advanced Placement testing near the end of the school year. At the elementary level, there might be Cognitive Abilities Testing for first grade students in the fall, Otis Lennon testing for second grade students, and statewide standards testing for third and fifth grade students in the spring. In most schools, just about the time one test is sent, another one is in need of preparation. Considering the preparation time and implementation time that is devoted to testing, it is understandable that if the school counselor is the testing coordinator, there is less time available for providing counseling services.

Professional Practice

RENEE (ES)

I have been the test co-coordinator in a school, assuming responsibility for scheduling, training examiners, and administering and packaging all standardized tests in our building. It is a very time-consuming job that requires a great deal of attention to detail. On the positive side, it has given me a great base of information about each of the tests that our school system uses. This allows me to speak knowledgeably to parents who may have questions regarding their child's test scores.

TESTING AND THE SCHOOL COUNSELING PROGRAM School counselors who are test coordinators must manage the demands on their time. However, even in schools where the counselor does not assume the testing coordination duties, testing detracts from the time that could be devoted to providing more comprehensive counseling services.

Professional Perspective

ESTHER (HS)

The counselor's role in testing takes a lot of time away from individual and group counseling and contact with students.

We have already discussed the fact that teachers may resist having students taken out of class for counseling purposes. This is especially true when teacher performance is based, in part, on how students perform on standardized tests. For this reason, teachers want as much time-on-task as possible with students to make sure they are prepared for the tests, and rightfully so. School counselors must be flexible and try to work collaboratively with teachers in order to minimize student time out of class, yet also provide effective counseling services.

The resistance to allow students to leave class for counseling services seems to diminish slightly if the reason is academic in nature. For example, small groups that promote effective study skills do not get the same negative reaction as other groups because teachers typically refer more students for this type of group than any other. In addition, school personnel and parents may receive classroom guidance that deals with topics such as test-taking skills or test-anxiety strategies more positively because they are related directly to the academic needs of students. The conflict arises when counseling activities focus solely on academic issues and fail to address personal/social concerns. While school counselors work to help students achieve academically and become effective learners, there must also be emphasis on the importance of addressing personal and social issues that might impede the educational process.

State and local education authorities and policymakers often change the education requirements and policies that govern schools. Testing policies are no different. Whether it is the type of test, the material being tested, or the manner in which the test is administered, the rules are always changing. It is important for school counselors to be knowledgeable about testing policies that affect the students. What areas must be passed in order for students to be promoted or to graduate? What is the minimum score required to be promoted? How do parents/teachers/students interpret results? Is the test being piloted or is this the one that counts? School counselors should attend information sessions, ask questions of administrators or directors, and understand what the testing means for the students. This requires time on the counselor's part, but is useful knowledge if school counselors are to be in the best position to advise or counsel students in areas related to academic progress and testing.

THE ROLE OF THE SCHOOL COUNSELOR IN TESTING— ARE THERE OPTIONS?

> Some counselor educators and counselors may believe that involvement in assessment . . . is not legitimate for school counselors because those functions are designed to achieve instructional and administrative goals. The counselors' ability to change these circumstances in most school systems in the near future, however, is very limited. (Baker, 2000, p. 272)

When the time comes to interview for a school counseling position, it is important to ask and understand what the role of the school counselor is in the school testing program. If the testing program falls under the job responsibilities of the school counselor, you may want to negotiate for assistance with the clerical responsibilities involved (e.g., counting tests, preparation for mailing, etc.). Office staff or parent volunteers could perform these tasks; it is appropriate to use parents as long as the test results are not part of the information. Confidentiality should be maintained throughout the testing process.

If testing is one of the school counselor's responsibilities, it is crucial to continue to intersperse counseling duties with testing duties. Depending on the time needed to perform testing duties, school counselors must continue to perform individual and small group counseling, classroom guidance, and consultation with parents and teachers. School counselors must make time for these important counseling services. Effective time management and good organizational skills will be necessary to do this. In addition to fulfilling responsibilities to the school counseling program, counseling also gives the school counselor a break from the stresses related to testing.

An integral component of the school counselor's role regardless of testing responsibilities is to provide support for teachers, students, and parents who often find testing very stressful. Teachers are anxious because they want students to do well; students are anxious because they feel pressure to do well. Even parents feel the pressure. School counselors can do several things to help.

- Provide support groups for students with anxiety.
- Provide small groups that focus on testing issues.
- Offer to visit classrooms prior to the test to provide strategies to reduce anxiety.
- Post positive messages for teachers and students in areas that are visible to all (e.g., "You can do it! Try your best!").
- Provide breaks for teachers who are testing for long-periods of time; it's amazing how far a bathroom break goes.
- Encourage students to participate in fun, stress-releasing activities after school or after testing.
- Provide strategies for parents to help their children maximize their performance on the test.
- Once the testing is over, celebrate in some small way, but acknowledge in a big way the accomplishment of finishing the testing.

Baker (2000) provided advice to school counselors who find themselves taxed with the testing program or some component of it: "If refusing to participate is not an option, helpful participation demands competence" (p. 271). In other words, if life gives you lemons, make lemonade. It may be that participation in testing is a role you will enjoy and, more importantly, is a role in which you can provide a valuable service to your school and your students.

REFLECTION AND DISCUSSION

1. Testing is a noncounseling duty for school counselors. What types of evidence might you provide that indicates that this role is an inefficient use of your time as a school counselor? Who do you think might need to be convinced?

2. You are in a job interview for a school counseling position. During the interview, the administrator indicates that he or she would like for you to assume the role of co-coordinator of the testing program. How would you respond? How would this information affect your decision about working in that school?

CONCLUSION

Perhaps the unique feature of the recommended roles of the school counselor is that they not only complement each other, but also in some situations are inextricably connected. Coordination and consultation are both components of counseling and classroom guidance. Coordination of a special counseling activity or event might begin with consultation with outside resources to begin planning. The articulation of these roles as separate and distinct is somewhat misleading and does not reflect the interaction and overlap inherent in these roles. Even noncounseling duties offer the opportunity to implement the counseling roles and responsibilities of school counselors. Evidently, the roles of the school counselor keep life active, perhaps even hectic; but it is nonetheless exciting, challenging, frustrating, exhilarating, and necessary for the good of students in schools.

REFLECTION AND DISCUSSION

1. The role of the school counselor in consultation and coordination may be interrelated. Think of and discuss situations in which you might perform both roles at the same time.

2. What would you do if you felt that some of your assigned duties and responsibilities were detrimental to your role as a school counselor? Who needs to know? How would you approach the situation? What if the situation didn't change?

3. Part of the confusion about the role of a school counselor is due to a general lack of awareness and understanding of what school counselors do. In what specific ways could you educate others? What types of public relations activities might help clarify the roles of school counselors?

CHAPTER 5

Supporting Students: Fostering Academic, Personal/Social, and Career Development

Many times, the school counseling office becomes a reprieve for students who are angry, are upset, or just need a place to vent. A school counselor's primary role is to support and advocate for students. The school counselor must often perform a balancing act in order to maintain a positive and supportive relationship with adults in the student's life while also advocating for the student's interests. Most importantly, it is critical to understand the conditions in which many youth live and to realize that life circumstances are not left at the school door.

Conditions of Youth in Schools

Recent data (Annie E. Casey Foundation, 2002a) indicated that the number of children younger than age 18 is more than 72 million. This is a 14% increase since 1990, due in large part to the number of children who have immigrated to the United States. In 2000, more than 53 million children were school age (ages 5 through 17). Funding for new schools and new social programs is struggling to meet the demands of this increase in the youth population. The report also indicated an improvement in the well-being of youth in the United States over the past decade; there has been a decline in infant mortality, child and teen death rates, and school dropout rates. Further, childhood poverty fell by almost 6%, and teenage pregnancy decreased 7% from 1990 to 1998 (Annie E. Casey Foundation). Even though there is good news, the Children's Defense Fund (2002) indicated that issues such as abuse and neglect, poverty, lack of health insurance, deficits in reading and math proficiency, lack of supervision, homelessness, and hunger are still prevalent conditions of youth today. These life circumstances, among others, may impact the educational progress and experience of school-age children. School counselors can help students with these issues either by accessing appropriate resources to meet basic needs or by providing essential services to students and families who are experiencing these struggles.

Despite obstacles, it would be unfair to paint a negative picture of youth today. Most students do want to perform well in school, have many friends, and plan for a promising future. Their reality, however, is very demanding and full of pressure. Youth today are on the fast track; living in a world of high-speed technology and immediate gratification has sometimes resulted in loss of patience and an unwillingness to take time to solve problems. Students may seek the quick fix, whether in the form of Ecstasy or other drugs or in the form of a person who will fix their problems for them. It is not solely the students' fault that their reality is hurried, even frantic. Our society has created its own challenges.

This could be truly worrisome, except this generation also has the potential to be the best and brightest. No other generation has the opportunities that today's students have and no other group has been so prepared for the technological advances of the future. Yet despite the advantages and opportunities, our kids often struggle. Part of the appeal of school counseling is the chance to become an adult who makes a personal connection with students and provides support when obstacles arise.

This chapter focuses on the students. It will examine the situations and circumstances that children and adolescents often bring to school. Further, it will explore examples of significant life events that might impact students' academic progress. Also, it is important to examine the academic, personal/social, and career issues that might present themselves. We will talk about the significant role of school counselors as they interact with the persons for whom they advocate the most—the students.

Each of the topics in this chapter could be a chapter or a book in and of itself. The information presented on each is not exhaustive, and the suggestions are not finite. It is always a good idea to research several sources to fully understand an issue and its effect on youth. While information and statistics might imply that certain age groups or ethnic groups could be stereotyped, each statistic represents a group of individuals as diverse as our society. Regional differences, language differences, socioeconomic differences, and life experience differences will vary between and within groups of students. Thus, students should not be grouped into one category. However, it is important to comprehend the problems many students are dealing with today, as well as the implications of these problems, in order to effectively provide school counseling services for them.

Counseling for Academic Success

By now it should be clear that one of the major roles of school counselors is to help students achieve academic success. There are two major ways that school counselors can intervene to help students succeed academically. First, school counselors can be proactive and help create a school climate that promotes academic success. Second, direct counseling interventions can be used with individual students or groups of students for whom academics are a challenge.

Creating a Climate for Learning

Purkey and Schmidt (1996) identified several characteristics of inviting school environments, but only one was specific to students. They found that students are more likely to want to perform well academically in a school where they are recognized for their accomplishments and encouraged to fulfill their potential. Brown (1999a) indicated that school counselors can be a part of developing this climate by conducting awards programs and recognizing student achievements.

> ### My Story
>
> In my elementary school, I started a program called "Super Students." Each week, a student was selected from every classroom; the names were announced over the P.A. system on Monday morning and each student received a certificate to take home, a Super Student pencil, and a special certificate to be displayed on a bulletin board in the front hall of the school building. The criteria for the Super Student award were often academic, but not always. I asked teachers to make sure that each student in their classes received the Super Student award sometime within the school year. This request accomplished two things: (a) making sure that every student received the reward at least once, and (b) requiring teachers to look at their students in different ways, since it was not always easy to come up with a reason for each student to receive the award. When working with middle school or high school students, it is equally important to reward outstanding effort and achievement, especially in academics. As a high school counselor, I would always make sure that if a student received a scholarship or award, it was in the morning announcements. In addition, we had a Scholarship Night during which each senior who had received an award was recognized. It was very reinforcing for these students to have their outstanding work recognized and appreciated.

It is easy to encourage and reward students who are motivated to succeed. But the school experience is not always perceived as positive. Some students detest the structure and demands of school curricula and find it difficult to conform to the school environment and the expectations of others. School counselors should focus on students who struggle academically and who are simply trying to get through the day at school. Direct counseling interventions are needed to support whatever goals are important to the students, and successes, no matter how small, should be celebrated. Creating a climate for academic progress includes engaging students in their own learning. School counselors can be instrumental in identifying the factors that facilitate learning for all students.

Counseling Interventions

ASSESSING THE PRESENTING PROBLEM School counselors should be aware that issues that present as academic may, in fact, be symptomatic of other issues. The purpose of the school counselor's initial intervention should be to determine the source of the academic problem. Is the issue solely academic, or is it more psychological, social, or emotional? Is the source of the issue outside of the school environment? The answers to these questions will influence how the school counselor proceeds with intervention.

Professional Perspective

BETH (MS)

Students' academic problems often alert people to other issues. I find that, typically, students don't begin doing poorly in school when nothing is wrong in their lives. Some students are slow learners and will always have academic difficulties. For students whose problems are purely academic, we can provide strategies to help studying become a little easier. We also occasionally have students who are developmentally young; they do not care much about school, so they are not focused academically. Beyond that, there are students with more severe issues, such as learning disabilities, ADHD, and many other problems that can affect academic performance. If we look beyond the academic, it may be that the problem is more social and emotional, such as family issues that are manifesting as poor grades. Sometimes poor peer relations upset students, and they don't focus as well on academics. School counselors really have to explore the sources of the issues when students are having academic problems.

SETTING GOALS When students have educational and career goals, they are more likely to be successful academically (Brown, 1999a). Therefore, school counselors must focus on helping students establish goals. This is not always easy, as some students have difficulty determining what they want in life. Goals may need to be short-term and very concrete, such as, "My goal is to turn in all of my assignments in algebra this week." Goals must be concise, precise, and most of all, meaningful. The counselor could ask, "How would turning in all of your math assignments help you?" The student might respond, "Well, it might be the difference between a D and an F, and I need the math credit to graduate." This is a meaningful subgoal for the student if graduation is the ultimate goal.

When setting goals for student academic success, it is critical that the student is committed to the goals. School counselors must determine whose goals are being addressed in counseling sessions. When students struggle academically, they usually see the counselor through teacher or parent referral. At the secondary level, students may self-refer, or the counselor may identify academic problems when reviewing report cards. If a teacher has tried to help a student with class work but has seen no improvement, the school counselor will likely be consulted. There may be a tendency to establish goals based on teacher or parent opinion rather than student needs. While parent and teacher input is invaluable, it is the student's commitment to the academic goals established that will ultimately determine the student's success.

SELECTING APPROPRIATE COUNSELING SERVICES TO FACILITATE LEARNING When a student struggles academically, it is imperative that intervention begins as soon as the difficulty is identified. If the struggle goes untreated for too long, a student's self-concept and social interactions may be negatively affected. A group referral may suffice when a student is having minor academic problems, whereas individual counseling may address more serious academic difficulties.

Brown (1999a) identified several types of direct interventions to use when trying to improve learning and/or achievement: behavioral contracts, study skills groups, time management training, classroom guidance units aimed at improving test-taking skills, achievement/motivation groups, standardized testing preparation courses (SAT, ACT), peer/volunteer tutoring programs, and homework support networks (p. 4). Planning and implementing each of these interventions will require a commitment of time and energy, and the school counselor is integral in providing these services.

Professional Practice

ESTHER (HS)

I am often asked to assist children who have difficulties with staying on task, organization, or time management. I run groups addressing study skills, and I teach some classroom guidance lessons on study skills and test-taking strategies. If a student's academic problems are not being resolved, he or she may have a learning problem. If a learning problem is suspected, I become one of a team of professionals who may evaluate the student and determine if he or she is eligible for special services.

At the elementary level, the school counselor, in collaboration with teachers and other school personnel, has the important task of helping students understand the value of academic success. Classroom guidance lessons on goal setting and the steps for reaching those goals help students focus and plan for the future. Individual and group counseling with students provides more specific attention to those who need academic support. At the secondary level, goal setting is still the focus, but students' commitments to achieve their goals as they begin to consider life after high school is also a critical issue. Secondary counselors can ask students about their interests, educational or occupational plans, and the steps they will take to achieve their goals. Classroom guidance sessions on college exploration or vocational interests will help students identify and understand the academic requirements of their chosen paths. Individual and small group counseling can help address specific needs of students and provide support for students with little or no motivation.

Professional Perspective

ESTHER (HS)

There is a wide variety of academic issues that must be addressed at the high school level: inappropriate placement in an academic class, poor study skills, poor academic background, need for remediation, and learning/information processing problems. High school counselors help students, teachers, and parents deal with all of these issues by finding or providing appropriate support resources.

School counselors are in a key position to reward the academic successes of students and to support students who are academically challenged. Being involved in the academic lives of students is a key element in the school counselor's quest to promote effective lifelong learning and maximize student success.

REFLECTION AND DISCUSSION

1. School counselors' primary goal is to help students become effective lifelong learners. A major component of this goal is academic success. As a school counselor, how would you motivate the unmotivated student? What specific strategies would you use to engage students in their education?

2. Often, school counseling services might conflict with academic programs/classes. How would you work with teachers and students to address students' counseling needs while not interfering with the academic program?

Counseling for Personal and Social Development

In an ideal world, we would be able to protect children from life events that cause them stress and pain. The reality is that students' lives are affected by significant life events that are usually unexpected. School counselors might identify extreme changes in student behavior or attitudes as a result of a significant event or change in the student's life. Students frequently seek out school counselors because of upsetting or stressful life events. School counselors must help students address the thoughts, feelings, and behaviors that result from the stressful events in their lives.

Children's Stress and Life Events

Borden (1992) defined three categories of events that may occur throughout the developmental life span:

- Normal events that happen at certain ages that are determined largely by biology and have similar timing and duration for all people. Although these are typically perceived as normal events, they may cause stress for some youth. For example, puberty can certainly be a tumultuous time for students.

- "Normative, history-graded events that are experienced by most members of a cohort" (p. 136). For example, war or terrorism would be considered an adverse life experience. Students might respond to these events in a stressful way, either due to the events or their perceptions of the events as they relate to their current situations.

- Non-normative events that occur infrequently and are uncommon for many people (e.g., sudden illness or death, job loss, or moving). These events may cause a young person to be in a state of distress and can result in changes in behavior and/or academic performance (p. 136).

Regardless of the type of event, the effect can be overwhelming. It is heart wrenching to learn about the circumstances in which some students live. Often, school personnel don't discover students' problems until they have been occurring for some time, if the personnel ever discover them. A meaningful part of being a school counselor is intervening and supporting the student when a situation is realized. The school counselor can orchestrate a plan to provide the best services available to help students. The professional practices of our veteran counselors indicate the variety of services that school counselors provide to address students' personal and social problems.

Professional Practice

RENEE (ES)

In elementary school, I primarily deal with personal/social issues. Elementary school children are beginning to develop separate identities from their parents. Peers are a large part of that process. As children move through elementary school, they are trying to learn how to interact with their peers and how to resolve conflicts. A great deal of my time is spent helping students work out problems with their peers. I also get referrals for students who are experiencing difficulty demonstrating appropriate classroom behavior. If a student is preoccupied with personal or social problems, it often affects his or her academic performance.

BETH (MS)

At the middle school level, student issues are more personal/social. Peer relationships are critical for middle school students. They really begin to gossip and are very conscious of what their peers think. It's very important to be accepted. Middle school students are not likely to be individualistic. They want to be accepted and liked, and are hurt if they are rejected. School counselors help students make sense of changing friendships. Students assume that their friendships from elementary school will continue. But friendships will often fall by the wayside, particularly because of changing classes, and that usually hurts students. They can't make sense of why friendships fall apart, and school counselors can intervene and help.

ESTHER (HS)

High school students' personal/social issues usually pertain to conflicts with friends, teachers, and parents; loss, transition, and adjustment problems; gender issues; substance abuse issues; pregnancy; decision making; dating and sex; and self-concept and self-consciousness. At the high school level, you must be prepared to deal with whatever issue comes through your door. Individual counseling, group counseling, classroom guidance, and consultation are all useful services, depending on the nature of the problem.

The School Counselor's Role in Personal/Social Issues: Two Examples

To demonstrate how school counselors work with specific personal/social issues, the next sections will explore two examples of loss events that are common to many youth today: divorce and grief. While these issues result in similar feelings of loss, they are unique life events that might require different types of counseling services.

DIVORCE/CHANGING FAMILIES

Facing the Facts and Feelings   With half of all marriages ending in divorce, it is expected that many students will either witness or be part of a changing family situation. School counselors may need to provide services for students at any point in the experience:

- the decision to separate,
- one parent moving out,
- custody arrangements,
- filing for divorce,
- establishing visitation schedules,
- going to court,
- the first holiday after the separation,
- living in two places,
- parent(s) beginning to date other people,
- parent(s) remarrying, or
- step-situations (stepparent, stepsiblings, stepgrandparents).

So many issues surface during separation and divorce that students often find it difficult to focus on anything else. The world as they know it is in upheaval, and even if divorce or separation is for the better, children are typically not happy when it happens. Most children harbor some hope that their parents might reconcile. What they don't realize are the issues that might arise in the event of reconciliation—counseling, how their parents change, the atmosphere at home, and what happens if it doesn't work.

My Story

Having worked with students through all stages of the divorce process, I can honestly say that most youth handle the changes very well. For many, divorce is the end of a battle that has been going on for a long time. Some are just glad that the fighting has stopped; others feel abandoned by the parent who left. Each student has a different experience, yet the feelings are often the same—sadness, anger, relief, and maybe even excitement about the changes. For some students, being successful in school is no longer a priority; when your personal life is in chaos, it seems odd to focus your energy on schoolwork. Often, concerns about the family and what is going to happen engulf the student, making concentration in school very difficult.

Students' responses to divorce are as varied as the circumstances that lead to divorce. Many students, especially those who are younger or are almost finished with high school, seem to maintain a life-as-usual attitude. This is probably because at this point in their lives, school is a constant. Whether because school helps them forget about their home lives or the consistency and structure of school comforts them, many students maintain attendance and grades once their initial responses to divorce are over. Other students struggle with the changes in their families. Emotions range from depression to anger to confusion throughout the phases of divorce. Sometimes children feel responsible and express their emotions through destructive behaviors, such as self-mutilation, eating disorders, and sudden acts of violence or fighting. It is not unusual for students to exhibit behaviors that are totally out of character. Students sometimes believe that if their behaviors are extreme enough, their parents will focus on them rather than the divorce.

When one parent simply disappears, it is not out of the ordinary to see the child exhibiting extreme behaviors as a result of feelings about the divorce and feelings of abandonment. The reality is that divorce changes the family dynamic for the short- and long-term, and these changes do affect students, whether they deny or confront them.

Direct Counseling Services   There is a natural progression of children's emotions and needs throughout the divorce process. It typically begins with the need to talk about their personal situations and, as they understand that the divorce is a reality, becomes a need to be with other students who are going through similar experiences. For this reason, counseling should progress to meet those needs as they occur. Once a school counselor learns about a student whose family is going through either a separation or divorce, the counselor should connect with the student as soon as possible.

A student may be resistant to talk about the divorce for several reasons. First, the student may be in denial about the split, and not talking about it makes it easier to believe it isn't really happening. Second, the student may feel confused and overwhelmed by the feelings he or she is having, which can result in a "I just can't deal with it" attitude. Even when the student acknowledges that the divorce/separation is happening, the feelings may be too much handle. Third, the student may feel that discussing the situation is involving others in private family business. For example, many students are taught that sharing information about family problems is wrong or inappropriate. Sometimes, students just do not want to share things about their private lives, especially with school personnel who they are not sure they can trust. Fourth, if a student does not already feel some connection with the school counselor, it may be difficult to share something so personal. In the event that the student shows no desire to talk to the school counselor, the best recourse is to not force it. It is unethical for students to be forced into counseling services. Finally, the student may not want to talk about the divorce if he or she is happy about improvements in life since the divorce occurred. Regardless of the reason, when a student does not want to talk about the situation, the counselor should do the following:

- Let the student know that the counselor is aware of the situation. The source of the information does not need to be revealed. Don't say, "I heard . . ." because students can become defensive if they feel they are being talked about.

- Make the student aware of the ways in which counseling might be helpful. For example, "Other students have found that talking about how they are feeling about changes in their families is helpful."

- Remind the student that counseling is confidential. For example, "I was thinking that it might be good for you to have a place where you could vent about all that's happening, and I would keep our conversations confidential."

- Let the student know about counseling services. For example, "If you do not want to meet individually, I am also running a small group for students who are going through changing family situations. You are more than welcome to participate in the group instead of individual sessions."

- Remind the student that counseling is available in the event he or she becomes ready to talk. For example, "Please remember that I am available and willing to talk with you if you decide you want to talk about this or anything else. Do you know where my office is or how to let me know you would like to talk?"

When students are ready and willing to talk, it is important to connect with them as soon as possible. Feature 5.1 offers ideas for topics that might be discussed during an individual session with a student whose parents are divorcing.

FEATURE 5.1

*Issues to Address in Individual Counseling
With Children of Divorce*

- Feelings about the changes that are occurring as a result of the split
- Logistical changes that are occurring as a result of the split (alternating households, visitations, etc.)
- Educational impact of the changes ("How have things been going in school since you found out your parents were separating?")
- Friendships/support systems that are available to the student ("Who are the people you can talk to?")
- Future implications ("How are you feeling about the divorce becoming final?" "How are you feeling about going to court?" "What do you think your family life will be like in 5 years?" "What might it be like if either your mom or dad starts dating someone else?")
- Group counseling ("Would you like to participate in a small group with other students whose families are also changing?")

Whether students whose families are going through divorce participate in individual or group counseling, or do not participate at all, continue to check in with them. Even when students indicate they do not need counseling services, make contact to see how things are going. This communicates on-going concern and empathy for their situation.

GRIEF/LOSS In addition to divorce, there are other significant grief/loss experiences that children and adolescents may experience. Students may experience the following types of loss:

- death of a relative or friend,
- moving to a new house or community,
- parental or family member incarceration,
- alteration in family structure due to an event other than death (i.e., divorce),
- friends moving away, and
- parental change in or loss of job.

Most students will experience some loss event, and school counselors should be prepared to help them work through the related issues.

Stages of Grief Depending upon the source of grief/loss, reactions can vary. Capuzzi (2002) identified 10 stages one may experience following a loss: shock, emotional release (such as anger), depression, physical symptoms of distress or psychosomatic problems, anxiety, hostility or bitterness, hesitancy to resume normal activities or the immediate return to normal activities, guilt, healing memories, and finally, the acceptance of one's new role in life. A student's progression through these stages may be quick or it may take a long time.

Direct Counseling Services There are several factors that may influence how a school counselor counsels a student who has experienced loss. First and foremost, the counselor must determine how willing the student is to participate in the counseling process. Is he or she ready to talk about the loss? Second, the counselor must find out what support structures and services are already in place. Is the student in outside counseling to address similar issues? If so, the school counselor can certainly provide support for the student while he or she is at school, but should not duplicate services that are being provided in therapy. Finally, the counselor must determine what stage of the grief process the student is experiencing. The answers to these questions will determine how the school counselor should intervene.

The school counselor should also pay attention to other indicators that the student is in need of counseling services. If there is a change in attendance, grades, class participation, or friendships, the school counselor should acknowledge these changes as a sign to intervene. One way to decide if counseling should occur with a student who has experienced loss is to assess potential problem areas. Have there been changes in the student's behavior at school or at home? Does there seem to be a change in the student's general attitude about life? Is the student maintaining social relationships and friendships? Is the student connected to a family member or adult who can provide support? An informal assessment with parents, teachers, or the student will indicate how the loss is affecting the student. Once the assessment is complete, the school counselor will have a better idea of how to most appropriately progress in the counseling relationship.

As indicated in the discussion on divorce, if a student is in denial about the loss or is not prepared to deal with the emotions related to the loss, it would be ineffective to force counseling services on him or her. It is appropriate, however, to remind the student that you are available and that counseling may help him or her work through this difficult time—even if it is about something seemingly unrelated to the loss. Sometimes, as a school counselor, the best way to get at the real issue is to come through the back door. Engaging the student in another way or on another topic may make it easier to approach the feelings and issues related to the loss.

Hopefully, the student will be willing to talk to the school counselor about the loss. At the elementary level, most students are willing to participate in counseling, depending on the level of rapport the students have with the school counselor. At the secondary level, students may be either very open or completely opposed to talking about the loss. One exception to this seems to be when the loss is sudden, such as the death of a teacher or peer. Students seem to be much more willing to talk about feelings related to a more public loss. They are more likely to seek help if they observe their peers also seeking help. It normalizes the experience of seeking help from the school counselor if others are doing the same.

Regardless of how a student comes to the school counselor, it is important to acknowledge how difficult it is to talk about a loss. While it is advantageous to identify with the student, it is typically not effective to say, "I know how you feel," or to spend time self-disclosing about a personal loss. Loss is a very private experience, and initially, the student needs to feel validated for having unique feelings and responses. Self-disclosure about a similar type of loss may be appropriate at some point, but the student is typically more involved in the feelings he or she is experiencing.

Once the student becomes comfortable and starts talking about the loss experience, it is important to assist the student through the *process* of grieving. Initial individual sessions might focus on the loss itself by having the student talk about life prior to the loss, the experience of the loss, and feelings immediately after the loss. Middle sessions could deal with the student's current feelings about the loss and the impact it is having on his or her life. Final sessions begin the healing process by dealing with the loss in the context of the future (e.g., "How do you think you will feel about this loss next year? In five years?" or "What are some ways you might keep the memories alive as you go through school and get older?"). When dealing with loss situations, school counselors should perform the essential function of guiding students through the grieving process.

A student who may not be ready to participate in the one-on-one interaction of individual counseling might agree to participate in group counseling with peers who have also experienced loss. One word of caution about grief/loss group counseling is to make sure that group participants have experienced similar levels of loss; see the "My Story" box for further discussion of this issue.

When dealing with intense issues in group counseling, such as grief/loss, school counselors should allow time for processing any emotions that emerge in the group. Feelings related to grief and loss may be very intense when

My Story

I was screening members for a grief/loss group and realized that I had four students who had lost a parent or sibling and one student who had lost a pet. While pet loss is a significant loss and should be addressed and processed, I did not feel it was appropriate to have this student in with other participants who had experienced the loss of an immediate family member. It is worthwhile to screen all group participants to make sure the degree of loss is somewhat similar. This will promote group cohesion and healthy empathy among group members.

discussed or confronted. Group members in schools are expected to return to the regular educational program and to respond appropriately to the normal functions of the school day after they leave the group session. If a session has been particularly emotional for one or more members, it is critical to include time to help them compose themselves before they return to class. For example, if a student is overcome with anger or sadness and exhibits strong behaviors in the group, it is not wise to send that student back into a situation that could trigger an extreme response while he or she is emotionally vulnerable.

Specific group counseling activities might include dealing with feelings of anger, hurt, sadness, guilt, and fear. Talking about the loss experience, creating memory books or journals, and facing future challenges are also important components of grief counseling. For students, being counseled through the grieving process and the various feelings associated with loss can be very meaningful and even life altering. The group counseling experience provides an appropriate forum for students to connect with others who are also experiencing grief.

Children and adolescents experience loss in a personal, meaningful way. School counselors can guide them through the many feelings that result from loss. Loss, no matter how big or small, means change, and change is a challenge. School counselors can engage students in the counseling process in order to help them learn to deal with the challenges of loss and change that will inevitably occur in their lives. It is a life skill that will be invaluable to them throughout their lifetimes.

OTHER PERSONAL/SOCIAL ISSUES: GENERAL GUIDELINES   There are many other personal/social issues that school counselors deal with: anger, sibling issues, jealousy, frustration, lack of motivation, friendship issues, gang involvement, relationship issues, sexuality, self-concept, drug use and abuse, family issues, racism, and peer pressure, to name a few. One aspect of being an effective counselor is identifying and understanding the students' issues. Based on experiences and input from practitioners, the following general guidelines may be useful when counseling students with personal and social concerns.

- *Listen to the story.* Students need to be heard, and maybe they need to hear themselves. Often, they just need someone who will objectively listen without interference.

- *Help students identify their concerns.* There may be multiple issues to be addressed. What seems to be the most pressing? Which is interfering most with the student's life?

- *Meet the student where the student is.* If a student is not ready to talk or not ready to work on a problem, do not force it. Counseling services are to be offered, not imposed.

- *Help the student set goals.* If the student is ready, talk about the goals the student has for dealing with the problem. What would be different as a result of these goals? What would the student need to do differently to reach these goals?

- *Consider challenges along the way.* Discuss the possible consequences of the student's decisions. What if something does not go as planned? Are there alternatives?

- *Be available, and check in with the student.* Often, after something is resolved, the student may not come back to the counselor. It is important for the counselor to find the student and check in to see how things are going.

- *Consider referral.* Depending on the nature of the problem, it may not be possible for the student to address this problem at school, or the school counselor may not be trained to help with a particular issue. In this case, outside referral would be needed. Consulting with colleagues may offer valuable input when deciding about outside referral.

It is inaccurate to assume that there is no relationship between a student's personal life and academic behavior. We cannot assume that students leave their problems at the school door and become completely focused on the academic tasks at hand. The school counselor can be a bridge between personal and social concerns and academic progress. Viewing a student's personal, social, emotional, or academic development as if it exists in a vacuum or in isolation is a narrow vision that will ultimately neglect the full potential of the student. School counselors must take a holistic approach. The unique training that school counselors receive enables them to discover how each developmental area is intertwined with the others, understand how each issue interacts or interferes with development in other areas, and help students problem solve and work through important issues that will ultimately affect their overall functioning.

REFLECTION AND DISCUSSION

1. Select a personal/social issue that a student might have (at any level). Discuss the problems or possible areas of concern that surround this issue. Develop a counseling intervention strategy that will address this issue.

2. As a school counselor, what will you do if the counseling interventions you provide do not seem to be helping a student? What resources will you use to try to help the student?

Counseling for Career Development

The school counselor's role in the career development of students is one of the foundations of the school counselor job. Since vocational counseling was the central focus of counseling services in schools in early school counseling history, it is only natural that career counseling is still a primary responsibility of school counselors. The connection between career development and the school counselor is evidenced by the inclusion of career development as a strand of the ASCA National Standards for School Counseling Programs (Campbell & Dahir, 1997).

Prior to the 1980s, career counseling focused solely on helping students discover what jobs or careers they wished to pursue, and then helping them decide what paths they might take to achieve those goals. Career counseling at the high school level included interest inventories, computer software packages that explored various careers, college information as it related to careers, and other student career resources. In 1985, the American School Counselor Association took a position on the school counselor's role in career development, or *career maturity* (Herring, 1998), suggesting that career growth was a process rather than a decision to be made at a specific time in one's schooling. In 1987, the National Occupational Information Coordinating Committee (NOICC) launched the National Career Development Guidelines initiative "to support and encourage activities designed to strengthen and improve comprehensive, competency-based career guidance programs" (Miller, 1992, p. 1). The guidelines were based upon three areas of development: self-knowledge, educational and occupational exploration, and career planning. Specific objectives targeted each of these areas throughout students' development, from elementary to middle to high school.

The most recent ASCA Position Statement on this topic united educational planning with career planning, which is supported by the career development section of the National Standards. The statement posits that: "Professional school counselors play a critical role in assisting students in the development of a comprehensive plan allowing for exploration of their educational and career opportunities . . . [and] advocates for developmental guidance programs involving individual and group activities stressing educational planning (i.e., decision making, career awareness, and exploration)" (ASCA, 2000a, p. 1). The National Standards (Campbell & Dahir, 1997) present specific competencies that students should achieve through career development counseling. The specific practices that school counselors use vary depending on school level.

Elementary School: Career Awareness

At the elementary level, career development begins with an exploration of self and others. Activities that explore likes and interests, as well as similarities and differences with others, help promote the idea of uniqueness or special talents. Another area that is important is awareness of the world of work. This can occur through experiential activities, such as hosting career speakers from various occupations or taking field trips to a variety of work places (e.g., fire station, hospital, or restaurant). In the lower elementary grades (kindergarten through second grade), the emphasis is not deciding what one wants to be when one grows up, but is mainly helping students become aware that after their student careers, they are probably going to engage in an occupation. Making students aware of the many options is part of the career awareness experience.

Professional Perspective

RENEE (ES)

Career development at the elementary level is primarily focused on exposing the children to the world of work and the variety of career opportunities available, as well as developing the students' understanding of their interests and abilities and how they may relate to future career choices. Career education can be a fun and dynamic experience for the elementary student—it is never too early to start. Even kindergarteners enjoy brainstorming about all of the different jobs in which a worker would need a hammer, or a pair of scissors, or a bandage.

In later elementary years (grades 3 through 6), students begin differentiating between careers and may also be able to picture themselves in certain jobs. They also become aware that working is a means to an end; people usually have to work in order to make a living so that they can buy houses, raise families, buy cars, and generally support themselves. A good activity that school counselors can do with upper elementary students is to have them interview people from various occupations. Often, this creates important dialogue between students and adults, such as parents, neighbors, and community leaders, about the many opportunities and challenges in the working world. This awareness will help them as they move into the next phase of career development.

Professional Practice

RENEE (ES)

I address career development through classroom guidance lessons and by hosting a Career Fair. I believe that the students will find career education much more meaningful if it is presented by people actually performing the jobs they are learning about. So I gather guest speakers to come to school to tell the children about what they do. The students seem to get excited about the different jobs they learn about. At Career Fair, I give the children interview questions to ask the guests. For example, "How do you use math in your job?" or "What types of skills would I need to do your job?" There are also great computer programs and Web sites that provide interactive ways for the students to identify their career interests and careers that they may want to learn more about.

Middle School: Career Exploration

As students reach middle school age or early adolescence, they become more aware of their personal interests, aptitudes, abilities, and values. This develop-

My Story

It is often in the upper elementary grades that students fantasize about certain careers. When I was an elementary counselor, I would go into the sixth grade classes and conduct a career lesson that involved having students project themselves 10 years into the future. I would ask: "What do you see yourself doing in ten years?" Without fail, many of the students saw themselves as professional athletes—playing for the NFL, the NBA, professional baseball, professional soccer. I found it was difficult to sway them from their positions. I did not discount their future dreams (perhaps one of them would become the next Michael Jordan). However, I would often say: "You know, Michael Jordan got a degree in Geography in case the basketball career didn't work out. Just in case the sports career doesn't work out, what do you think you might do instead?" It is important to let students fantasize and dream, but it is also good practice to help them consider options in case the dream isn't realized.

mental period is an ideal time to begin exploring possible career fields or areas of occupational interest. Lankard (1991) asserted that at this level, students should learn more about careers, the education or skills required to work in specific careers, and the lifestyles that certain jobs represent. In particular, activities should have: (a) more emphasis on self-knowledge and developing competencies, (b) more involvement of community members representing various occupations to students, (c) increased attention to the benefits of doing well academically and the relationship between education and occupation, and (d) increased emphasis on the skills necessary to seek and obtain jobs. It is not unusual for students this age to begin working in some capacity, for example babysitting, mowing lawns, or delivering newspapers. Therefore, making the connection between the world of work and the personal implications of working is a good way to begin the exploration process.

School counselors at the middle school/junior high level are in a unique position to facilitate career exploration. A middle school counselor may lead classroom guidance activities, perhaps in a computer lab, where students have access to career exploratory programs. These interactive software programs typically include several questionnaires that ask students to respond to questions regarding their personalities, interests, abilities, and values. Based on the input received, the students receive a profile or information regarding potential occupational matches. Students can explore specific occupations by accessing information about how much education is needed, the salary range, and the outlook for job opportunities. Students typically enjoy this activity because they are not only learning about themselves, but are also beginning to think about their futures. School counselors can initiate dialogue that helps students explore the results of the programs and how well they believe the results match their self-perceptions.

Professional Practice

BETH (MS)

We are now using a program called Bridges that is designed specifically for middle schools. We usually do classroom and computer guidance lessons and sometimes piggyback with the work and family (home economic), history, or other classes as appropriate. For example, if a language arts class is learning about writing a reference letter or resume, we'll help them. We also conduct a parent presentation on "Helping Your Child Plan for the Future," during which we talk about scheduling issues and what classes to take to prepare for the future. We also make students aware of programs in the county for minority achievement and opportunities for women.

Another way the middle school counselor may foster career development is through consultation with other school personnel, most likely teachers, as they conduct lessons on work ethics or interpersonal skills. By working with teachers on collaborative lessons, school counselors can be involved in curriculum and also offer individual services to students as the need arises.

A final example of how school counselors can provide career development opportunities at the middle school/junior high level is by having a Career Day or Week, as in the example in chapter 4, during which students in a particular grade level or all grades have the opportunity to learn about career options. The counselor may also want to encourage students to volunteer in areas where they might have occupational interests. Fostering and having personal interaction can be very influential in the career decision-making and planning process that begins as students transition to high school.

High School: Career Planning and Decision Making

Career counseling at the high school level is somewhat more of a priority than it might be at either the elementary or middle school levels for one obvious reason: The students will soon be entering the world of work. For most, this means college or further education; but for many, high school is the transition to the world of work. Lankard (1991) recommended that high school career activities should: (a) place increased emphasis on activities related to awareness of how life roles are interrelated, (b) emphasize the understanding of the role of work in the economy and how work influences the way we live, and (c) provide opportunities for students to improve social skills when interacting with others (p. 6).

Professional Practice

ESTHER (HS)

Counselors present grade-appropriate career units every year. They interpret and administer career inventories, use computerized college and career information databases, maintain a job bank for part-time and summer employment, and conduct activities on resume writing and interviewing, which develop career-seeking skills.

A unique characteristic of career development at the high school level is that career counseling may not be the responsibility of the school counseling program. Often, there is a career center and a person with specialized training in career counseling to assist students with college and vocational searches. Also, most high schools provide internship, apprenticeship, or work-study programs through which students actually spend portions of each day in training on job sites or in work places. These opportunities are often organized and implemented by business departments or other departments of the school. This is not to say that the high school counselor does not have a role in career development. In fact, the high school counselor is essential in helping students begin and complete the decision-making process. For example, in ninth grade, students may begin to develop a portfolio that will follow them through the planning and decision-making process. This portfolio might contain the following:

- school activities,
- grades and testing scores,
- work and/or volunteer experience,
- educational program or courses completed,
- hobbies or interests outside of school, and
- projected future plans (i.e., college, technical or vocational school, work).

Each year, these plans should be updated. The high school counselor is typically responsible for keeping the portfolio information up-to-date. By the time a student reaches the 12th grade, there should be enough information to help the student either through the college application process or the job application process. It was my experience that these one-on-one meetings were a worthwhile opportunity to also check in on the academic and personal/social issues or concerns of students.

Much of the high school counselor's role in career development is consultative and supportive. If a student has a question or concern, the school counselor must be aware of resources where the student can find answers. When a student is struggling with a decision or does not have a clear plan, the school counselor can explore options with the student and help the student come to an acceptable conclusion. Working with teachers and administrators, the high school counselor can provide a comprehensive approach to the all-important question: *What am I going to do after high school?* This can be an overwhelming question for some students, and the school counselor's role is to assist in any way possible to alleviate the anxiety and worry that often comes with making major life decisions.

REFLECTION AND DISCUSSION

1. Some students may not be interested in considering what they will do in the future. How would you motivate students to begin exploring career options?

2. A student comes to you and tells you his career plans. Based on the student's academic performance in school, you doubt that the student will be able to achieve what he wants. As a school counselor, how do you respond to the student? Do you encourage him to continue to pursue the goal, or do you try to present the reality of the situation? Discuss the implications of either decision.

CONCLUSION

School counseling activities and services can help students develop qualities that will prepare them to deal with life's challenges and opportunities. In schools today, there are many safety nets, and much has been done to ensure the physical safety of our students. It seems reasonable to also give students the internal mechanisms and skills to overcome the personal challenges that they will inevitably face. Students have questions that cover a broad range of issues: Will I be able to refuse drugs if my peer group begins to make drug use a criteria for membership? Can I continue to do well academically when my family is falling apart? Should I quit the basketball team and ruin my chances for a scholarship because my mother needs me to work to support the family? Could I have intervened with the girl in my third period class so that she didn't feel alone and commit suicide? How can I be myself and still be what everyone else expects me to be? What if my grades aren't good enough to get into the school of my choice?

School counselors have the unique opportunity to get beneath the facade; to explore the unique personalities, strengths, and talents of the students in our schools; and to help them flourish as they develop academically, personally, socially, and in their life choices. Schools are responsible not only for facilitating learning throughout students' lives, but also for helping them learn to live in and become effective members of our society.

This chapter has been devoted to the population to whom school counselors have the greatest commitment—the students. This chapter specifically addressed each area of development covered by the ASCA National Standards (Campbell & Dahir, 1997) and focused on the role school counselors have in fostering the growth of all students. While not exhaustive, the chapter provided general guidelines for working with students on a variety of issues and offered specific examples and strategies from professionals in the field. By focusing on the academic, personal/social, and career needs of students, school counselors help children become more productive in their school careers and more resilient in their personal endeavors. This role may be the most important one of all for school counselors.

REFLECTION AND DISCUSSION

1. What are some ways you plan to connect with students at the elementary, middle, and high school levels? Are there special considerations for counseling students at each level? What are they?

2. Students may bring very significant stories of adversity to the school counselor's door. How would you, as a school counselor, empathize with students while remaining emotionally objective?

3. This chapter has discussed the three areas of student development that school counseling services should emphasize. Which area do you think should have priority? Think of an example in which all three areas might need to be addressed with a student.

CHAPTER **6**

Supporting Students: Working With Diversity and Special Needs

*T*he student population in schools is constantly changing. What does not change is the need for school counselors to be responsive to the needs of diverse populations. This chapter will focus on the school counselor's role in working with diverse students and those with special needs. Diversity includes an entire spectrum of issues related to gender, sexuality, age, and ethnicity. Entire books are devoted to these important topics in counseling. While cultural considerations must be given to all students, for the purposes of this discussion, we will focus on diversity as it relates to students for whom English is a second language (ESL), as this is a population that is growing rapidly in schools. A second focus will be students with special needs and the school counselor's role in the processes and practices of special education, including a discussion of inclusion of special education students within the mainstream classroom. The chapter will refer to the special needs team as the "Child Study Team" for consistency, although the title may vary from school to school. Finally, a discussion of the school counselor's role in working with sexual minority youth is necessary, as this population is in dire need of support in schools.

Multiculturalism in Schools

It is no secret that the population in the United States is becoming more and more diverse. Researchers project that by the year 2010, the Caucasian population will have grown only slightly, while African American and Latino population growth rates will have accelerated (U.S. Census Bureau, 2001a). Another statistic that will certainly influence education is the influx of English as a Second Language (ESL) students in our schools. According to the Federal Interagency Forum on Child and Family Statistics (2001), in 2000 the statistical breakdown of children by race/ethnicity was as follows: 64% White, non-Hispanic; 16% Hispanic origin; 15% Black, non-Hispanic; 4% Asian or Pacific Islander; and 1% American Indian or Alaskan Native (p. iii). Hispanics/Latinos have increased more rapidly than other ethnic groups in the United States; they comprised 9% of the child population in 1980 and 16% in 1999. Projections are that by 2020, one in five children will be of Hispanic descent (Federal Interagency Forum on Child and Family Statistics). The issues that arise as a result of this influx of multicultural students must be addressed in this new millennium, which is characterized by great diversity.

According to Shore (2001), there are more than 180 different language groups among the students in American schools. Further, "it is estimated that this population is growing two and a half times faster than that of native English-speaking students" (p. 30). In order to counsel diverse populations effectively, Capuzzi and Gross (2003) emphasized that school counselors must consider cultural issues such as language, identity, generation, cultural customs and styles, geographical locations and neighborhood, and family history and traditions. At the most basic level, the first consideration must be the barriers related to language. The Census 2000 Data provided a language profile for the United States that indicated that almost 3.5 million children between the ages of 5 and 17 speak English less than very well. This means that, in terms of speaking English, 5.1% of the school-age population is linguistically challenged (Annie E. Casey Foundation, 2002b).

Schools must rise to the challenges presented by the increase in diverse student populations, and school counselors can be at the forefront of these efforts. One way that school counselors can be prepared to work with students from diverse ethnic backgrounds is to develop *multicultural competence*—to understand and develop the attitudes, beliefs, knowledge, and skills that are needed to work with culturally diverse populations. While most school counselor preparation programs require coursework in multicultural counseling, school counselors-in-training should also seek out professional development opportunities through workshops, seminars, and conference sessions that include discussions on working with culturally diverse students. The diversity within student populations will increase in the coming years. It behooves school counselors to be responsive to these challenges.

Culturally Responsive School Counselors

While there are many services available for ESL students, the acculturation process is nonetheless difficult. School counselors can help ease the pain of these often difficult transitions and respond in a culturally sensitive way that values the child's heritage and helps him or her acclimate to the school environment.

Professional Perspective

RENEE (ES)

Primarily, I see my role as fostering a school climate that is accepting of our many differences and embraces many cultures. This is done by coordinating school-wide activities and classroom lessons, modeling behavior, and creating a comfortable space that is representative and respectful of different cultures.

Lee (2001) recommended that culturally responsive schools take a "salad bowl" rather than a "melting pot" perspective of education (p. 258). This implies that instead of considering diversity as a separate entity that sort of melts into the mainstream, we should consider each diverse student group as a separate but necessary part of the entire student body (i.e., the "salad"). School counselors have important roles in this process. Specific strategies might include individual or group counseling sessions that focus on self-awareness and self-concept so that students feel positive about their identities within and outside of their cultural arenas. Also, school counselors can help organize or sponsor multicultural activities (e.g., Multicultural Night or a Multicultural Awareness Week) in which students from all cultures have the opportunity to share customs, traditions, dress, foods, and items from their cultural heritage. This could lead to a greater understanding of and appreciation for diverse cultures.

In some cultures, education is not valued as much as it is in the mainstream U.S. culture. Therefore, students from a culture that does not emphasize education may be less motivated to achieve academically. Individual, small-group, or classroom guidance activities could focus on the usefulness of education and the purpose of getting a high school diploma or equivalent. This would be particularly effective at the middle and high school levels, where the connection between education and the working world becomes more apparent.

Shore (2001) offered specific counseling strategies that focus on success for ESL students, including assessing needs, empathizing, fostering a sense of belonging, valuing bilingualism, and encouraging family involvement. School counselors should determine as quickly as possible the student's English-language proficiency and help determine the level of intervention needed. It will be important to discover words the student understands or learn words that help the student communicate. Also, pairing the ESL student with another student, preferably bilingual, will help foster a sense of belonging and prevent feelings of social isolation. It is also important that the school counselor encourage the student to continue to speak and write in his or her native language. Expecting the student to only communicate in English could be perceived as demeaning to the student's culture. Showing appreciation for and interest in the culture and language of the student demonstrates acceptance of his or her culture.

When addressing academic development, school counselors may need to consult with other school personnel to help diverse students with basic skill acquisition. In addition, small group counseling that focuses on study skills, test taking, time management, and organization might be helpful for students who have not been exposed to the American education system. School counselors should also advocate for needed services that address the unique barriers that many ESL students may experience. School counseling services differ slightly at each school level, although the goal of successful integration of ESL students into the education process is consistent.

When considering career development of ESL students, Herring (1998) identified issues, such as language and stereotypes, that must be confronted in order for students to begin successful career exploration and decision making. School counselors also need to seek positive role models for students from different ethnic backgrounds. Inviting a variety of career speakers who represent different ethnic groups might help spur an interest in a career or vocational path.

Professional Practice

RENEE (ES)

I work in a school with an ESL center, so we have a very diverse student population. We typically have up to eight translators present for Back to School Night. With such a diverse population, it is important for students to accept and appreciate each other's differences. We attempt to celebrate the diversity of our students. Our staff works together and we formed a committee with staff and parents to address this need. One example of this committee's activities is having students paint the ceiling tiles in the cafeteria to represent the countries of their origins. I help coordinate a multicultural night to which families bring desserts from their native countries. This is always a huge success. On a smaller scale, I try to make sure that my office is representative of the diversity of our school. I include posters, puppets, books, etc. that represent a variety of cultures. I don't want a student to come into my office, look around, and think, "She doesn't understand me at all." I teach classroom lessons on appreciating diversity. I also try to assist parents who may need a translator for parent conferences or Child Study meetings by referring the appropriate agency. Letters that are sent home are translated into different languages as often as possible.

BETH (MS)

We create schedules for the ESL students, and then we work with other support personnel on translation and helping the student transition to the school. Because most counselors are not bilingual, the language barrier can be a problem. We have peer mediators who are bilingual so that ESL students feel represented during mediations. Also, we try to close the gap with minority students by supporting the ESL teacher. We've tried hiring counselors who are bilingual, but they are few and far between, so it is not always easy. Many times you can pull in other resources, though, to nurture students and help them transition into the school. It's hard enough to enter a new school, and it's twice as hard for students whose first language is not English. We have outside resource professionals who offer groups after school to deal with making the transition.

Lee (2001) advocated that school counselors are in an ideal position to be advocates for diverse students. Not only can school counselors provide direct services that help and support the student, they can also intervene on the student's behalf, promote teacher and administrator awareness of the unique needs of diverse students, and reinforce "culturally responsive approaches to education" (p. 260).

Professional Practice

ESTHER (HS)

Counselors work hard to facilitate cultural understanding. At our high school, we have created a unique student enrichment seminar (counseling group) called the Diversity Leadership Group, which serves to promote cultural understanding, share cultural traditions, and train minority and culturally diverse students to become leaders in the school setting.

ESL students are placed with an ESL teacher for two days even before their schedule is formed so that both the counselor and ESL teacher can assess the students' abilities and skills for appropriate academic placement. The counselor works closely with the ESL teacher and other academic teachers on the scheduling for these students, monitoring progress to promote the academic success for each student.

Clemente and Collison (2000) recommended a collaborative dialogue between school counselors and ESL staff to include promotion of bilingualism rather than foreign language in school curriculum, indicating they should meet once per week to discuss how to improve services to ESL students and develop interventions to help students feel more successful in schools. School counselors can empower ESL students by providing and promoting activities that develop a variety of skills: "(a) problem-solving skills to develop self-confidence and cultural pride, (b) planning skills consistent with the student's family system to establish goal setting, (c) leadership skills that go across ethnic groups, and (d) integration skills to develop self-acceptance" (Clemente & Collison, p. 346).

Another consideration for school counselors is how to work effectively with biracial children. A natural result of the influx of many cultures in our country is an increase in biracial children. Nishimura (1995) suggested that developmental counseling programs should focus on themes that will be supportive of biracial children: family, cultural heritage, diversity, and identity development. These themes do not differ from those addressing all cultural groups.

> Addressing issues of biracial children as part of an expanded developmental counseling curriculum would increase awareness and sensitivity of all students regarding the appreciation of the many aspects of diversity. All students would benefit from such a program emphasis in that the many shades of diversity would be celebrated and acknowledged as intricate components of society that are all within the realm of normality. (Nishimura, p. 57)

Perhaps most importantly, school counselors need to keep their own perspectives on multiculturalism in check. Effective school counselors will acknowledge personal prejudice or bias and then decide how to work through it in a way that is beneficial to students. Constantine and Gainor (2001) suggested that school counselors participate in activities that allow them to consider their own cultural identities and how those might influence their interactions with students' cultural identities, particularly those that are different. In the event that bias cannot be resolved, it is the ethical obligation of the counselor to refer the student to other counseling services.

Working With Diverse Families and Communities

To maintain a holistic and systemic approach to supporting students, school counselors cannot only focus on multicultural students, but must also determine how to work successfully with diverse families and communities. The best efforts at acculturation in schools will not be supported outside of school unless families and communities are included in the process. One of the best ways to initiate positive interaction with parents from a diverse culture is to make sure there is a translator present at any meetings or events the parents may attend in the school. Imagine the frustration of coming to learn about your child's education only to be unable to comprehend what is being said. It is often difficult to find interpreters to represent all of the different languages, but school counselors can consult with community agencies or organizations that might provide interpreter services.

Professional Practice

ESTHER (HS)

Counselors work with translators to foster communication during parent and student contacts and to offer support to minority parent groups. At our school, we have the Concerned Parents Group (African American Parents), the Asian Parent Group, and the Hispanic Parent Group. Counselors offer programs and provide information regarding colleges, scholarships, parenting, and other requested topics.

Another way to foster a positive relationship with parents and community members is to find out if a parent or member of the cultural community has any talents or skills he or she might be willing to share with classes at the school (Shore, 2001). School counselors could initiate contact with parents and community members of varying cultural backgrounds and ask them to participate in cultural awareness events or activities. Partnering with diverse communities is certainly a positive way to foster good relationships, as well as promote a sense of collaboration between the school and community.

Lee (2001) recommended that school counselors consider actually taking the school counseling program to the parents and community. Some parents may not be comfortable with or may be intimidated by the school building or school environment itself. Counselors could provide services in the communities by using community centers or other spaces where counseling programs (e.g., parenting programs) could be held. If parents perceive school activities and school counseling services as inviting and nonthreatening, they are more likely to be active participants in their children's educations. While this takes some effort on the school counselor's part, it establishes a working alliance with parents and promotes greater interaction between schools and culturally diverse communities.

A final way to promote a collaborative and collegial relationship with parents and communities of diversity is to be aware of the differences between the mainstream culture and others. For example, time is perceived differently by different cultures. It is important to be cognizant of the differences that are inherent to specific customs, traditions, and lifestyles of various cultures. It is equally important, however, to never make stereotypical assumptions about cultural groups simply because of past experiences or information. There are as many intercultural differences as there are cultures.

This section has briefly explored the school counselor's role in working with diverse populations. Individual counseling, small group counseling, classroom guidance, consultation, coordination, and collaboration are all roles that the school counselor will play to ensure that the needs of culturally diverse students are met. These interventions must be immediate and ongoing so that students have consistent support and encouragement to be successful in academic, personal/social, and career development.

REFLECTION AND DISCUSSION

1. In most schools, there is a wide range of diverse cultures represented. As a school counselor, what are some obvious ways to indicate that you embrace diversity?

2. The most obvious challenge when working with ESL students is the language barrier. If there is no translator present when a school counselor is counseling an ESL student, what are other ways that the school counselor might communicate caring and concern for the student?

3. Imagine that you are a school counselor who is planning to present a parent workshop in a multicultural community. Discuss the planning and implementation of the workshop and special considerations you would need to keep in mind as you prepare for the workshop.

Counseling Students With Special Needs

According to Census 2000 Data, the number of people age 5 and over with a disability is nearly 20% of the entire U.S. population. Of this population, 5.2 million people are between the ages of 5 and 20, or 8% of the total population in this age group. More specifically, in 1997, 11.2% of children ages 6 to 14 had some type of disability (U.S. Census Bureau, 2001b). Given this information, it seems relatively safe to assume that approximately 1 in 10 school-age children have some sort of disability.

There is a wide range of disabilities and needs related to special education services. Often, gifted education is considered a special needs category, but it will not be addressed in this text. The focus of this discussion will be on students who are served under the categories established by Public Law 105-17, the Individuals with Disabilities Education Act (IDEA) of 1997, which was formerly known as Public Law 94-142, the Education for All Handicapped Children Act. This act provides for free and appropriate education for all students, regardless of disability. There is some discrepancy in the terms used to describe students who qualify for special services. The terms *special needs students* or *challenged students* are sometimes used; however, proponents of special education use the term *students with special needs* to emphasize the person-first orientation—the student is a person who has special needs. Therefore, this text will refer to this group as *students with special needs,* which includes students with one or more impairments or disabilities that affect their educational performance. Special education categories may vary in title, but tend to fall under the broad categories of autism, visual impairments, hearing impairments, emotional disability/disturbance, specific learning disability, speech or language impairment, mental retardation, orthopedic impairments, severe disability, multiple disabilities, traumatic brain injury, and other health impairments. These categorical names may vary from school district to school district, but the criteria are consistent.

The Special Education Process

The process for receiving special education services under IDEA involves several steps. The Office of Special Education and Rehabilitative Services (2000), a subdivision of the U.S. Department of Education, has published a guide for the special education process, from referral to development, of the Individualized Education Plan (IEP) that describes the following basic steps:

Step 1:   A student is identified as possibly needing special education and related services. When a teacher or parent has concerns about a student and several strategies have been implemented and are unsuccessful in remedying the problem, the student is referred to a Child Study Team. The persons involved in this meeting are parents/guardians, regular education teacher, special education teacher, individual(s) who can evaluate the student and interpret results (usually an educational diagnostician and a school psychologist), school administrator, and any individuals with knowledge of the child or special expertise. Often, any school personnel who provide related services to the student (e.g., speech pathologist, school counselor, etc.) might be invited to offer their insights on the case. At the middle and high school levels, the student may also attend this meeting.

Step 2:   In the meeting, a decision is made regarding whether or not the student should be evaluated. There must be ample evidence that several strategies have been tried and a documented history of difficulty in order for evaluation to be considered. The evaluation typically includes a social history provided by the parents, intelligence or ability testing, achievement testing, observation of classroom performance, and a teacher report. This information must be gathered and presented to the committee within 60 working days.

Step 3:   Based on the results of the evaluation data, eligibility is decided. Team members typically come to consensus about a student's eligibility for services. If parents disagree with the decision, they may ask for a hearing to challenge it.

Step 4:   If a student is found to be eligible for services, an Individualized Education Plan (IEP) team has 30 calendar days to create the IEP.

Step 5:   An IEP meeting is scheduled, usually by a person trained in special education.

Step 6:   At the IEP meeting, the IEP is written and signed. Members present at this meeting will include the parents/guardians, the student (when appropriate), the special education teacher, an administrator, and any school personnel who will be providing related services. At this meeting, the members will decide upon the level and intensity of services. Students are to be served in the *least restrictive environments* that will still meet their special needs. The parents must give consent before the school system can provide any services to the student.

Step 7:   Services are provided. The IEP spells out specifically how services will be provided. Teachers are made aware of the IEP. The IEP must be strictly followed and all services must be provided to the extent and for the duration indicated.

Step 8:   Progress is measured and reported. The student's progress is measured and noted so that when the IEP is reviewed, there is evidence of any improvements or changes. Parents receive progress reports on a regular basis (typically with report cards).

Step 9:   An annual review of the IEP is conducted. The IEP team meets at least once per year (more often if parents or school personnel ask for a review) and revises the plan to meet student needs. Any concerns may be discussed, and an updated IEP is written and filed.

Step 10:   After no more than three years, each special education student is reevaluated. This evaluation is called a "triennial review" and its purpose is to assess if a student continues to qualify for special services. A review is typically scheduled to determine what components need to be evaluated. Based on the results, the Child Study Team makes a decision regarding eligibility, and if the student continues to be eligible, the IEP process continues.

The School Counselor's Role in Special Education

Though it varies among schools, the counselor is often considered an essential member of the Child Study Team. The counselor benefits from participation in two ways: (a) If the counselor has had any interaction with the student, he or she can share relevant information with the team (within the boundaries of confidentiality), and (b) the school counselor may learn information about the student that warrants interaction with the student. The school counselor could be part of the strategy or a related service, depending on the student's needs.

The level of involvement of school counselors in the special education process may vary from school to school and may range from limited to extensive. At the secondary level, school counselors are often involved with special education personnel to assure that special needs students are appropriately placed in classes and to assist in post-secondary planning.

Professional Practice

RENEE (ES)

As the school counselor, I may know the student in question from a different perspective and may have insight into circumstances that may be contributing to his or her difficulties. Sometimes, issues are brought to light in a Child Study meeting that would indicate that counseling would be an appropriate intervention. I may offer counseling services myself or provide referrals to qualified professionals. If a child is found eligible for services, counseling may be part of his or her Individualized Educational Plan (IEP) and must be provided as indicated in the plan.

BETH (MS)

We often handle the scheduling of the special needs students to make sure they are in the classes they need to be in. We also try to take special care to address their individual needs. For example, we wouldn't schedule students with ADHD with the most demanding teacher, nor would we want to place them with the teacher who is the least structured; they would probably flounder in either of those settings. So the first thing I try to do for special needs students is give them an optimum schedule, and that eliminates some problems right off the bat.

I sit in on all of the Child Study meetings for my grade level. I also talk to the parents at some point, as well as the student. In the meetings, I am the student advocate because the other specialists may only know the child on paper. I typically know the student and have been around him or her (for several years sometimes), so I have insight that others don't have. I may have personal input or information that may not come out on a standardized test. I feel that I am often the binding piece that pulls the information together.

ESTHER (HS)

High school counselors are very involved in the special education process. Counselors coordinate the referral of students to Child Study committees. They collect teacher comments, existing testing information, grades, and transcripts for the child study team to review. They also observe the student in the classroom. They issue and collect teacher narrative summaries about the student and serve on the Child Study Team as the student's advocate.

Your graduate program in school counseling should include a course or extensive exploration of the needs of students with specific disabilities. The American School Counselor Association (1999b) identified several ways that school counselors can intervene on behalf of students with special needs, including serving on the child study team, collaborating with other support personnel to provide services, and working with students and families throughout the special education process. The following counseling interventions, based on practical experience working with students with special needs, might also be useful:

- individual counseling to address academic problems;
- individual counseling to help the student learn to cope with his or her disability and the changes that might result from eligibility (i.e., being pulled from regular classes for resource services, etc.);
- group counseling for students who share similar concerns about their disabilities or for students who have common exceptionalities;
- classroom guidance to help build tolerance for students with special needs and increase awareness and understanding for unique learning styles so that special education students are identified as learning differently, not unable to learn;
- participation in inclusion models of special education by helping classes become more team-oriented and foster collegiality and acceptance for individual differences in the mainstream classroom; and
- consultation with teachers and parents as they attempt to meet the needs of students; sharing strategies or ideas for helping students experience success is an important function of the school counselor in general, and this is especially true when assisting students with special needs.

While every student has special needs and special talents, it is important for the school counselor's role to be one of involvement and advocacy, as well as support.

The School Counselor and Inclusion

In the last decade, one of the most controversial trends in schools has been the inclusion of special needs students in regular education programs. Although students with special needs are to be served in the least restrictive environment, only recently have identified students been spending more time in regular education classrooms and receiving special accommodations within the regular education curriculum. Full inclusion means that students with disabilities are in general education classrooms full-time and receive necessary support in order to succeed academically (Tarver-Behring, Spagna, & Sullivan, 1998).

Proponents of inclusion feel that students with special needs benefit from the social interaction and exposure to nonchallenged students. Willis (1994, as cited in Quigney & Studer, 1998) suggested that the academic exposure to more difficult content and higher expectations within the mainstream classroom may be most beneficial to special needs students.

Opponents of inclusion argue that it is not feasible for educators to meet such a vast range of abilities within the regular education classroom without the entire academic program suffering. Further, Kaufman, Lloyd, Baker, and Reidel (as cited in Quigney & Studer, 1998) expressed concern about the special needs of students with behavioral and emotional disorders within the regular education program, and they doubted "that the regular education setting will be appropriate for all students with these types of disabilities" (p. 78). Regardless of the arguments for or against inclusion, this movement appears to be permanent. Professional school counselors must decide how they will participate in and support inclusion in their school counseling programs. According to Quigney and Studer:

> By virtue of their training and experience, school counselors should play a vital role in the collaboration and planning involved in inclusive education. These professionals have knowledge and formal preparation in human relations, group development, interpersonal skills and counseling dynamics. (p. 78)

Carpenter, King-Sears, and Keys (1998) identified several roles for school counselors as members of transdisciplinary teams: collaborator, community liaison, family liaison, case manager, group process facilitator, and counselor. The degree to which a school counselor performs these roles may vary from case to case and school to school. It is important that as you look for school counseling positions, you ask what level of involvement you will have as a member of the special education team.

DIRECT SERVICES TO STUDENTS WITH SPECIAL NEEDS

Counseling and Classroom Guidance   Regardless of the level of involvement, school counselors provide services to students with special needs because they are, first and foremost, students in the building. Quigney and Studer (1998) emphasized that school counselors work with students in two ways: (a) They work with nonchallenged students to help them understand the unique qualities and needs of challenged students, and (b) they work with special needs students to help them deal with the academic, personal/social, and career challenges that may present themselves as they are included in the regular education process (p. 79). These interventions seem to be applicable across all levels—elementary, middle, and high school. Sometimes classroom guidance may be an appropriate forum to work with the nondisabled students. Lessons that focus on understanding and appreciating differences might help with the acceptance of disabled students in the classroom. Individual or small group counseling is an effective way to work with students with special needs and their peers to address specific areas of concern. Issues such as social skills, study skills, impulse control, stress management, and feelings can be appropriately addressed in small group or individual counseling. One elementary counselor found: "Small group counseling provides a time when students come together in a nonacademic atmosphere, teaching one another and learning with their peers. The camaraderie and acceptance felt in the group seems to have as great an effect on the students as the interventions" (Deck, Scarborough, Sferrazza, & Estill, 1999, p. 152).

Individual counseling sessions with students with special needs can address very specific concerns, thoughts, and feelings. The forum of individual counseling sessions provides a safe place for students to verbalize their feelings and rehearse specific situations or scenarios that may be troublesome. Often, students with special needs simply need a support system, or someone who will not judge them or treat them differently because of their disabilities. School counselors can provide tremendous support for students with special needs and develop strategies to help them experience success academically and socially as they are included in the regular education program.

Consultation and Collaboration The school counselor works with administrators and teachers in the inclusion process. Consultation with teachers and administrators may involve training or providing resources for the successful inclusion of students with special needs. The school counselor may work specifically with teachers on strategies to effectively educate students with special needs within the regular education classroom setting. School counselors collaborate with special education and regular education teachers by being informed about information and resources regarding special education and sharing counseling skills that will facilitate successful inclusion (Tarver-Behring, et al., 1998).

School counselors also play an important role with families and community agencies that may be involved in the special education process and inclusion. Parents often need to be reassured or need to have the special education process explained in a personal, individual way. The school counselor may also be aware of special family circumstances or situations that might affect a student's placement or participation in inclusion. For this reason, school counselors should seek out the parents of special needs students in order to provide the most comprehensive services for the students. In addition, school counselors can facilitate important parent-teacher collaboration on special education services and inclusion, including encouraging parents to involve themselves in classroom activities and providing opportunities for parents of challenged and nonchallenged students to work together as much as possible (Tarver-Behring, et al., 1998).

The school counselor may interact with community agencies to "seek the expertise and knowledge of community members to enhance the personal growth of all students, particularly students with special needs" (Quigney & Studer, 1998, p. 79). For example, if a high school student with special needs is looking for summer employment, the school counselor might intervene on the student's behalf and help the student find work in an area that will support his or her special needs and provide meaningful employment.

In general, the school counselor's role in special education and in working with students with special needs is a necessary investment of time and resources. It is important to educate oneself about the federal, state, and local laws regarding special education. Further, it is beneficial when school counselors have an understanding of the characteristics and specific needs of children with disabilities. In addition to supporting other school personnel, the school counselor has a professional obligation to educate themselves and others about circumstances surrounding special education. Being a consultant for parents and teachers, collaborating as a member of the multidisciplinary team, and providing direct counseling services such as individual and small group counseling for special needs students are just a few of the important roles school counselors fill in working with special education and special needs students. Serving as a support, a resource, and a liaison is essential to the success of all students, and this is no less true for students with special needs.

The School Counselor and 504 Plans

Beginning in the early 1990s, more and more students were being diagnosed with Attention Deficit Hyperactivity Disorder (ADHD) (American Psychiatric Association, 2000) or disorders that did not fit into any category of special education (labeled other health impaired, or OHI). Initially, students with ADHD were not required to have accommodations in the classroom to deal with the challenges of the disorder in the academic setting. The huge increase in diagnosis of ADHD in the last decade and the related problems prevalent in classrooms became a major area of concern for parents, educators, and specialists, in addition to concerns about the students themselves. Students who did not qualify for services under a particular disability were still struggling in schools. According to the Parent Advocacy Coalition for Educational Rights (PACER Center, 1994):

> Section 504 of the Rehabilitation Act of 1973 is a civil rights statute which provides that "No otherwise qualified individual with disabilities in the United States . . . shall, solely by reason of his/her disability, be excluded from participation in, be denied the benefits of, or be subjected to discrimination under any program or activity receiving federal financial assistance or activity conducted by any executive agency." (p. 3)

In short, no organization (including public schools) can discriminate against persons with disabilities. The definition of an individual with disabilities means "any person who has a physical or mental impairment which substantially limits one or more major life activities, has a record of such impairment, or is regarded as having an impairment" (PACER Center, 1994, p. 1). This definition includes many categories, such as impairments related to orthopedics, vision, speech, and hearing; physical disabilities; emotional illness; AIDS or HIV-related disorders; Multiple Sclerosis; heart disease; cancer; ADHD; and so on. It also applies to short-term disabilities, such as a broken arm or leg, or injuries that interfere with physically or mentally performing academic work. Section 504 therefore makes it possible for students to receive accommodations and help as long as the level of impairment meets the criteria just described, regardless of whether or not the student has been identified within a special needs category. As one might guess, many students in school qualify for these types of plans.

In some schools, the special education chairperson or a team member may also be in charge of the development, implementation, and maintenance of 504 plans. The documentation of 504 plans is less tedious and detailed than that of IEPs for special education students, but the accommodations may look quite similar. Typical accommodations for students with a 504 plan might include:

- Preferential seating,
- providing a written schedule or an assignment book,
- supplementing verbal instructions with written instructions,
- reduced assignments,
- extra time to complete assignments,
- use of tape recorders or computers to complete assignments or take class notes, and
- peer or volunteer assistance in class.

While most of these accommodations are specific to the classroom, it is critical that the school counselor serve as a support system for the student and teacher(s) that are affected by the 504 plan.

Working with students with 504 plans is similar to working with students in any special needs category. Often, students who are identified as needing accommodations or special services deal with feelings of inadequacy, low self-concept, or various other feelings that result from being treated even slightly differently than other students. School counselors must rise to the challenge of helping students deal with their disabilities and challenges in ways that promote positive images of self and positive interactions with others.

The American School Counselor Association took a strong position about the school counselor's role in working with 504 plans: ". . . the school counselor should not be responsible for the coordination of the 504 planning team or supervision of the implementation of the 504 plan" (ASCA, 1999b, p. 2). While this clearly discourages school counselors being over-involved in 504 planning and implementation, it does not discount the role that the school counselor plays in helping support students with 504 plans.

Tarver-Behring et al. (1998) suggested that school counselors focus on promoting social adjustment, fostering peer acceptance, and providing direct counseling services to address difficulties, such as impulse control, conflict with classmates, and coping strategies. Individual counseling may be appropriate when addressing the specific needs of a student related to his or her unique disability. In addition, providing classroom guidance sessions on tolerance and acceptance of others is important to developing the nondisabled students' empathy for students with special needs. The reality is that all students benefit from these types of services because the lessons learned are lessons that will help students throughout their lives. Accepting oneself, accepting others, capitalizing on strengths, and confronting challenges are all important life skills that are useful and beneficial to everyone.

REFLECTION AND DISCUSSION

1. Consider the conditions of special needs students at each level (elementary, middle, high school). What would be some of the concerns of each group in terms of academic, personal/social, and career development?

2. Are there any special needs categories that intimidate you? If so, which one(s) and how will you confront your feelings about this population?

3. What accommodations or counseling services seem to be most needed by special needs populations? What are your thoughts or observations about the school counselor's role in special education, inclusion, and Section 504 plans?

The School Counselor's Role in Working With Sexual Minority Youth

Counseling gay, lesbian, bisexual, and transgender youth (GLBT) is an area of counseling that runs the gamut in terms of services provided. The response to this population of students is varied. Some schools and school districts provide extensive support programs for adolescents as they begin to explore and identify their sexual orientations. Other schools and school districts have policies against promoting or supporting any sexual orientation other than heterosexuality. Even in a society that claims to be moving toward greater tolerance for diversity, sexual orientation is a forbidden topic in many schools and great efforts are made to avoid the subject (Herring & Furgerson, 2000; Marinoble, 1998). According to Fontaine (1998), from 1987 to 1998, only five articles regarding counseling sexual minority youth were published in the two primary school counseling journals. The fact is that an estimated 10% of the population in the United States is lesbian or gay (Jucovy, 2000; Marinoble), which indicates that at least a portion of the students in our schools are GLBT youth. Therefore, school counselors cannot deny the needs and issues that often result from the sexual orientations of students.

While there has been evidence of students claiming a certain sexual orientation to their elementary school counselors (Fontaine, 1998), it should be no surprise that awareness of sexual orientation is more likely to develop in middle and high school. Developing sexual identity and identifying with one's sex are normal developmental tasks in adolescence.

It is important to clarify the definitions of and relationships between *sexual orientation* and *sexual identity*. According to Eliason (1996), sexual orientation refers to the predisposition of a person to be attracted to or be sexual partners with one gender or the other. The exception would be bisexuality, in which a person can be sexually attracted to and involved with persons from either gender. Ryan and Futterman (2001) indicated that most of the research that is conducted on bisexuality is with adult subjects; while bisexual behavior may occur as a result of exploring sexual orientation, self-labeling as a bisexual tends to occur at a later age. *Sexual identity* is an encompassing phenomenon that includes biology, gender, sex role, and sexual orientation. Therefore, sexual identity is the entire perception of one's sex and sexuality, while sexual orientation focuses specifically on romantic attraction and behavior.

While a school counselor may have a personal conviction about sexual orientation and sexual behavior, it is important to have an informed understanding of some of the issues that sexual minority youth face in sometimes intolerant school environments.

Issues Sexual Minority Youth Face

There is a large body of research that has explored the unique issues that sexual minority youth encounter. Belonging to the sexual minority can put students at great risk for harassment and verbal and physical abuse. It appears that our schools mirror society on this issue; there are major variations in the levels of tolerance and acceptance of sexual orientations other than heterosexuality.

Research indicates that youth who self-identify as homosexual often have feelings of isolation and stigmatization (Black & Underwood, 1998; Marinoble, 1998), peer relationship difficulties, and family conflicts as a result of "coming out" about their sexuality. Cooley (1998) also identified isolation as a reality for gay and lesbian adolescents, in addition to educational issues, family issues, and health risks that might result from homosexual relationships. This feeling of isolation often is a result of homophobia exhibited by students, school personnel, and family members. Jucovy (2000) defined homophobia as "the irrational fear, disgust, or hatred of gays, lesbians, or bisexuals. Homophobia refers to the discomfort one feels with any behavior, belief, or attitude that does not conform to traditional sex-role stereotypes" (p. 9). Addressing the homophobia that is often present in schools and society can be challenging and extremely isolating for sexual minority youth. Herring and Furgerson (2000) identified other realities that sexual minority youth must face: invisibility, lack of support systems, violence, sexual abuse, and the risk of sexually transmitted diseases.

Most research addresses the external issues that confront the sexual minority student. Often, internal factors can be equally, if not more, distressing. Omizo, Omizo, and Okamoto (1998) noted that sexual minority youth may experience several serious emotions about their sexuality, including confusion and not being understood, fear and negative reactions from others, concerns about the future, and internalized hostility. Jucovy (2000) labeled the last emotion as *internalized homophobia*, which is the belief of the GLBT youth that their sexual orientations are inferior to heterosexual orientation. Internalizing these negative emotions can result in poor self-esteem (McFarland, 1998), difficulty with self-acceptance, and even more harmful behaviors, such as substance abuse (Russell, Driscoll, & Truong, 2002) and suicide (Fontaine, 1998; McFarland; Russell & Joyner, 2001).

While this paints a seemingly negative picture for sexual minority youth, it is essential to note that the awareness and acknowledgement of one's sexual orientation and the recognition of sexuality is an awesome and meaningful milestone for a young person. School counselors should try to not label a student's coming out as a negative experience. There should be a balance between discussing the realities and the opportunities inherent in a particular sexual orientation.

School Counselors and Sexual Minority Youth

Professional school counselors are committed to facilitating and promoting the fullest possible development of each individual by reducing the barriers of misinformation, myth, ignorance, hatred, and discrimination based on sexual orientation. (ASCA, 2000c, p. 1)

One of a school counselor's first considerations when working with GLBT youth should be his or her personal values and feelings about different sexual orientations. Some people have very strong feelings about sexual orientation, either based on religious teachings or personal values. As a school counselor, it is important to remember that one must be a support system for the student in school, regardless of the student's sexual orientation. Openness, tolerance, and acceptance are a large part of the mantra of school counselors. If for any reason a school counselor does not feel they can provide appropriate services for a student, he or she has an ethical obligation to refer the student to another counselor.

Fontaine (1998) conducted a survey of 101 school counselors at the elementary and secondary levels to explore counselor experiences with sexual minority youth. Significant findings from the study indicated that more than half of the secondary school counselors reported having worked with at least one student who was confused about sexual orientation, and 42% reported having worked directly with a self-identified gay or lesbian student. Further, the most common problems cited by school counselors of homosexual students were fear of peer and parental rejection and inner conflict about sexual identity (Fontaine). Bailey (2003) indicated that some GLBT students also fear for their safety in schools. The issues faced by sexual minority youth are extensive and include both external and internal factors. School counselors should consider both when planning how to provide comprehensive support for GLBT youth.

It is a good idea to become aware of the stance that the school district or school takes regarding sexual minority youth. Again, the level of tolerance and acceptance will vary from place to place. If the policy or position is not in alignment with your personal philosophy or beliefs about GLBT youth, it is critical to learn this upfront in order to make an informed decision about being employed in that school district.

HELPING THE STUDENT   Recommendations for working with sexual minority students are extensive in school counseling literature. This section will present some of the suggestions offered specifically to school counselors.

One of the important steps for the sexual minority youth is the desire to express their sexual orientations, or "come out." This is an extremely crucial time for the school counselor to provide guidance and support. "While coming out can produce psychological well-being, it can also be dangerous. . . . Coming out should be postponed until the adolescent gains a reasonable amount of self-worth and a support network" (Black & Underwood, 1998, p. 17). The school counselor should discuss the possible consequences of coming out to peers and parents. Individual counseling sessions can help prepare the student for reactions and also provide opportunities to consider how to address possible responses from others. Further, school counselors can support students and their families by facilitating dialogue and addressing the issues that may be present for the student and the family.

Black and Underwood (1998) also suggested specific guidelines for the school counselor in terms of direct intervention strategies, including being sincere, respecting confidentiality, allowing the student to express feelings, and being aware for the potential for depression or self-destructive behaviors. Cooley (1998) recommended that school counselors allow for expression of feelings and engage in dialogue with students about these feelings; help secure a safe and nonthreatening educational environment for the students; help students deal with family issues as they pertain to sexual orientation; and address the health issues that may be present as a result of sexual practices or behaviors.

Muller and Hartman (1998) offered group counseling as an appropriate counseling service for sexual minority youth. The specific goals of the group focus on discussing feelings related to sexuality, developing coping skills, and identifying support systems for sexual minority youth. The use of group counseling with sexual minority youth provides a safe forum in which students can express their feelings openly. It might also be appropriate to include heterosexual students in the group in order to open the lines of communication and foster greater tolerance of diversity.

CREATING A TOLERANT CLIMATE   The school climate influences how sexual minority youth feel about their sexual orientation. A school environment that celebrates diversity and demonstrates tolerance might be a supportive environment in which a student can come out without fear. On the other hand, in a school where the majority feels that any deviation from the mainstream is wrong or inappropriate, students may feel less comfortable being themselves. The school counselor can be a positive catalyst to foster the unconditional acceptance of students. This school-wide effort should begin with administration and faculty.

Black and Underwood (1998) indicated that staff development in schools should focus on helping faculty and staff appreciate diversity. This could be done through in-services that provide information about sexual minority groups and confronting the assumptions and misconceptions as they relate to students. Faculty and staff must also consider their own prejudices and phobias in order to ascertain that students are not being unfairly treated or discriminated against. Further, Bauman and Sachs-Kapp (1998) suggested that school-wide programs that promote the acceptance of diverse sexual orientation should be a goal for school counseling programs.

Creating a climate of tolerance and acceptance for sexual minority youth must include assuring student safety. If verbal and physical harassment are occurring, the administration should be prepared to respond in an appropriate manner. Sexual harassment policies typically include references to sexual orientation, so any infraction related to a student's sexuality should be reprimanded.

Sexual orientation can be a sensitive issue in society in general, and being a sexual minority youth presents unique struggles. The school counselor's role is first and foremost to support students. While there are many considerations and issues that must be confronted when working with sexual minority youth, student needs and academic progress are a key focus for school counselors. As long as this priority is kept in the forefront, school counselors have responded professionally and appropriately.

CONCLUSION

This chapter has explored the school counselor's role in working with diversity and students with special needs. As schools become more diverse, it is imperative that school counselors become involved with the unique needs of these populations. It is evident that the four Cs—counseling, consultation, coordination, and classroom guidance—are all direct service interventions that are viable and useful methods for promoting the development of diverse populations of students. As counselors-in-training, you have an advantage in understanding the significance of the school counselor's role in providing effective services to students with unique needs.

REFLECTION AND DISCUSSION

1. Within a school population, there will be many multicultural groups and special needs populations. As a school counselor, you may find it challenging to try to meet the needs of all groups. How would you organize your time and manage to work with all of these groups?

2. On a piece of paper, draw four columns. At the top of each one, put one of the four Cs (counseling, classroom guidance, consultation, coordination). In each category, list the types of services that you, as the school counselor, will provide for culturally diverse students and special needs students.

3. "I believe that all students have special needs." What are your thoughts about this statement? Do you agree or disagree?

4. Some believe that by promoting tolerance of GLBT youth, schools are actually promoting alternative sexual lifestyles. As a school counselor, how would you respond to this accusation? How would you describe the ways that school counselors support sexual minority youth?

5. Consider this scenario: *In the high school where you are working as a school counselor, there are several organizations that support the interests of various minority groups (e.g., African American Students, Hispanic/Latino Club, Gay/Lesbian Coalition). As the school counselor, you learn that animosity is developing between groups and that there may be a rally at which each group could become militant about issues that are specific to its unique circumstances.* How might you intervene and promote greater tolerance and acceptance between these groups? What role does a school counselor have in creating a tolerant climate for all groups? What ethnic and cultural considerations might affect your intervention?

CHAPTER 7

Collaborating With Teachers: Building Positive Working Relationships

*R*ather than protecting turf, attempting to carve out recognition, and being solo players in the school, all professional educators and community experts must work together to increase the strength of services for students. (Niebuhr, Niebuhr, & Cleveland, 1999, p. 678)

Teamwork fosters cooperation, collaboration, and commitment. Schools, as part of a system, often seek to foster the atmosphere of teamwork so that school personnel feel a shared responsibility for the students in the building. The importance of school counselors' alliance with faculty and staff in schools cannot be overstated. For school counselors—who, it is hoped, epitomize teamwork, collaboration, and cooperation—being team players, working with others, and being catalysts for unity are crucial roles that will inevitably affect the educational program.

This chapter will focus on the school counselor as a team player when working with teachers in the school. As part of this exploration, we will examine two questions that might affect the perspective of the school counselor: Should school counselors have experience as classroom teachers prior to becoming school counselors? Are those with teaching experience more effective than those without? In addition, we will provide tips for how school counselors can approach their role in discipline and explore the school counselor's role in teaching and classroom management. Finally, we will conclude with a discussion about how school counselors can project the image of team player and work collaboratively with teachers to ensure student success.

To Teach or Not to Teach . . . That Is the Question

Twenty-two years of training teachers and non-teachers alike to be school counselors has convinced me that the teaching requirement is an unnecessary criterion for entering the profession. In my opinion, the person and the training . . . are the major factors in training competent and effective school counselors. (Baker, 1994, p. 314)

Historical Research

As early as the 1930s, teachers were the primary candidates for school counseling positions (Allen, 1931, as cited in Baker, 1994). During this time, the selection of teachers to serve as school counselors was heavily based on the success of the individuals as teachers. There was no debate about the need for teaching experience, and there was general consensus that a teaching background was advantageous to working in the education environment.

Throughout the 1940s and 1950s, experts began to debate the question. Baker (1994) cited several research studies that argued that teaching experience is necessary for effective counseling and some that suggested that having teaching experience could actually be detrimental to a school counselor's

performance. Arbuckley (1961, as cited in Quarto, 1999) made a strong statement against the teaching requirement: "Evidence tends at least to point to the
possibility that teaching gives one so many bad counseling habits that a major
function of counselor education is to help former teachers to unlearn most of
what they learned as teachers" (p. 378). This strong statement is diametrically
opposed to earlier thinking.

In the 1960s and 1970s, the debate continued and became more pro-
nounced. The proponents of teaching experience as a certification requirement
for school counselors argued that prior experience in education would give
school counselors a greater knowledge of how schools operate, as well as necessary empathy for school teachers. Opponents focused on other issues because
imposing a teaching requirement could both prevent effective counselors from
entering the school counseling profession and allow ineffective teachers to
become school counselors as a way to get away from teaching (Baker, 1994).
The conclusion was that although both sides had evidence to support their
positions, one side seemed no more convincing than the other. There was a call
for research findings that might help resolve this issue once and for all. Baker
synthesized the results of studies throughout the 1960s and into the 1970s and
found no significant differences between school counselors with and without
teaching experience. Any differences that the studies suggested seemed to be
based on perception rather than on objective data.

There is a gap in research studies addressing this issue between the early
1970s and the early 1990s. While states were still considering the teaching
requirement during this period, and some were even changing it, empirical
research is absent. There was, however, a shift in the focus of counselor education programs. Programs began to emphasize field-based work, including more
intensive and extensive internships, as a way to provide more in-school experience for school counselors. Higher standards for programs, such as those proposed by the Council for Accreditation of Counseling and Related Educational
Programs [CACREP] (2001) helped ensure that school counselors, regardless of
teaching experience, were adequately prepared to work in school settings.

Recent Research

A resurgence of interest in the issue occurred in the 1990s. There has been a
steady decline in the number of states requiring teaching experience for school
counselor certification. As of 1992, 21 states still required teaching certificates
and at least a year of teaching or related experience in order to become a certified school counselor (Kandor & Bobby, as cited by Quarto, 1999). That number
decreased to 16 states by 1997 (Randolph & Masker, 1997). According to ASCA
(personal communication, August 29, 2003), fewer than 10 states currently
require school counselors to have prior teaching experience. The most current
research has focused on others' perceptions of school counselors with or
without teaching experience—specifically principals, teachers, and counselor
educators.

My Story

When I first became a school counselor, it became evident rather quickly that my teaching experience was perceived positively by my administrator and the teachers. At the time, it seemed that teaching experience was definitely a plus in my role as a school counselor. However, the half-time counselor in my building did not have teaching experience or an education background. Over time, I observed that the teachers and administrators did not show any resistance to or hesitation about working with my colleague. It was obvious that once school personnel observed and experienced that we were both effective counselors, the teaching experience (or lack thereof) was no longer a factor.

PRINCIPALS' PERCEPTIONS   A study by Olson and Allen (1993) was at the forefront of efforts in the last decade to address this seemingly endless debate. Principals who supervised 138 school counselors from all levels were asked to respond to a questionnaire that reviewed several general categories of school counselor responsibilities in a comprehensive program. The results of the study were significant (Olson & Allen). Elementary and high school counselors with or without teaching experience were perceived to be almost equal in their effectiveness in carrying out counselor functions. Middle school/junior high principals perceived school counselors with teaching experience to be more effective in only three of the categories. The principals' responses to the classroom guidance function of the counselors were even more enlightening. There were no significant differences between the principals' perceptions of counselors with or without teaching experience at any level in terms of effective classroom guidance performance (Olson & Allen). This is surprising because one of the arguments against school counselors without teaching experience is that they are not as skilled in classroom guidance or classroom management. The study concluded that greater consideration should be given to the training of effective school counselors rather than the issue of teaching experience.

TEACHERS' PERCEPTIONS   School counselors without teaching experience did not fare as well in a study by Quarto (1999), who explored the perspectives of teachers. Quarto created the "Teachers' Perceptions of School Counselors Questionnaire" and administered it to 152 teachers at all levels. The questionnaire included sections on general counselor effectiveness, as well as specific functional effectiveness. Participants were asked to rate counselors in terms of knowledge, skills, and experience. In addition, the teachers were also asked to indicate a preference for working with certain counselors based solely on provided descriptions of counselors. Specific results of the study

(Quarto) indicated that (a) teachers rated school counselors with teaching experience as more effective in general and in dealing with specific issues, and (b) 93% of teachers preferred to work with school counselors with prior teaching experience.

The results were overwhelmingly supportive of school counselors with teaching experience. This contrasts the results of the Olson and Allen (1993) study of principal perceptions of school counselors with and without teaching experience. Quarto (1999) provided a possible explanation for this:

> Principals are not as likely to have the same day-to-day, intimate contact with and/or knowledge of students like teachers and school counselors. Teachers may be in a better position to evaluate the effectiveness of counseling inter- ventions because it is likely to impact them (teachers) more directly. . . . On the other hand, it could be argued that teachers' perceptions are clouded by their inherent bias toward school counselors with teaching experience. . . . In fact, principals may be better qualified to evaluate the effectiveness of school counselors in a way that does not favor school counselors with teaching expe- rience. (p. 382)

There is still no obvious answer to this debate. However, one important factor seems to be the quality of school counselor preparation programs. Thus, the perspective of counselor educators should also be considered.

COUNSELOR EDUCATORS' PERSPECTIVES   As mentioned previously, the standardization of counseling practices might be an answer to the question of whether school counselors should or should not have teaching experience. CACREP accreditation standards are very specific and regulated, so school counselor preparation programs are continuously being reviewed and improved upon in order to ensure that school counseling practices are appro- priate and relevant to school settings. In addition, the National Council for Accreditation of Teacher Education [NCATE] (2002) standards also include specific objectives and requirements for school counseling programs, ensuring the quality of school counselor preparation. While accreditation credentials are not mandatory for quality counselor training programs, they certainly lend credibility and professionalism to the programs. Holding school counselor preparation programs to a high standard for practice and training is one way to assure school personnel that school counselors are ready for employment in a school setting.

Since quality of training is certainly a consideration in this debate, it is important to consider what position counselor educators take. Smith, Crutchfield, and Culbreth (2001) surveyed 136 counselor educators to under- stand their perspectives on a teaching requirement for school counselors. Impressively, 75% of counselor educators felt that prior teaching experience is not necessary for school counselors to be effective. However, more than half (59%) also felt that school counselors without teaching experience might need additional experiences in the school setting to get a better idea of how schools operate. There is evidence of this opinion in school counseling preparation programs, many of which require extra coursework or assignments that expose nonteaching counselors-in-training to educational foundations, policies, or processes.

Smith, Crutchfield, and Culbreth's (2001) sample was a representative sample of counselor education programs from 36 states. At the time of the study, 13 states still had the teaching requirement. The result of the study is quite clear. While a majority of counselor educators do not feel teaching experience is necessary to be an effective school counselor, most do believe teaching experience or extended exposure to school experiences can be beneficial. This study, as well as the others mentioned, indicates that this issue does not seem to have an easy resolution. One way to address the issue is through school counselor training and quality preparation programs. "Regardless of their teaching experience, all school counselors need to be educated in how to address personal, political, and family issues within a school context. . . . Former teachers as well as nonteachers should receive the type of training that allows them to meet this goal" (Smith et al., p. 223).

Professional Perspective

ESTHER (HS)

I was a teacher prior to becoming a school counselor. However, many of my younger colleagues were not. I feel that it is an asset to have taught in the classroom before becoming a school counselor. At each grade level, the counselor works with groups of students, and experience in classroom management and effective presentation of information in front of large groups is very important. The counselor also speaks in front of parent groups, and the experience of being in the classroom gives the counselor self-confidence in public speaking. If counselors have some teaching experience, they can really understand and appreciate the needs of classroom teachers. However, if counselors can be sensitive to the challenges classroom teachers face, then they can be just as supportive in assisting classroom teachers with discipline and learning problems, as well as consultation.

BETH (MS)

I taught grades 6 through 12 at various times. I taught high school for about 3 years, grade 6 for four years, and grades 7 and 8 for 2 to 3 years. I don't think that it's necessary for school counselors to have teaching experience, but I think it can be helpful, depending on the person. What I found helpful was being able to relate to the things that teachers said were going on in their classrooms. I feel like my teaching experience gives me a sense of the various things that can go on in a classroom that can make life difficult for teachers. I also feel that I have the ability to control and relate to large groups. When I'm presenting a guidance lesson, I feel very confident and able to maintain order and making the lesson interesting at the same time. I have seen some counselors without

TABLE 7.1
School Counseling With Prior Teaching Experience

Benefits of Prior Teaching Experience	Challenges of Prior Teaching Experience
More clout with teachers (having "been in their shoes")	The tendency to lapse into teacher "voice" and behavior
Greater awareness and knowledge of school operations, policies, and procedures	A skewed perception of student issues (tendency to overemphasize the academic)
More practice with classroom management skills and techniques	Difficulty being viewed in the counseling role (especially if teacher position was in the same building)
Greater experience working with parents	Taking an unpopular position due to priority role as student advocate
Confidence in working within the educational setting	

teaching backgrounds who feel uncomfortable in the classroom setting because it is a different experience than small-group or individual counseling. The downside to teaching experience is that counselors who have been teachers sometimes fall back on teaching rather than counseling, which is something that they will have to address.

RENEE (ES)

I have never been a classroom teacher. I don't feel that counselors need teaching experience in order to be effective as school counselors. However, they must understand and appreciate what classroom teachers do. As a school counselor, you are part of an educational team and will be teaching and performing some of the duties that teachers perform. There are many things that a good counselor can learn from classroom teachers, such as classroom management skills. You will need to develop an understanding of classroom teachers' experiences so that you have an idea of what interventions or strategies you can realistically ask teachers to implement. If the teachers sense that you are capable and competent in the classroom, they are more likely to trust your opinion and will be more willing to work with you. It is imperative that you have the respect and trust of the classroom teachers in your school.

Benefits and Challenges: Both Sides of the Debate

A clear factor in the debate seems to be the perspectives of the personnel within the school in which the school counselor works. There are certainly benefits and challenges for school counselors with and without teaching experience. These are listed in Tables 7.1 and 7.2. While the benefits of prior teaching experience

TABLE 7.2
School Counseling Without Prior Teaching Experience

Benefits of No Prior Teaching Experience	Challenges of No Prior Teaching Experience
Greater focus on students' personal/social needs	The need to learn the inner workings of a school (process, policies, procedures)
Unskewed perception of education process	Lack of understanding and empathy for teaching
Greater openness and willingness to work "outside the box"	Lack of skill or experience in classroom management techniques
A flexible and unbiased attitude toward working with all school personnel	Possible lack of professional confidence due to inexperience in education setting

may be an asset, they are certainly not mandatory in order to be an effective school counselor. Having a background in teaching may be helpful in terms of working with colleagues, but it may also result in a difficult adjustment to the new role as a school counselor. There are comparable advantages and disadvantages to not having teaching experience. Some of the benefits and challenges identified in Tables 7.1 and 7.2 will be addressed in the next sections on the school counselor's role in teaching and working with teachers.

REFLECTION AND DISCUSSION

1. If you have been a teacher or are currently teaching in a school, how do you think this background will benefit or limit you as a school counselor? If you have never been a teacher, how might this lack of teaching experience benefit or limit you?

2. Whether or not you have teaching experience, how will you address the concerns that administrators, teachers, and parents might raise regarding your experience, or lack thereof?

The School Counselor's Role as School Personnel

As members of the school faculty, school counselors often have to accept roles that are not necessarily related to school counseling, but are associated with the education process or general school faculty responsibilities. The nature of the school environment often requires counselors to assume roles and responsibilities that are not complementary to the counseling process. School counselors may have to function in disciplinary roles in order to protect and provide safety and security for students.

Discipline: The School Counselor's Role

School counselors are adults who work in the school building. This reality automatically makes them partially responsible for the safety and security of students and for providing an effective learning environment. Stickel, Satchwell, and Meyer (1991) stated: "The administration of discipline is not considered a function of the school counselor; however, counselors as school-based professionals do become involved in some way in the discipline process. Counselors may need to challenge themselves to look at this involvement, particularly in light of the role of the counselor as student advocate" (p. 111). In fact, the American School Counselor Association (2001) established a clear position on the school counselor and discipline:

> The professional school counselor works with school system personnel and other stakeholders to establish and maintain policies that encourage appropriate behavior so that schools can be a safe place where teaching and learning can be effectively accomplished. Such policies promote the use of the school counselor as a resource person with expertise in the area of discipline plan development for prevention and intervention, not as a disciplinarian. (p. 1)

The difference between being involved in the development of discipline policy and actually providing discipline is an important one. Consider a scenario:

> *You are a school counselor in a middle school. In terms of protocol, the chain of command identifies you as the person in charge in the event that all administrators are out of the building. It is a Friday morning and you know that all of the administrators are attending a professional development meeting in a city 2 to 3 hours away. The office secretary calls you. "We've got a problem," she says. "Mrs. Smith has sent Toby down to the office with a note that says he called her an inappropriate name during her science class. What should I do with him?"*
>
> *As you ponder this situation, you know that you are going to have to respond to this behavior. It certainly isn't appropriate to allow students to swear at teachers and you are sure this teacher will want to know what consequences the student will face because of his actions. On the other hand, as Toby's counselor, you know that he has a long history of anger issues and that his inappropriate behavior usually stems from a rough night at home. You are supposed to be acting as an administrator, but you can also understand Toby's particular issues. What should you do?*

Serving as an administrative designee and acting in a disciplinary role certainly present repercussions for the school counselor. ASCA (2001) indicated that school counselors should not be placed in the role of designating or implementing punishment, but should be involved in affecting overall behavioral change. In fact, placing the school counselor in a disciplinary role impedes the counseling process by associating the school counseling program with punishment or being in trouble. When I was a high school counselor, it was not uncommon for a student to ask, "What did I do wrong?" when I would request a visit to my office. Despite our best efforts to dispel the image of the school counseling office as a discipline center, there still seems to be the misconception that students who are asked to visit or seek out a counselor are in trouble. Efforts should continue to contradict this opinion.

Stickel et al. (1991) conducted a study of 160 counselors at all levels in three western states to assess the involvement of school counselors in the discipline process. The results of this study were informative:

- Most of the counselors' involvement in discipline was direct service through individual intervention at the request of principals (54%) and teachers (64%).
- Principals more often requested counselor consultation than direct intervention, but the focus of the consultation still tended to be discipline regarding individual students rather than overall school discipline policies.
- While 57% of counselors frequently consulted with teachers about individual student discipline problems, only 18% consulted with teachers about general classroom discipline.
- Counselors reported being involved with parents on discipline issues; 51% reported consulting about discipline problems at home, and 35% reported consulting about discipline problems at school.
- Nineteen percent of the counselors perceived a conflict between their roles in counseling and their roles in discipline, but 38% desired a greater role in helping develop school-wide policies and procedures for discipline (pp. 112–114).

This study indicates that school counselors are often consulted after misbehavior has already occurred, which suggests that intervention has been reactive rather than proactive. In addition, it appears that school personnel typically consult with counselors about individuals who are misbehaving rather than creating an environment that fosters positive behavior.

School personnel have an obligation to correct misbehavior, especially if it threatens the safety or security of students or interferes with the learning process. School counselors are specifically trained to provide individual, small group, and classroom interventions in order to help students learn to behave appropriately and follow rules (Beale & McCay, 2001).

While disciplining students is not a desirable role for the school counselor, it may be necessary on occasion in order to ensure student safety and security. School counselors are certainly capable of developing discipline policies, as well as consulting with school personnel on disciplinary issues. Although it may not be a favorite role or responsibility, involvement in disciplinary procedures is a part of working within a school environment. Hopefully, school counselors will be involved in the development of discipline policies aimed at prevention rather than in reactive disciplinary action.

My Story

As a school counselor, it was not unusual to dismiss my small group members from our session and then stop one of them from running or being disruptive in the hall on the way back to class. Both roles are essential in being a student advocate—one advocates for social and emotional health and the other for the physical safety and integrity of the educational environment. Both are necessary and in the best interest of students.

REFLECTION AND DISCUSSION

1. How do you feel about being a disciplinarian? Does the traditional concept of discipline in schools conflict with your personality? If so, in what way?

2. Think about the school counselor's role in discipline. How will you approach a situation with students in which you might have to intervene in a disciplinary way?

3. School safety and student security are primary goals of schools today. If your role as a school counselor intersects with your role as a school employee who should promote student safety above all else, how will you respond?

4. List the ways in which you might involve yourself in the development of the school discipline process.

The Teaching Role of School Counselors

Because one of the traditional roles of the school counselor is classroom guidance, it is inevitable that school counselors will eventually be in charge of large groups of students, faculty, or parents. Although school counselors may not aspire to be teachers, they may be required to impart information and provide instruction at all levels. From presenting a first grade classroom guidance lesson on sharing to reviewing registration procedures in high school, a school counselor's role is likely to include teaching.

Because the school counselor works in an education setting, the expectation and reality is that working with groups of students is a natural part of the job. For some, the skills of effective teaching come naturally; others have to work at it to be effective. One issue that always arises, especially for school counselors without classroom experience, is managing the classroom. What happens when you walk in and 28 sets of eyes are on you? Or *not* on you, which may be a bigger concern.

My Story

It was my experience that large classes or groups of students were usually cooperative and manageable. This is not to say there were no challenges; after all, students will test the limits with any new or unfamiliar adult until they understand the boundaries. I found that the simplest way to manage the classroom was to adhere to the behavior policies established by the teacher. If there were any problems with particular students, I would first try to talk with the students myself, and if the problems persisted, I would mention the behavior to the teacher and he or she would proceed with disciplining the students. While I was always willing to give students second chances, I also let them know what my boundaries were. For example, if a student was continuously disrespectful to me or to other classmates, I might remove him or her from the group and then talk with the student while the rest of the class was engaged in an activity. An important rule of thumb to remember is to always talk to students about their behaviors privately rather than embarrassing them publicly. I might say, "Tim, it seems to be difficult for you to respect what others are saying. Please return to your seat (or to a different area) and we'll talk about this in just a minute." The message this statement sends is two-fold: (a) Your behavior is disrespectful to others, and (b) there will be a private discussion about your misbehavior.

CLASSROOM MANAGEMENT Managing a class of students, regardless of age, can be overwhelming and intimidating if a person is not prepared. Managing different age groups requires different techniques, and some classes or groups are more easily managed than others. In teacher preparation programs, significant time is spent preparing potential teachers to manage student behavior. School counseling programs may spend time addressing classroom management, but this topic certainly does not receive the same amount of attention from school counselors-in-training as it does from teachers-in-training. For this reason, it seems important to talk about strategies for classroom management and provide some consideration for successfully implementing classroom guidance.

At the secondary level, large group lessons or guidance may be a bit more intimidating. This is not to say that the students are more frightening, but managing large groups of adolescents can be somewhat daunting. Consider the following scenario:

One morning at 7:30 a.m., Ms. Suarez presented a session on PSAT results to four classes of high school juniors in the auditorium. She prepared a slide presentation to show the students how to interpret results and how their results might relate to their SAT performance. She had planned an interactive

and dynamic presentation that would have them all swooning with enthu-
siasm and energy! As she stood in front of the group, she realized two facts—
it was 7:30 in the morning and she was addressing teenagers. While most
seemed somewhat interested, there were those who were catching up on
gossip from the weekend and others who wanted to catch up on sleep. Many
of the students were interested in the information, but only wanted to know
how their scores would affect their acceptance into colleges or clubs. Those
who believed in living in the present were more focused on the homework they
had not completed for second block.

While the presentation was somewhat successful, Ms. Suarez learned important lessons:

- When a group is too large (e.g., 50 to 100 students), it is hard to connect with students and address their individual needs; smaller groups may be a more effective way to disseminate information and provide instruction.
- Make sure the setting is conducive to interaction with the students. The auditorium setup made it difficult to have close proximity with the students. Walking around the room and interacting with the students one-on-one may have been a more efficient way to keep their attention and provide the necessary information.
- If possible, try to schedule meetings at a time that may be more conducive to interaction and involvement, for example during or right after lunch.

This scenario addresses some of the circumstances school counselors may need to consider while directly involved in teaching situations. However, there are some strategies for classroom management that aim to prevent disruptions or interruptions before they can occur.

Specific strategies for classroom management offered by the Florida Department of Education (2002) focused on the areas of organization, communication, monitoring, and delivery of instruction. Using these categories, school counselors can employ similar strategies when conducting large group or classroom sessions.

Organization and Monitoring

- Arrange the seating in order to ease movement among and interaction with the students.
- Post an agenda for the scheduled session. For younger students or nonreaders, verbally explain what is going to happen.
- Identify words or gestures to get students' attention. For younger students, use phrases such as "1-2-3, Eyes on me," and for older students, use a simple and direct word or gesture.

- Use student helpers to pass out papers or materials so that you can give instruction.
- Move around the room and use proximity to correct misbehavior.
- Give clear directions about what should happen if there is a transition. For example, "Once you have the drawing paper, please return to your desks and begin your picture."

Communication

- Talk directly to the students, speak courteously, and focus on present behaviors and activities.
- Be aware of V-C-T (voice-cadence-tone). The louder you are, the louder they will be. Talking too fast can be agitating and distracting; talking too slowly may seem patronizing or boring.
- Consider the developmental age of the students and try to match it. Talking below or above the level of understanding of the students can lessen their focus.
- When correcting behavior, describe the misbehavior with a statement: "I think it's hard for everyone to hear over the talking that's going on. Let's work on listening to each other one at a time." Questions such as, "Why are you all talking so much?" make students defensive.
- Use empathic, nonjudgmental listening skills. Pay attention to non-verbal cues, and monitor student involvement and interaction.
- Consider any cultural barriers to effective communication. ESL students can be paired up with students who are bilingual. If there are hearing or visually impaired students in the class, prepare materials beforehand or ask for assistance from the special needs teachers.
- Thank students for their participation and willingness to share. Let them know how much you appreciate and value their input: "I have really enjoyed spending this time with you. Thank you so much for all of the important things you had to say and for your willingness to share."
- Begin by praising positive behaviors; observe and reinforce positive behaviors from the beginning.
- Establish ground rules, and remind students about a rule if it is about to be broken. Sometimes, the reminder is enough to thwart the behavior.
- Be consistent in your implementation of consequences for misbehavior. Make sure to treat each student fairly. While many advocate for treating each student the same, there may be a student with special needs or circumstances that affect his or her ability to behave appropriately. Individual conditions and needs should be taken into consideration. Sameness does not always equal fairness.

- If a group of students is acting out or not participating, it is best to deal with the group (or the individuals in the group) in private if possible. The influence of the group is often usurped when its members are dealt with individually.

Delivery of Instruction

- Engage the group as quickly as possible; ask about their understanding of certain concepts or their thoughts on the topic to be discussed. This will often serve as the springboard for discussion and dialogue.
- Vary the media used when teaching. Use visual aids, auditory questioning, and hands-on tasks to help provide information. Because student learning styles vary, approaches for effective teaching must also be varied.
- Apply information and discussions to experiences in the students' lives so that learning is meaningful and relevant. Create situations, scenarios, and role plays that are representative of students' experiences.
- Activities should be interesting and fun so that students are engaged, interested, and invested in the lesson.

While the recommendations for classroom management provide general guidelines, they don't address how to respond to difficult students. Interruptions or disruptions may be caused by the misbehavior of a small group of students or just one student. Following are some strategies for working with a disruptive student or group of students:

- *Investigate the cause of the disruption.* Does the student understand the lesson or activity? Is the student experiencing distress for another reason, such as being hungry or being upset?
- *Focus on building positive qualities.* For example, if a student tends to lead in a negative way, have him or her be a small group leader or help monitor the activity in order to channel leadership in a positive way.
- *Give students choices rather than threatening them with punishment.* A school counselor might say, "Alex, you have two choices. Either you can participate in the group and enjoy this activity, or you can sit at your seat and observe the rest of the group. Which would you prefer?" This gives the student ownership of the situation and the opportunity to make a choice and accept the consequences of that choice.
- *Explore personal expectations for student misbehavior.* Some people are much more lenient or less structured and ignore, or casually address, students' disruptive behaviors. Other people have a low tolerance for

disorder or interruption and may need to have more control over the behavior of students. It is important for adults who work with youth to decide what their management styles will be. What level of disruption is acceptable? Where is the boundary that a student must cross before being reprimanded?

Hopefully, you will have the opportunity to practice your classroom guidance skills throughout your counselor training program. Another recommendation is to observe the classes of teachers who have successful classroom management strategies. It might also be valuable to co-facilitate a large group activity with a teacher prior to conducting a lesson alone. The more time spent in classroom settings, the more comfortable school counselors feel when working with large groups of students.

REFLECTION AND DISCUSSION

1. On a scale of 1 to 10, describe your comfort with teaching large groups of students. What steps might you take to increase your comfort level?

2. As a school counselor, you may also present to or teach large groups of teachers and/or parents. What issues might arise when presenting to large groups of adults? How will you handle these issues?

3. Imagine the following: *You are a school counselor in your first year at a new school. You are doing a great job, but have been told that some of the teachers feel they must be present during your classroom sessions to manage the behavior of the students because they feel the students will take advantage of you.* How would you respond to this situation?

Collaboration With Teachers: Providing Support

Probably the most significant relationships school counselors have in their schools, other than with students, are with teachers. Although working collaboratively with administrators and other school personnel is important, it is the relationship with teachers that truly influences the efficacy of the school counseling program. Rice and Smith (1993) stated:

> Working with teachers can be the counselor's most important contribution to the school staff. Because teachers are alone with students most of the day, they sometimes feel isolated from their peers and administration. By sharing skills, the counselor helps teachers realize that others care about the frustrations, ideas, resourcefulness, and success of each of them. (p. 202)

School counselors have a major obligation to initiate and maintain supportive and reciprocal relationships with teachers.

Professional Practice

RENEE (ES)

You need teacher support to coordinate and implement activities. After September 11, I was working with students on character education. We wanted to focus on caring. I worked with a team of third grade teachers, and we developed a set of classroom guidance lessons in which the students read *Sadako and the Thousand Paper Cranes.* I led the class discussion on caring and the students came up with the idea of folding 1,000 paper cranes to send to the Pentagon as a sign of peace and hope. It became a major project for the students. They checked out books on origami and spent part of their lunch and recess time folding cranes. When they finished the cranes, we packed the cranes up and sent them to the Pentagon. We were told that they would be displayed in the new section of the building when it reopened. We couldn't have done this project without teacher support. It was a springboard for many discussions about conflict resolution and what it means to be a caring individual. The teachers were very patient and supportive as the students used this project as a healing and educational activity.

The School Counselor's Role in Supporting Teachers

SKILL ENHANCEMENT Rice and Smith (1993) noted that school counselors are the obvious school personnel to help expand the teachers' repertoires of skills. Anderson and Reiter (1995) identified one of the roles of the counselor as working as an ally with teachers in order to help teachers handle the demands of the classroom. Teachers need empathy and support in dealing with student issues, relationships with parents, and the demands of a challenging academic curriculum. School counselors are key personnel to assist teachers as they provide the educational best for our students.

Professional Practice

BETH (MS)

One teacher I worked with seemed to have a negative perspective; I think he was already burned out, although he was relatively young. My sense was that he had unrealistic expectations of what kids are like in school, possibly because he was relatively new to teaching. One time he came running into my office and said, "You've gotta get this kid out of my class, he's horrible." I shared with him that the student had told me that this teacher's class was one of his favorite classes. That really turned the tide. The teacher was frustrated and felt that he wasn't reaching this student, and what he needed to know was that he was reaching this student, and making a difference. Once the teacher knew he was having a positive effect on this student, he was able to build on that.

One way school counselors can aid teachers is by helping them finesse their teaching skills. School counselors can provide in-service opportunities for groups of teachers or for individual teachers who request new or innovative ideas to improve teaching skills. Pelsma (2000) recommended a solution-focused model for helping teachers assess their teaching strengths and identify challenges. These steps include helping the teacher identify what has worked in the past, identify what needs to change, set goals, and evaluate the change. Sometimes teachers are resistant to change because they feel they have to alter their practices or perspectives. One way school counselors support the efforts of teachers is by helping teachers identify things they do well and encouraging them to continue. When teachers feel that they are doing several things effectively, it is easier to focus on areas that might need improvement in order to be even more successful.

Another way school counselors can connect with teachers is by providing training that links effective counseling and teaching skills. Rice and Smith (1993) emphasized that teachers not only need content training, but also need to be able to communicate effectively. In-service training could include having school counselors demonstrate the verbal techniques of (a) probes, (b) interpretations, (c) restatement (of content or feeling), (d) reflective statements, and (e) summarization (pp. 204–205). These are not skills that are typically taught in teacher preparation programs. School counselors can demonstrate and give teachers the opportunity to practice these effective communication skills in order to advance effective working relationships with students, parents, and peers.

STUDENT INTERVENTION Most of a school counselor's interaction with teachers will be through consultation about students. This is always a challenging role because teachers may be frustrated, almost pushed to the limit, before asking for assistance. Intervention with students at the request of teachers usually requires a process, although the process is not always the same. The following steps could be one way to approach intervening with a student upon a teacher's request:

Step 1   When a teacher approaches the school counselor about a child, it is imperative that the school counselor listen to the teacher, try to identify the teacher's concerns, and establish an initial plan. An important component of this conversation is the exploration of the strategies that have been tried with the student. If the teacher has not tried interventions with the student, the counselor may want to help generate potential problem-solving solutions so the teacher can try them prior to intervention by an external source.

Step 2   If the teacher interventions have been unsuccessful, the counselor may schedule a time to do an observation of the student or may make a plan to meet with the student individually to get his or her perspective of what is happening in class. An important discussion to have with the teacher is the level of involvement of the parents in this problem. Because the school counselor will most likely need parent permission to see the student, it is helpful to know whether or not the parent is aware of the problem. Hopefully, the teacher has communicated his or her concerns to the parents and has acquired their consent in working toward solutions.

Step 3   If observing in the classroom, it may be necessary to ask the teacher to both not single out the student and not totally ignore him or her. The observation should take place in as normal a situation as possible in order to make sure the counselor is getting an accurate impression of the student's issue. One strategy to use when doing a student observation is to identify two or three students who are similar to this student in several ways (e.g., age, social interaction). By using other students as a baseline comparison, it is easier to assess how extraordinary the student's behavior is. While the counselor may want to concur with the teacher's assessment, it is always essential to remember that the school counselor's role is to be first and foremost the student's advocate. Having an objective assessment of the student's behavior will be an essential component of an intervention plan, if needed.

Step 4   Once the observation is completed, the school counselor should process what he or she saw and develop a report to share with the teacher. If the counselor does not agree with the teacher's assessment, he or she will need to approach the teacher very tactfully. For example, "I know you expressed concern about Maria's excessive talking. When I compared her with two or three other students in the class, I didn't observe her to be talking any more or any less than the other students. Do you think what I observed was typical?" This gives the teacher the opportunity to ponder the observation and respond to it. The teacher may say, "Well, you didn't really see her in action. She is usually ten times worse than that." Another response might be: "You saw her for 30 minutes. It's different when you're with her for 6 hours (45 minutes, 90 minutes) every day." It is certainly not desirable to disagree with a teacher's perception of a problem. However, the teacher's perception of the problem may, in itself, be the problem. A good response to the above statement is: "You're right. Perhaps I didn't see what you see everyday. Based on what you have seen, how would you like to approach this problem and how can I help?" It is at this point that the school counselor might offer to meet with the student individually or in group counseling, or to develop a behavior contract with the student (see the following discussion). Remember to involve the teacher and the parents, if possible, in the development of the plan. Approaching the problem from a systemic perspective is much more likely to result in long-term behavior change.

Behavior Contracts One of the tasks that typically becomes the responsibility of school counselors is the development of behavior contracts. Because teachers are responsible for entire classes of students, the school counselor is an obvious resource to help develop individual student contracts that address behavioral, social, or academic issues that may manifest in class.

School counselors may develop behavior contracts with students to address a variety of issues, although classroom behavior is a very common problem. One strategy that counselors may find helpful is to have students sit at the computer and help develop their contracts. Middle and high school students may type the contracts themselves. This can increase their sense of ownership and responsibility for working on the desired behaviors. In general, the following steps are helpful to the development of a student behavioral contract:

- Decide what behavior(s) need to be changed. If there is more than one, it is important to start with just one or two because it may be too overwhelming for the student to try to change multiple behaviors at once.

- Specify a reasonable goal regarding the number of instances of the undesirable behavior that will be allowed in a certain period of time, or the length of time the student must go without performing the behavior. Write this in positive terms, for example, "Sally will complete classwork in at least 60% of her classes daily." It is important to start small so that students are able to succeed; this will help reinforce the positive behavior.

- Decide on the incentives/rewards that will be given when the student achieves or exceeds the goals established in the contract. It is important to have the student help identify the rewards so he or she will be motivated to succeed. Also, check with all stakeholders to make sure the incentive can be provided. For example, if the student wants to be a P.E. assistant, make sure the P.E. teacher is amenable to the agreement.

- Identify the time when the student will receive the reward. Will the contract be checked daily or weekly? Try to provide the reward as close to the completion of the contract as possible. Immediacy will also reinforce the positive behavior.

- If behavior is disruptive or dangerous, specify the consequences of extreme negative behavior and circumstances under which the contract may become null and void.

Once the student agrees to the terms of the contract, acquire the signatures of all stakeholders (student, teacher, counselor, parent, administrator, etc.) and give each a copy. This makes the contract official.

Behavior contracting is an effective way for school counselors to work together with teachers to address behavioral problems with students. The tripartite interaction between the teacher, student, and school counselor is essential in order for the behavior plan to be appropriately implemented, monitored, and evaluated.

PARENT CONFERENCES School counselors also have a role in helping teachers and parents work together. Although school counselors should not unnecessarily insert themselves in teacher-parent relationships, it is often appropriate and advantageous for school counselors to serve as liaisons between parents and teachers, such as during parent-teacher conferences. Our veteran counselors provide insight into this supportive counseling practice.

Professional Practice

ESTHER (HS)

Counselors play an important role in conferences involving classroom teachers. They facilitate and coordinate face-to-face meetings with parents, students, and outside resource personnel. In these meetings, counselors heighten the awareness of students' special needs. They also can establish a mutually agreed upon system for follow-up on student progress. With the advent of computer technology, and especially teacher to parent e-mail, communication and follow-up become easy. Teachers and parents can correspond about strategies to support future assignments and the clarification of deadlines and guidelines for student work and include the counselor in their communication loop.

BETH (MS)

I find it is best to talk with teachers before a conference so that I have a sense of what their concerns are. I think the challenge is to have teachers feel that you are supporting them while you are also advocating for the student. I try to acknowledge what they are going through and empathize with them. I also ask for their input, because I think counselors can come across as trying to be experts. In fact, the teachers are the experts; they see a child's behavior in the classroom setting on a daily basis, so they can compare the student to the other students they teach. Their input, in that way, is valuable.

The school counselor can help facilitate important dialogue between parents and teachers that will foster student progress. Serving as an objective but interested party may help all invested members stay focused on the primary goal—enhancing the education of the student.

School Counselors and Teachers: A Winning Team

The efficacy of teamwork involves some specific components, such as mutual respect, empathy, understanding, cooperation, and a common goal. All of these are based on a key factor—*effective communication*.

EFFECTIVE COMMUNICATION BETWEEN SCHOOL COUNSELORS AND TEACHERS Communication is the key determinant of the effectiveness of interaction between school counselors and teachers. The following dichotomies illustrate the differences between effective and ineffective communication with teachers.

Intervention Versus Interference There are times when a school counselor is asked by an administrator or other school personnel to intervene with a teacher about a situation. The school counselor must tread lightly in this area. When approaching a teacher about a situation in which there may be a need for change, it is important to present the situation as an intervention that is going to be beneficial to all persons involved. If the teacher is unaware of the problem, the involvement of the school counselor may be viewed as interference. Therefore, the school counselor must be professional and tactful when approaching a teacher about possible intervention in a situation. For example, a school counselor might simply start the conversation by asking how things are going and then move more specifically to the area of concern. Once the topic has been broached, the counselor may want to say: "It sounds like this problem has made it challenging for you to accomplish your goals with the student. I would be happy to help you figure out a way to work on this situation, if you're comfortable with that." With this comment, the counselor has (a) acknowledged the challenge for the teacher and (b) offered to intervene without interfering. This gives the teacher the option of agreeing to the intervention or not.

Suggestion Versus Criticism Sometimes the school counselor may disagree with the teacher or, conversely, a teacher may resist a suggestion to try to improve the situation. What might be offered as a useful suggestion might be perceived as a criticism, which could lead to defensiveness and negative feelings. Also, the school counselor may differ philosophically with how a teacher interacts with students or the teacher may not perceive the school counselor as an essential part of the educational process. When these types of conflicts occur, it is best to always remain professional. One way to do this is to acknowledge the supposed impasse: "It seems we disagree on this particular issue, but I think we both want to do what's best for Patty. Do you have any suggestions for how we can work together?" This question demonstrates a willingness to overcome the obstacles and to focus on the student.

Synthesis Versus Metamorphosis Change is challenging. There may be some innate or embedded quality or characteristic of a teacher that does not mesh with a student's personality, or a teacher may have a weakness in a particular area, such as discipline. For this reason, it seems best to approach teachers with the idea that they do not necessarily have to change what they are doing. Instead, perhaps they need to adapt what they are doing in order to evoke positive changes in students' behavior and the classroom. This is an extension of the solution-focused strategies for working with teachers, which was mentioned earlier. School counselors should encourage teachers to maintain those techniques that are working and acquire the flexibility to adapt and synthesize new strategies to improve a situation. Change is frightening; school counselors can alleviate the fear by reassuring teachers that things may not have to change, they may just need modification or adaptation.

Professional Perspective

RENEE (ES)

Teachers and counselors need to work as a team. Each has a unique perspective on students that can be crucial to helping them be successful in school. As a counselor, you may have worked with a student and the student's family for several years before a teacher gets to know them. You may be able to provide valuable input that will help the teacher interact effectively with a student and aid in that student's success.

General Guidelines for Beginning School Counselors: Becoming a Member of the Education Team

Davis and Garrett (1998) made several recommendations for helping school counselors bridge any gaps in their relationships with teachers, including meeting the faculty, consulting with teachers consistently, observing classroom dynamics, and co-facilitating with teachers in order to foster collaboration, which was mentioned earlier. School counselors should try to connect with teachers when possible and ask them for their input, as well as make themselves available to help meet teachers' needs. Teachers often just want to have their opinions valued and acknowledged. When an issue about a student arises, the school counselor can make sure the teacher has had the opportunity to voice concerns and offer input. Acknowledgement goes a long, long way.

It is reinforcing and encouraging to students when teachers and counselors work together. School counselors should involve teachers whenever possible in teaching lessons, explaining concepts, and other activities, and vice versa. Again, the teacher is with the students much more than the school counselor. An effective way to reinforce teamwork and collaboration is to model it.

The guidelines offered in this chapter, while general, provide important ways for school counselors to begin to develop relationships with teachers as soon as they begin working in a school. Making the connection early on will help facilitate a positive working relationship in the future.

CONCLUSION

In this chapter, we have explored the roles of school counselors and teachers in the school setting. We began with an examination of an age-old issue: Should school counselors have prior teaching experience? While there is no obvious answer, there are benefits and challenges to either position. An examination of some of the teaching roles of school counselors indicated that school counselors should not be put into disciplinary roles; however, there will be times when school counselors need to be well-versed in classroom management techniques in order to ensure the safety of students.

An essential component of this chapter was the discussion of how school counselors support teaching personnel. Through enhancement of skills, collaboration about student behavior, and supportive consultation with parents, school counselors build a positive working alliance with teachers. Finally, the key component of a good working relationship—effective communication—provides the foundation for the development and maintenance of essential relationships with teachers. General guidelines for becoming a member of the educational team were provided as a springboard for helping new school counselors adapt quickly to the school environment.

School counselors and teachers obviously have a great deal to contribute to educational programs and the success of the students' academic experiences. Pooling the unique skills and abilities of teachers and counselors can only benefit students. It is important, above all, to understand the contribution of each to the student's well-being, and the positive power of the collaborative relationship between the two.

REFLECTION AND DISCUSSION

1. This chapter has emphasized the importance of a collaborative working relationship between school counselors and teachers. How might you approach a teacher who is resistant to refer students to counseling or who is hesitant to have you provide services in his or her classroom?

2. What boundaries separate teachers and school counselors? Although there may be differences, what goals unite the two?

3. One of the best ways to promote the school counseling program is to demonstrate how school counselors and teachers work together. This message should be clear from the first day of your job as a school counselor. What types of things might you do to engage teachers and inform them that you are there to support them?

CHAPTER **8**

Collaborating With Administrators and Other School Personnel: Working as a Team

Working With the Team Captain: The School Counselor
  and School Administrators
> *Tasks for Building Alliances With School Administrators*

The School Counselor's Role in Working With Support Personnel
> *Secretaries and Office Personnel* • *Student Services Personnel* •
> *Student Assistance Personnel* •
> *Working With Other School Personnel*

Contributing to the Winning Team: The School Counselor's Role

CONCLUSION

REFLECTION AND DISCUSSION

Chapter 7 focused on the significance of developing positive and collaborative relationships with teachers. Teachers are key members of the education team, and it is essential that school counselors work with them in an effective and proactive way. This chapter will focus on school counselors' working relationships with other school personnel—administrators, student support personnel, and a variety of other faculty and staff members who work in schools. It should be noted that not all school districts have these personnel in each building. Some school personnel are itinerant or have job responsibilities at multiple schools. Others may serve as consultants to the school and may not be available every day. Regardless of the level of interaction, school counselors should strive to foster effective working relationships with all members of the school faculty and staff. Building successful relationships is an essential factor in providing effective and comprehensive counseling services.

Working With the Team Captain: The School Counselor and School Administrators

It is often the relationship with school administration that establishes the general perception of the function of school counselors in the education program. Therefore, it is a relationship that deserves exploration. When asked to describe the "ultimate school counselor," one experienced administrator responded that the ultimate school counselor should possess the ability to work with *all* kids, the ability to work with *all* teachers, the ability to develop a close working relationship with administration, a working knowledge of community resources, and the desire to advocate for students. Interestingly, this response is in alignment with effective programs and practices of school counselors.

Professional Perspective

RENEE (ES)

I have always worked very closely with my school principals. I have found that we often consult with each other on how to handle various situations. Quite often, the counselor may become the principal's designee when he or she is out of the building. The principal will often ask me to sit in on parent meetings to support both teachers and parents. The counselor often is in a position to hear the perspectives of the educators and the families and to assist in mediating uncomfortable situations.

The working relationship between school counselors and principals can be a major influence on the success of a comprehensive school counseling program. In a study by Lehr and Sumarah (2002), school counselors acknowledged the critical role of administrative support for comprehensive school counseling programs. "School counselors reported that principals' involvement in (a) the initial professional development of the concepts, (b) implementation, and (c) delivery of the [program] contributed to the program's success in their schools" (p. 295). Another interesting finding in the study was that the counselors who were in secondary schools felt they had to work harder than elementary counselors to articulate their school counseling roles. This was due, in part, to the perceived historical roles of secondary school counselors and more recent attempts to redefine roles based on the ASCA (1999c) role statement.

Niebuhr, Niebuhr, and Cleveland (1999) recommended a proactive and collaborative relationship between principals and counselors. An example of this type of interaction would be using data to assess the school climate in order to develop counseling services to address problem areas or concerns. Often, collaboration is needed to develop important school programs, such as character education or the school's crisis management plan. Another proactive strategy for school counselors is to make sure administrators understand the counseling services that are priorities for school counselors. Informing school administrators of the transformed role of school counselors would be an effective way to educate administrators about the integral services school counselors provide.

Professional Perspective

BETH (MS)

To the best of our ability, school counselors should educate administrators about what we do as school counselors. Sometimes it comes down to dollars and cents. It is important to point out that the school's money can best be spent by having school counselors perform counseling services that support the academic program. Sometimes, I've agreed to perform duties that are not in my job description so that I can build rapport with the administration. Then, when asked to perform other noncounseling tasks, I may say, "This really should not be the responsibility of the school counselor." Hopefully, the response will be: "You know, the counselors are willing to do their fair share in the school, but there are limits to what we should ask of them."

Administrators at all levels often rely on their counselors to help deal with challenging student, parent, and faculty situations. Because school counselors are trained in effective communication and counseling skills, administrators can feel confident that counselors can rise to the challenge of difficult situations.

Professional Practice

ESTHER (HS)

School administrators are asked to attend difficult conferences for students with serious discipline problems or other issues. Counselors share important background information with administrators on an as-needed basis, or when something threatening or potentially harmful occurs. Counselors facilitate communication with administrators and encourage administrators to keep them in the communication loop as well. Counselors meet with administrators to plan and coordinate grade-level parent meetings and share in programming responsibilities.

Tasks for Building Alliances With School Administrators

When working with school administration, the school counselor can establish a strong alliance by focusing on several specific tasks: (a) sharing a vision, (b) communicating openly, (c) inviting input, and (d) demonstrating mutual respect.

SHARING A VISION   It may seem obvious that a shared vision is a critical attribute of successful schools. When faculty and staff share a vision and focus on the same goals as the administration, better student performance and higher productivity is likely. When administration and faculty are working against each other, the overall morale of the school may suffer, and that can affect student performance and behavior. Having a shared vision, or at least a common goal, is one way to communicate that everyone is on the same team. This may not always be easy. Consider a possible situation:

> You are a new school counselor in a school. You have come to this school with lots of program ideas and effective ways to provide counseling services. In your interview for this position, you and the administration were in agreement about the roles and responsibilities of the school counselor in the educational program. You felt that this administration would support your role as a school counselor.
>
> On your first day, you arrive to learn that there has been a change. Some of the administrators were transferred to other buildings or positions, and new administrators have been assigned to your school. You have no idea how the new administrators feel about the school counseling program. Will they support you? What if they don't?

Given this scenario, the school counselor has groundwork to do regarding how he or she will work with administration. Primarily, it will be critical for the school counselor to meet with the administration as soon as possible in order to establish a collaborative relationship and a shared vision.

Specific ways the school counselor and administration might work together on a shared vision follow:

- Schedule meetings between counselors and administrators to discuss the school environment. This dialogue is important because the administration must focus on academics, but the school counselor can provide valuable input about the personal/social elements in the school that might be impeding the academic process.

- Develop specific objectives that focus on the holistic education of students. While administrators deal with discipline and making sure the curriculum is ensuring academic development, the school counselor can include objectives that foster emotional and social development and enhance the academic component of school.

- Keep each other aware and informed of changes in policy, procedure, or law, especially as they affect students. The school counselor and administrator can meet to discuss any revisions that should be made to current practice in the academic and school counseling programs. The school counselor may need to offer more support in a certain area (e.g., more study skills small groups to address state testing requirements and improve test scores) in order to support changes to the overall educational program.

The school counselor and administration need to have productive dialogue and open lines of communication in order to advance the development of students in the school.

COMMUNICATING OPENLY   In an ideal world, every school administrator or principal-in-training would take an entire course on how to work with school counselors. This course would include a detailed description of school counseling practices and the types of services school counselors provide. Conversely, it would be beneficial for school counselors-in-training to have an opportunity to explore and discuss the roles of administrators in the school building. However, there has been evidence that administrators are becoming more aware of the essential services school counselors provide. In a study by Fitch, Newby, Ballestero, and Marshall (2001), 86 principals-in-training were asked to respond to a survey about the most significant school counselor duties. In general, the results provided good news for school counselors. The principals-in-training appropriately prioritized school counselor duties in accordance with the ASCA (1999c) Role Statement. There seemed to be common knowledge and acknowledgement of the importance of the primary school counselor roles: counseling, classroom guidance, consultation, and coordination. However, almost 30% of the potential administrators also prioritized discipline as a primary school counselor responsibility (p. 98). They also listed record keeping, administering tests, and registering students among the priorities of school counselors. One might conclude that while principals-to-be understand the major roles of school counselors, they also may assign noncounseling duties that can dominate the counselor's time and detract from the counseling program.

It is critical for school counselors to inform administrators about what they are and should be doing in order to maintain their appropriate roles in schools. Information that should be shared with administrators includes:

- the National Model for School Counseling Programs;
- the National Standards for School Counseling Programs;

- the ASCA Role Statement and ASCA Ethical Standards;
- the yearly plan for the counseling program, which should include information about *goals, services, and plans for evaluation;*
- a list of "fair-share responsibilities" (Gysbers & Henderson, 2000, p. 76), which describes duties that are manageable and will not be detrimental to the provision of counseling services;
- clarification of role boundaries to avoid confusion and overlap;
- notification of what the counseling department is doing, such as giving the principals a written copy of any correspondence to teachers or any information about upcoming counseling programs and services;
- information about the role of the school counselor in special education; and
- anticipated level of school counselor involvement in school-wide programs and specific services for at-risk students.

In addition to keeping administrators informed about the school counseling program, it is important to ask a few questions of the school administrators: What are the expectations for the school counselor? Are there duties that the school counselor has performed historically that might be handled by other school personnel? Does the principal understand how the school counselor supports the education program—not as an appendage, but as an integral part of the whole? Further, school counselors should seek information about the work of school administrators. An understanding of the roles and duties of school administrators will foster empathy and understanding. This exchange of information is necessary if a positive working alliance is to be formed.

INVITING INPUT   One of the best ways to build collegiality and shared responsibility is to ask for the principal's input and opinion. This communication can be as informal as sending a note or asking, "Can I get some feedback on an idea?" It may be that the school counselor does not integrate the administrator's input, but to ask for thoughts or opinions on an issue shows that the administrator's input is valued. Another example of utilizing the insight and expertise of the administrator might occur if a school counselor is struggling with classroom management and knows that he or she is due for a performance evaluation. Rather than waiting and dreading the observation and evaluation, the school counselor can be proactive and ask an administrator to sit in on a lesson in order to give feedback or tips for improving classroom management.

DEMONSTRATING MUTUAL RESPECT   This task is possibly the most necessary in the development of a collaborative relationship between school counselors and school administrators. In addition to a clear understanding of the roles of each position, there must be a shared respect and appreciation for the unique responsibilities and practices of the other's profession.

My Story

In my experience, there were times when I knew what I wanted to accomplish with students, but I wasn't quite sure how to accomplish it. It was during these times that I appreciated the input of my administrators. School administrators are trained in problem solving and decision making, and it is often true that "two heads are better than one." As long as the confidentiality of the student is maintained, it is appropriate to ask for help when it is warranted, especially if a situation is unfamiliar or new. I found that seeking input from administrators provided me with a different perspective and helped me make more informed, effective decisions than if I had not asked for input.

Professional Perspective

RENEE (ES)

In order to establish a good working relationship with your administration, it is important that you develop a sense of mutual respect and trust. I have found that the best way to do this is to demonstrate your skill and professionalism in dealing with parents, teachers, and students. It is also important to define appropriate duties for a school counselor. There is a delicate balance between being a "team player" and maintaining the integrity of your role as a counselor. Working with an administrator who is supportive and understands your role as a counselor goes a long way toward making your job easier, more enjoyable, and more effective.

School principals and counselors should work together. There should be a mutual acknowledgement of and appreciation for the role of each in the educational success of students. Administrative issues and counseling services should go hand in hand in terms of supporting and facilitating learning. Seeking out the administration and initiating important dialogue can have a positive effect when developing and implementing a successful counseling program.

REFLECTION AND DISCUSSION

1. What seem to be the biggest obstacles to an effective working relationship between school counselors and administrators? What strategies would you use to overcome these obstacles?

2. There is often more than one administrator in a school building and there may be conflicting thoughts or opinions about the role of school counselors in schools. How might you approach the various perspectives of administrators who do not seem to agree on the role of school counselors?

3. Imagine that you are making a presentation to the administrators in your school about the role of the school counselor in the school program. What would be important components to include?

The School Counselor's Role in Working With Support Personnel

There are many school personnel who provide support for the educational process and progress of students. School counselors are in a pivotal position to interact with support personnel. Collaborative working relationships with key faculty and staff members will significantly enhance services to students, parents, and community members.

Secretaries and Office Personnel

In most schools, if you were to ask, "Who really knows what is going on in this school?" the answer would include the administrative assistant or secretary. Secretaries are personnel who are full of information and who often keep the school running smoothly. Organization, time management, and the ability to keep calm in a crisis are necessary abilities when working in a school office.

Professional Practice

BETH (MS)

The guidance secretary's job is extremely stressful, so whenever I feel that I can protect her from additional stress, I do. She is absolutely the school counselor's greatest ally. A good guidance secretary can relieve the counselors of duties that are really not counseling functions. School counselors need to support guidance secretaries and show them how much they are appreciated. They should be viewed as essential members of guidance and counseling teams.

The counseling or guidance secretary is a person who must be aware of everything that is going on in the counseling department and how it relates to what is going on in the entire school. Though elementary schools may not have secretaries assigned specifically and solely to the counseling programs, it is likely that school counselors will have close working relationships with the secretaries in the administrative offices. The nature of this relationship will depend on the level of interaction between the counseling office and administrative office.

Professional Practice

ESTHER (HS)

Our office support personnel coordinate and schedule conferences, student registrations, programs, publications, and updates of publications; handle student registration, paperwork, and mailings; and process transcripts. They are often underpaid and overworked, so we make time to appreciate them!

School counselors and secretaries have important and multidimensional relationships. Often, the secretary may have more information or know more about a student's situation than the counselor does. For this reason, working with the secretary becomes a significant task for school counselors. Secretaries who are specifically assigned to the guidance department are usually responsible for essential tasks, including maintaining student files, assisting with student record keeping, working with test materials, and providing copies of student transcripts. In addition to these tasks, it is also critical that guidance secretaries have the ability to connect and work with students. Often, the secretary is the first person with whom a student or parent interacts, and the first impression of the guidance or counseling department can play a significant role in setting the tone for future interactions. For example, if a parent comes to the office and is upset about a situation and the counselor is not available, the guidance secretary may intervene to calm the parent down and reassure him or her that every attempt will be made to resolve the issue. Guidance secretaries or front office support personnel can provide valuable information and insight that helps school counselors decide how to proceed in a situation.

Professional Practice

RENEE (ES)

Developing a positive relationship with support personnel can make a monumental difference in how you do your job. I have found that the support personnel have a unique perspective on the school and students. For example, it is often support personnel who register a new student in the school. They have a chance to meet the parents of the student and watch them interact. The personnel in the front office know who the "frequent flyers" to the clinic are, which students are chronically tardy or have histories of absences with shaky excuses, or which students do not have money for lunch or for field trips. These are all red flags that the support personnel can share with the counselor. I try to make sure that I express my appreciation to the support staff and do not ask them to perform administrative tasks that I can do myself.

Another important role of the guidance secretary is to police the traffic that comes into and out of the counseling offices. When there is a secretary or assistant who is very effective at taking care of administrative tasks, counselors have more time to provide counseling services. This type of efficiency helps in the effective provision of counseling programs and services.

In the event that there is not a secretary specifically assigned to work with the counseling program, school counselors will need to develop good working relationships with the secretaries, administrative assistants, and other office personnel in the main school office so that the counseling program runs smoothly. One way to work with secretaries is to inform them of the roles of the school counselor and goals of the program. Another discussion should focus on the ways in which the office staff and counselor can work together to meet the needs of students. One example might be deciding on the types of problems that should be handled administratively rather than through counseling. Consider this situation:

> A student walks into the high school counseling office and reports that two other students are planning to fight in the bathroom at lunchtime. The student making the report does not want to be identified as the informant and therefore has chosen to come to the counseling office instead of the administrative office. The counseling secretary can consult with the counselors or guidance director about the situation, but fighting is clearly an administrative issue. The secretary can then inform the administration of the pending altercation and also maintain the confidentiality of the student. The secretary might also mention the incident to the counselors in case they should intervene or meet with the students after administrative action is taken.

Other topics that might be discussed in order to develop a collaborative working relationship would include how phone calls will be handled, the school counselor's schedule, and whether or not the office staff is willing to help the counselor with paperwork or copying materials when needed. The earlier this dialogue can occur in the relationship, the better chance each party has of understanding the boundaries of the relationship and how they will work together.

One of the best ways to develop a positive working relationship with secretaries and office staff is to recognize the tremendous amount of work they do and the contributions they make to the school program. Often, teachers and other faculty who interact with students daily are recognized for their contributions to the school, but it is equally important to acknowledge the day-in, day-out efforts of office support personnel who keep schools running efficiently. Building positive, reciprocal relationships with secretaries, registrars, financial officers, and other office personnel will be an asset to the school counseling program.

REFLECTION AND DISCUSSION

1. What specific duties do you think might be the responsibility of the school counseling support staff rather than the counselor? Does this seem like a fair division of duties?

2. If you are the only counselor in the school, you may not have a secretary specifically assigned to help with your responsibilities. Identify other options (or people) for completing the noncounseling functions that often emerge in school counseling programs.

Student Services Personnel

School counselors also work with the persons who make up the Child Study Team for special needs students. As mentioned in chapter 6, these teams could include, but are not limited to, school psychologists, educational diagnosticians, school social workers, and special needs teachers. Murphy, DeEsch, and Strein (1998) noted: "Current realities make it abundantly clear that it is no longer possible for school personnel to function effectively in isolation" (p. 85). Developing effective relationships with these individuals is imperative for the school counselor because these personnel are often necessary to consultation and coordination of services for students.

Professional Perspective

RENEE (ES)

It is important to have a good working relationship with other personnel, such as social workers, school psychologists, and other specialists. These professionals can be an excellent source of support for counselors, especially in an elementary school, which may have only one counselor.

WORKING WITH THE SCHOOL PSYCHOLOGIST Murphy, DeEsch, and Strein (1998) noted that while school counselors and school psychologists have compatible training and knowledge, there are also some differences between their functions in schools. "School counselors possess skills in small group counseling, large group developmental interventions, and vocational and career development. School psychologists possess knowledge in applied behavioral analysis, personality assessment, and organizational consultation" (p. 86). In addition to testing students, school psychologists may be involved in individual and group work with students. The collaborative nature of the school counselor–school psychologist relationship involves consultation about student behavior. For example, if a student is involved in self-mutilation or other self-destructive behavior that seems to be psychologically motivated, the school psychologist is an appropriate person to evaluate the student's psychological functioning and help make a referral to outside therapy. While the school counselor is a part of this process, the school psychologist can provide additional information about psychological disorders and diagnoses, and may be able to administer an assessment in order to determine an appropriate intervention. It may also be helpful for both the school psychologist and school counselor to meet with the parent in order to emphasize the need for more extensive and intensive intervention outside of the school setting.

An example of effectively working with the school psychologist might be co-leading a group for a specific population of students, such as students identified as emotionally challenged. The school counselor and school psychologist can address a variety of issues that the students might encounter. Utilizing the experience and expertise of two professionals trained in counseling and psychology is an effective way to provide comprehensive services to students. The collaborative interaction of the school counselor and school psychologist provides a holistic approach to addressing the needs of students.

WORKING WITH EDUCATIONAL TESTING PERSONNEL   There are geographical and district-based differences in the process for testing students for educational services. In some areas, the personnel who conduct these tests are called *educational diagnosticians*. In other school districts, educational testing is the responsibility of the school psychologist. Regardless, the school counselor's relationship with school personnel who provide educational testing is important because the results may determine the academic achievement level of students, which could have implications for educational placement and counseling services. Personnel who conduct educational testing are a useful resource for students, teachers, parents, and counselors. They can offer suggestions based on test results that will help students become more successful in their schoolwork and improve their performance in the classroom. These strategies could include ideas for behavior management, time management, organization, and focusing.

WORKING WITH THE SCHOOL SOCIAL WORKER   Another important member of the student services team is the school social worker. The school social worker often works with the families of students who have academic or behavioral concerns. Part of the school social worker's role in the special education process is to conduct a social history, which is derived from an interview with the parent or guardian of the student who has been referred for special needs testing. Components of this report include a synopsis of the presenting problem or reason for referral, birth and childhood history, developmental milestones or developmental history, significant family academic, educational, or medical history, social and adaptive behavior development, and the parents' thoughts, concerns, or requests regarding their child's needs.

The school counselor and school social worker work closely together because it is often these two team members who have information about the student that might influence the decision about educational placement of a student. For example, if a child is struggling in seventh grade, but the school counselor and/or school social worker knows that the student's mother has recently been imprisoned, the committee might consider that the difficulty the student is having is related to what is going on outside of school and not a true learning disability. It is important to rule out external factors when making educational decisions about a student as these decisions have critical implications for educational placement (i.e., self-contained or inclusion within the mainstream).

Another critical part of the relationship between the school counselor and school social worker occurs when there is a potential Child Protective Services issue. Suspected abuse or neglect is a circumstance in which the school counselor and school social worker should collaborate, if possible, when making the report. School social workers usually have a thorough understanding of the referral process and often have worked in or with social services departments outside of the school setting. Therefore, he/she comes well equipped to help with cases that involve abuse and/or neglect.

School social workers may also conduct home visits or arrange for services for families. The school social worker can be a liaison between families and needs-based services, such as Medicaid, food, clothing, medical or dental care, and employment for parents. School counselors can collaborate with the school social worker to help make these connections when he/she learns that a student or family is in need.

Not every school in a school district has a school social worker that is assigned to only one school. Often, particularly at the elementary level, a school social worker may share several schools and serve as a consultant for school counselors in critical cases. This relationship, even if not readily available, is an important connection for school counselors to make, and school social workers provide an important link between the school and the community.

This section has focused on a few members of the Child Study Team. In most schools, the school counselor is an important member of this team and building a relationship with other team members is beneficial to everyone. The school counselor's role on this team is to serve as an advocate for the student while also providing important information about the student that will be helpful in making decisions about the educational services the student might need. Chapter 6 included a more in-depth discussion of the school counselor's role in special education and the importance of professional training in this area.

Student Assistance Personnel

Although the positions may vary from school to school, there are various student assistance personnel who provide essential services for students. These include the school nurse, school resource officer, attendance officer, and other student assistance personnel who may be community liaisons to the school or personnel employed by federal grant programs (e.g., Safe and Drug-Free Schools). The school counselor will interact with these persons and a collaborative relationship should be established to address multiple areas of student issues. While not all student assistance personnel will be discussed in this chapter, there are a few that school counselors may have the opportunity to work with, at least intermittently.

WORKING WITH THE SCHOOL NURSE School counselors call on the services of the school nurse more than one might expect. The school nurse is involved in medical and physical concerns related to student health, and the school counselor deals with issues of mental, social, and emotional health. The two often find that trauma in one area often affects the other. Students with somatic complaints of headaches or stomachaches are often dealing with emotional or social problems that manifest themselves in physical ways. Conversely, students with emotional or social problems often display physical symptoms of stress or anxiety. Therefore, the school nurse and school counselor will often interact in order to determine the origin of and a plan for the presenting problem.

Another way that the nurse and school counselor work together is collaborating about a Child Protective Services referral. Often, the school nurse may be the first to see physical evidence of abuse or neglect. While also a mandated reporter, the school nurse may ask the school counselor to talk with the student to try to ascertain what happened before reporting the incident. On the other hand, a student may tell the school counselor of an abusive or neglectful incident. If the incident created a physical mark or bruise, the school counselor might ask the school nurse to examine it to determine its origin. Because the school nurse is trained in this area, the school counselor can be more confident in his or her decision to make a referral. In addition, the school nurse might also ask the student what happened to check for consistency in terms of how the injury was acquired. Regardless of who makes the referral, it is reassuring that

My Story

At the elementary level, I worked closely with the school nurse. We were constantly consulting with each other on student cases. Our working relationship was reciprocal. Sometimes, students would come to me with an issue, and I would immediately consult with the nurse, particularly about physical or medical issues. On the other hand, a student might first go to the nurse for treatment of an injury, and after investigation, the nurse might refer the student to me to talk about an issue or concern. This collaborative relationship worked well for us and, more importantly, for the students.

As a high school counselor, I relied on the school nurse to help handle issues of sexuality. School board policy prevented me from counseling students on birth control issues and pregnancy. The school nurse, however, had greater latitude for dealing with these issues. Because the school nurse operated from a different code of ethics and worked from a medical model, she was able to be more involved with students and families about sexuality and sexual behavior.

at least two professionals, trained to look for different evidence, have come to the same conclusion.

At the secondary level, school nurses are an excellent resource and school counselors should utilize the expertise of school nurses when handling sensitive situations, such as teenage pregnancy, HIV, birth control, and sexually transmitted diseases. It is crucial that school counselors and school nurses work together for the optimal health of the student.

WORKING WITH THE SCHOOL RESOURCE OFFICER   Because of the incidence of violence and weapons in schools, there has been an increase in the number of uniformed officers and/or police personnel in schools. The presence of these officers is designed to prevent the escalation of potentially dangerous situations involving students. Having police personnel onsite may affect student behavior as students realize that threats to safety are taken seriously. For the purposes of this discussion, the school or student resource officer will be called the SRO.

The school counselor and SRO may work closely together in several ways. First, the school counselor may become privy to information that requires police intervention. For example, if a student tells a counselor of a party in which underage drinking or illegal drug use may occur, the counselor should inform the SRO so that he or she can take action or investigate the situation. Though this breaches confidentiality, it is the school counselor's ethical responsibility to report this activity, since there is the potential for harm to students. Further, underage drinking is illegal, so there is a legal component to consider as well. The school counselor may be able to provide the SRO with information while keeping the identity of the informant confidential; for example, the school counselor can inform the SRO of the location of the party or the student who is alleged to be hosting the party. This would not require that the counselor reveal the identity of the informant.

Second, the SRO might ask the school counselor to intervene and help resolve a conflict that has the potential to become volatile and violent. The counselor might be asked to conduct a mediation session with students who are fighting in an attempt to resolve the conflict peacefully. If the conflict becomes physical or an actual assault occurs, the SRO will intervene and proceed as legally appropriate. Finally, the school counselor and SRO may consult with each other about particular cases and try to determine what intervention might be helpful. Consider the example presented in the "My Story" box.

The working relationship between the SRO and school counselor can be effective as long as each person understands the roles and boundaries of each position. There are times when the law may override counseling ethics, and the SRO will be required to act in a situation. Conversely, there may be times when a counselor's responsibility or ethical code prevents the disclosure of information to the SRO. The ideal situation is a working relationship in which mutual respect and student well-being are the priorities and teamwork is the means to ensure both.

My Story

A student stole my wallet from my office. I knew the student had a propensity for stealing, and we had worked on this behavior for quite some time. Though the wallet showed up in a trashcan, the cash (about $22) was gone. Another student reported that my counselee told him about stealing the money. The first conversation I had was with the SRO. He wanted to arrest and charge the student for stealing, which is legally what should have happened. He asked if I wanted to press charges. I really had to think about this because I knew the student had a problem, and experiencing the consequences of his actions might teach the student a lesson and curtail future stealing. I was upset that he would take my wallet when I had been working so hard to help with this behavior, but I also had to consider that this was a real problem for him. After much thought and conversation, the SRO and I decided that he would not arrest the student. Instead, he would confront the student in order to get him to confess to the crime. We decided that I would not be involved at this point, but if the student confessed, we would need to decide what the consequences would be. Ultimately, the student came to me, confessed, and apologized. Unfortunately, the money was already gone, so we worked out a plan in which he would work after school, helping me with tasks, until I felt that the money had been paid back. The SRO and I felt this situation had ended positively for all parties, although the SRO also let the student know that this would be the last chance and the next incidence of stealing would result in arrest. The student and I were able to salvage our counseling relationship and continued to work on eliminating the stealing behavior. While I still had difficulty trusting the student, I felt I had professionally responded to the situation and could work to help him learn from the experience.

WORKING WITH THE ATTENDANCE OFFICER   The attendance officer is sometimes called the truancy officer. Typically, the school counselor will work with this person when a student's attendance has become a concern and is negatively impacting academic progress. Attendance officers might ask the school counselor to speak with the student to try to find out why he or she is missing so much school. Sometimes, the school counselor can intervene and help find a solution to the problem so that the student can attend school and be on time. On the other hand, the school counselor may ask the attendance officer to keep him or her informed of a student's attendance record, especially for students who have a history of attendance problems. When truancy is a persistent issue for a student and interventions do not work, it is typically the attendance officer, social worker, or SRO that will begin legal proceedings against the parent/guardian if the student is under 18. At this point, the school counselor may need to wait until the court system has ruled on the student's case to determine a plan of support. The court may rule that the student needs transition into another educational program or may develop a plan to help the student improve school attendance.

The relationship between the attendance officer and school counselor is typically very complementary. The attendance officer often learns information about students while investigating reasons for absences or tardiness and can refer the student to the counselor. Further, the attendance officer can let the school counselor know when a student's attendance or tardiness is about to influence academic progress. For example, when the number of student absences is almost at the maximum allowance and might result in failure, the school counselor should immediately inform the student and parents/guardians. Hopefully, the school counselor has intervened with the student and the family much earlier so that the situation does not become hopeless. The school counselor can work with the attendance officer, parents, and the student to try to alleviate problems that prohibit the student from coming to school. The working relationship of the school counselor and attendance officer is based on the common goal of keeping students in school, where they can develop as effective learners.

WORKING WITH COMMUNITY STUDENT ASSISTANCE PERSONNEL

The job roles and responsibilities of persons employed as student assistance personnel can vary. They can range from in-house suspension assistants to substance abuse counselors from the local community services board or community mental health facility. These persons can be useful in a school setting because they have specific training in areas that school counselors may lack (e.g., substance abuse rehabilitation). Regardless of the role of each person, the school counselor should make an effort to connect with any persons who are in direct contact with students, especially those who are providing services in which counseling might be a component. It is crucial to learn about each person and the role they play in student development. It is equally important to let each person know about the school counselor's role and to discover how these roles can best complement each other for the good of the student. Often, there are overlaps in student services because one does not know what the other is doing. Also, there may be "turf wars" that are perpetuated by miscommunication and misunderstanding. Simple communication and direct interaction can help prevent duplication in services and may clarify roles so that students have access to more comprehensive support services.

School counselors may also consult with student assistance personnel to gather information about community services. Often, student assistance personnel have knowledge of or connections with community agencies that can provide services that students need. This knowledge will be helpful for school counselors if they are consulted about potential outside services available for students and families.

Working With Other School Personnel

There are other school personnel with whom the school counselor will interact. Cafeteria workers and custodians are examples of school staff that provide immeasurable and valuable services to schools. School counselors benefit from positive working relationships with these staff members because the school counselor may need the services of the cafeteria and custodial staff. For example, if a school counselor is having a parent workshop in the evening, the cafeteria staff might be asked to provide light refreshments. If there is going to be a counseling department–sponsored assembly for teachers and students, the custodial staff may assist with set-up and clean-up, especially if there is a respectful, positive relationship between all parties.

Another group that school counselors often work with are parent volunteers. Many schools have active and involved parents who volunteer personal time to help the school in some capacity. It behooves school counselors to have positive relationships with the school volunteers because they can be an important resource for completing noncounseling tasks, such as copying handouts or organizing a student recognition assembly. Further, developing a positive working relationship with school volunteers, particularly parent volunteers, results in good public relations and advertisement for school counseling services.

The common thread in the school counselor's relationship with each of these personnel is the importance of a collaborative working relationship. The concepts of teamwork and cooperation are necessary in order for school programs to run smoothly and effectively. This is nonetheless true for school counseling programs. It will be detrimental to student success if school personnel attempt to isolate their roles and services. The more collaborative the working relationship between school personnel, the more effective the services offered for student achievement and success.

Contributing to the Winning Team: The School Counselor's Role

This chapter has explored the role of the school counselor in working with key members of the school faculty and staff. While the amount of interaction with each professional or group of people may vary, it is important to have positive working relationships with student support personnel, student assistance personnel, and other personnel throughout the school building. General guidelines for working with these essential school members are offered in Feature 8.1.

Perhaps the 3 Rs of teamwork that educators follow should be considered by school counselors: *respect + responsibility = rewards.* When school counselors respect the distinct roles and tasks of each member of the school team and take responsibility for the roles and duties of their positions on the team, they

FEATURE 8.1

*Guidelines for Developing Collaborative Working Relationships
With School Faculty, Staff, and Support Personnel*

- Within the first few days of working in a school, school counselors
  should introduce themselves to as many school personnel as possible
  and emphasize the desire to develop a collaborative and effective
  working relationship with each of them.
- School counselors should inform the school faculty and staff about
  the roles and responsibilities that are inherent in comprehensive
  school counseling programs. This could be accomplished through a
  letter, although connecting in-person may seem more personal and
  sincere.
- School counselors should provide information about the mission of
  the school counseling program to foster understanding of how school
  counselors help students with academic, personal/social, and career
  development. Copies of the ASCA National Standards, ASCA Ethical
  Standards, and ASCA National Model should be available to share
  with others.
- School counselors should meet with other student specialists in the
  building, including other members of the Child Study Team and student assistance personnel, to clarify roles and responsibilities. These
  meetings will prevent the duplication of services and will clarify each
  person's contribution to the education program and the students.
- School counselors may also meet with school faculty and staff to
  discuss what services will be provided and who will provide them.
  This clear delineation of roles and responsibilities will promote
  greater understanding of the functions of each position and will prevent role confusion and redundancy.

will be rewarded with a school faculty that collaboratively promotes excel-
lence in learning and maximizes student success.

CONCLUSION

This chapter has continued to emphasize the significance of the school counselor's collaboration and teamwork with school personnel. These important
interactions, if they are to be productive and positive, must be characterized by
understanding and respect for the work that each person does and the unique
contributions of each person to the school program. From the members of the

child study or local screening team to the custodian and cafeteria staff, everyone contributes to the overall climate of the school. In order to encourage student success, school personnel must model how effective teamwork benefits everyone involved. This it not to say that school counselors must love everyone they work with or compromise their own roles and responsibilities out of respect for those of other personnel. However, the message is clear: In order to provide effective and comprehensive services to students, which may require the input and expertise of many school professionals, school counselors should initiate dialogue and interactions that will benefit students. It is only through these effective working relationships and team efforts toward student development and success that everyone wins.

REFLECTION AND DISCUSSION

1. Obviously, there are many members of a school faculty with whom the school counselor must interact. Are there specific considerations when working with certain personnel? If so, what are they?

2. What could you do specifically to ensure positive interactions with all school personnel, particularly those you might not work with on a day-to-day basis (e.g., cafeteria workers, bus drivers, custodians)?

3. Some faculty and/or staff members may seek to work in a more individualistic manner and may be uncomfortable sharing or collaborating with others. What strategies might help you connect with a person who prefers to work alone? How would you address barriers that might interfere with developing a collaborative relationship with school personnel?

CHAPTER 9

Collaborating With Parents, Families, and Community: Making the Connection

*W*hen discussing teamwork and collaboration, it is necessary to explore the role of school counselors in working with parents, families, and community members/agencies. Taylor and Adelman (2000) acknowledged the significance of integrated relationships between schools, families, and communities:

> Schools can better address barriers to learning and teaching and promote
> positive development when they are an integral and positive part of the com-
> munity. Reciprocally, families and other community entities can better
> address barriers to development, learning, parenting, and strengthen the
> fabric of family and community life by working in partnership with schools.
> (p. 299)

An area of emphasis in the Transforming School Counseling Initiative (Education Trust, 2003) is the need for *systemic change*. Parents and community agencies are a significant part of the education system and are integral to promoting necessary change.

School counselors must consider all critical players involved in the education of students. Previous chapters have addressed the role of key school personnel in students' academic, personal/social, and career development. Parents of students are also an essential part of the education process. Academic programs that do not involve parents are likely to be less effective than those with parental support. Further, school counselors should acknowledge that students, though appreciated for their individuality, are part of their family systems. In addition, school counselors should make a concerted effort to connect with community services and agencies in order to provide consistent assistance for students and their families. When schools do not make an effort to collaborate with community agencies or to respond to community concerns, there may be little support for education when political or financial issues polarize a community. While parents, families, and community agencies are being discussed in the same chapter, we must explore the school counselor's role with each in isolation, as well as the collaborative efforts that can unite the groups. The common theme throughout this chapter is the integral role of the school counselor in gaining support for the counseling program through the development of collaborative connections among these groups.

The School Counselor as Parent Partner: Promoting Positive Interactions

Parents exert important influence in a child's life. It seems obvious that parents should be included in the academic development of their children. Further, parents should be consulted or informed about personal/social issues that may be affecting the behavior or performance of their children in school. Finally, parents should be involved in the career decision-making process that students engage in prior to leaving high school. Thus, from kindergarten until graduation day, parents should be involved. Cuthbert (2002) stated:

> Parents must be made aware of the fact that the emotional health of their child is directly related to that child's academic achievement and success in school. When parents understand the important relationship between emotional health and academic success, and become knowledgeable about the school counseling program, they will join with counselors in demanding that schools give the appropriate time to affective education. (p. 80)

Ideally, both parents will be invested in and committed to their child's academic and personal success. However, the ideal is often not the reality. In some cases, students may receive little support at home, not due to the parent's lack of desire to be involved, but because of the demands of day-to-day life. For example, if a parent must choose between helping Johnny with his homework or cooking dinner before he or she has to go to work to support the family, the parent will probably focus on the most immediate and basic need—food. While parents may want to be involved, their life circumstances may be such that they cannot sustain the level of involvement they would wish. School counselors cannot assume that parents who are uninvolved are disinterested.

Another issue that might arise with parents is resistance to the demands of the school system. Some parents may not have had pleasant school experiences, or perhaps they have had negative relationships with other governmental agencies and feel general animosity toward all government organizations, including schools. It is difficult to change attitudes and perceptions about the importance of education. If parents' perceptions are negative, they may unconsciously communicate this attitude to their children. Parents may also have had negative experiences with their school counselors, so they may project those negative feelings onto all school counselors, without giving them a chance to change that perception. The school counselor must try to guide parents beyond those preconceptions.

An important recent trend in school counseling is the shift from a hands-off approach to family counseling to an understanding that in order to be truly effective with students, school counselors may need to involve the entire family system. It does not make sense to try to change one part of the system without examining how the system might change to promote positive behavior in one or more of its members.

This section will explore the various school counselor roles in working with parents and families. In this chapter, the term *parent* will include parents and guardians of students, whether they are biological parents, extended family, foster parents, or other types of guardians. This chapter will explore approaches to educating parents about and promoting the school counseling program, strategies for getting parents involved in their child's academic, personal/social, and career development, and methods for working with families to help students be successful in school.

Promoting the School Counseling Program: Good PR With Parents

The most basic element of promoting the school counseling program to parents is educating them about the role of school counselors in the school program. There can be misunderstandings about what school counselors do, especially if parents have not had experiences with school counselors in the past. While parents may understand the roles of high school counselors, most parents did not have counselors in their elementary schools, so they may be uninformed or have misconceptions about the role of the elementary school counselor.

Promoting the school counseling program and demonstrating its importance in the overall school program is a large task. The basic formula for beginning this task is relatively simple. In order to promote the school counseling program to parents, school counselors must commit themselves to three basic behaviors: *visibility, accessibility,* and *flexibility.*

VISIBILITY One way school counselors can promote a positive image is to simply "see and be seen." It was my experience that some parents perceived school counselors as school personnel who stay behind closed doors, and who are often in meetings or on the phone. This perpetuates the misconception that school counselors rarely participate in the day-to-day experiences of students, faculty, and parents.

Most school counselors promote their school counseling programs in writing. Letters, brochures, or booklets may be sent home to inform parents about the counseling services in the school. Distributing publications can be an effective and efficient way to help parents better understand the school counseling program. However, school counselors can also overtly promote school counseling by being *physically* visible in the school setting. Techniques might include:

- being present in common areas at the beginning and end of the school day;
- stepping to the doorway and observing as students are changing classes or transitioning from one period/block to the next;
- assisting parents who are signing students in and out of school, if extra help is needed during high traffic times in the office;
- attending PTO meetings or volunteering to be a faculty representative to PTO;
- dropping in to the cafeteria to check in with students;
- attending school events or assemblies, especially those involving student recognition or awards;
- attending after-school activities, such as athletic events, music or drama presentations, club or volunteer events; and
- being a presence during unexpected school emergencies, such as fire drills, unexpected dismissals, or lock down.

My Story

Often, I would find myself with a few minutes between obligations or meetings. I would take a walk down the hallway or around the building and just observe what was going on. I called this my "walk-about." Sometimes I was able to briefly connect with parents who were entering the building or volunteering in classes. Sometimes I would see a student in distress or who was seemingly distraught, and I would intervene to see if I could be of assistance. Other times, I would see a group of students who were trying to skip class or spend extra time getting from class to class, and I was able to avert behaviors that might have had negative consequences for the students. Usually, I would see parents as they were making their way from one place to another, dropping off students, or checking on something in the office. My walk-abouts accomplished two goals: (a) They gave me a break from the intensity of a previous meeting or session, and (b) they gave me the opportunity to be a visible presence in the building and get a feel for how the school day was going.

When parents observe the school counselor being involved in the school process and actively engaged with students and faculty, they may better understand the counselor's effect on the academic program. Whether or not their children have individual or group exposure to school counseling services, this understanding goes a long way toward helping parents appreciate the benefits of having counselors in schools.

ACCESSIBILITY While the primary focus of school counselors is student well-being, there is an undeniable responsibility to the parents of the students in a school. For this reason, it is critical that school counselors are accessible to parents as much as possible. When a parent contacts the school counselor about his or her child, the school counselor should respond expediently, if only to acknowledge that the parent's request will be addressed as soon as possible. For example, a school counselor might respond to a parent request by saying, "I appreciate you sharing your concern with me, Mrs. Johnson, and I want to meet with you to get more information. However, I have obligations to other situations today. Would tomorrow or one day next week work for you?" Failure to respond to requests from parents may result in frustration and a lack of confidence in the school counseling program.

In addition to being accessible by phone and e-mail, school counselors should allow time in their schedules to meet with parents face-to-face. This might require meeting before or after school hours if this is more conducive to parents' schedules. While most parents may access counseling services only a few times in their children's school careers, school counselors will fare well if they are open and accessible to parent requests.

FLEXIBILITY   The need for school counselors to maintain a flexible schedule is obvious, since no day is ever predictable. School counselors should try to maintain a schedule, but there must also be time to respond to the unexpected. Further, school counselors must become masters of prioritizing and respecting the immediacy of some situations. For example, if a parent comes to the counseling office and seems in dire need of the counselor's attention, it may be appropriate to postpone another obligation in order to address the immediacy of the parent's concern. Depending on the nature of the issue, the school counselor can either (a) inform the parent that he or she would like to discuss the issue when they have more time to address the problem or (b) inform the people involved in the other obligation that the meeting or event will need to be rescheduled.

An important aspect of informing others about the role of school counselors is to make everyone aware of the need for flexibility in the school counselor's day. Most school personnel understand that an emergency demands a quick response from the school counselor, and that other events can be rescheduled. Also, teachers, parents, or administrators may request a change in a scheduled event with the school counselor for a variety of reasons. School counselors understand the need for flexibility and honor these requests as much as their schedules allow. School counselors are obligated to make sure that if something must be postponed, it should be rescheduled as soon as possible. This is also true in the school counselor's interactions with parents. Parents will usually respond positively if they are acknowledged and understand that the school counselor is committed to focusing on their concerns as soon as possible. Being visible, accessible, and flexible may require greater effort on the part of school counselors, but will help them be perceived as partners to parents in the education process.

Parent Participation: The Key to Collaborative Relationships

BARRIERS TO PARENT INVOLVEMENT   Life circumstances sometimes prohibit parents from being actively involved in their child's school career. Thompson (2002) identified several potential barriers to parent involvement: time conflicts between work and school schedules, uncertainty about how to become involved, cultural and language barriers, discomfort in working with the school, lack of support in the community, and lack of support from the parents' workplaces (pp. 171–172). Employment circumstances, external obligations, and situations at home may prevent parents from being as involved in their child's school life as they might wish. The basic issues of time, family, work, and daily routines can certainly limit the availability of parents to participate in meetings or discussions about their children. School counselors should be aware and sensitive to these constraints on parents' time.

Another barrier to parent involvement might be cultural differences. The most basic issue may be communication. Sending home a request for a meeting may be futile if the letter is written in English and the language in the household is not English. Another cultural difference is the value of education. In some families, the children may be the first family members to have the opportunity to complete formalized education in the United States. Parents may believe that their only obligation is simply getting their child to school and that the school assumes sole responsibility for the child's educational progress. This perspective is not unique to specific cultures; many people from a variety of cultures believe that once their children are on the bus or have arrived at school, any issues that arise are the school's responsibility. One challenge for school counselors is to help parents feel that their input and involvement is necessary to their child's success in school. Other significant cultural issues were discussed in chapter 6.

A notable barrier for some parents is that they feel intimidated by school personnel. For example, when parents come into a child study/screening meeting about their child, there are typically several school personnel already in the room, including an administrator, the school psychologist, the student's teacher, and other school personnel who are trained to work with specific student issues. Walking into a room with these "experts" can be uncomfortable for parents. Despite best efforts to create warm and welcoming environments in schools, parents may be overwhelmed by the situation or their lack of experience with school personnel.

One strategy that school counselors can use to alleviate these concerns is to offer to consult with the parents prior to the meeting to explain what is going to happen at the meeting. By providing parents with information about the process of the meeting and who is going to attend and why, the school counselor can help parents feel more comfortable about meeting so many unfamiliar professionals. Additionally, the school counselor can also offer to meet with the parents after the meeting to answer any questions or clarify any aspects of the meeting. It is important to engage parents as much as possible in educational decisions about their children.

Another issue that can be a barrier to effective communication between parents and school counselors is embarrassment or the tendency to deny that there is a problem either with the student or the family. It is important for school counselors to empathize and realize that it is difficult for most people to admit there is a problem or ask for help. One way that school counselors can help parents feel more open to counseling interventions is to normalize the situation and help them feel they are not alone. The counselor may say, "You know, I have found that having parents who are willing to talk about issues or concerns is one of the greatest assets a student can have. I appreciate your willingness to do what is best for your child." A little positive reinforcement goes a long way.

A final barrier to effective communication, and one that may not be as obvious, is the general belief that schools sometimes request greater parental involvement in activities or tasks that seem to be the basic responsibility of the school. For example, if schools send home a letter requesting that parents spend extra time helping their children with homework or working on tasks that were never covered in school, parents may not respond positively. While this may not be an issue directly related to the school counseling program, parents who have these types of concerns about the educational program may contact the school counselor. Thus, school counselors may be mediators for parents who express frustration with school requests.

DEALING WITH RESISTANT PARENTS   The reality in schools is that many parents are not involved with their children's academic careers. Despite many efforts to engage parents, some simply will not participate. Communication by phone or e-mail and home visits may also be unsuccessful techniques for engaging parents. For school counselors, these situations can be extremely challenging and frustrating.

What can a school counselor do when a parent absolutely does not want to be involved? One recommendation is to communicate to the parent that his or her input is necessary to put or keep the student on track. School counselors should reach out to parents and help them understand the value of their input to their children's educations. This comes back to the notions of *availability* and *flexibility*. In essence, if a school counselor can make contact with a resistant parent, he or she can make it almost impossible for the parent to say no by being overly helpful: "Can we meet at a time that is more convenient for you?" "Do you need transportation?" "Can we bring in an interpreter?" "Would you like to bring someone else with you?" "What can we do to make this possible because we really need you to help us help your child?" These questions indicate that the school is willing to persevere in involving the parent in the child's education. Although this approach does not guarantee parent involvement, the parent will recognize that the school is willing to work with him or her in any way possible.

Parents may also be resistant to allowing their children to participate in school counseling services. In Virginia, for example, parents have the right to opt-out students from any counseling service, whether it is academic, personal/social, or career-related. There may be good reason for parents to feel that counseling should not be provided for their children in schools, and they have the right to refuse services. School counselors should not take this personally. Cuthbert (2002) encouraged school counselors to utilize counseling skills and techniques to address criticism from parents. Specific strategies might include "[s]haring facts about the program in question, explaining the goals and objectives of the program, maintaining professionalism, and refraining from becoming defensive . . ." (p. 85).

Many parents, like many people in general, view counseling through a negative lens, and do not believe that counseling can be a healthy or life-enhancing practice. School counselors can dispel these perspectives by demonstrating that counseling is a support system to help students be successful in

---
My Story

In my nine years as a practicing school counselor, there were only five students whose parents opted for them to be removed from the counseling program, mainly due to religious reasons. Despite meetings with the families and clear explanations about the content of the counseling program and the delivery of services, the parents who chose to opt-out their children felt that the content covered by counseling would be better addressed at home. It was also not unusual for parents to refuse permission for group counseling. Again, much of this seemed due to a parent's misunderstanding of the group content or the parent's denial of the student's need for counseling. I would often call the parent and explain in detail the group process, the topics to be covered, and the goal of the group. If the parent still denied permission, I respected the decision and continued to support the student as much as possible within the education program.

---

school, regardless of the nature of the problem. An important way to demonstrate this to resistant parents is through positive interaction with the students. It is possible that the students themselves are the school counselor's biggest advocates. Building positive relationships with students can be a catalyst for building positive relationships with parents if students feel the school counseling program is beneficial and integral to a positive school experience.

Soliciting Parent Participation: General Guidelines

There are three general methods for building parental support for the school counseling program: seeking parental input on program design, providing activities to foster parental involvement, and offering opportunities for parents to evaluate the counseling program.

INPUT ON DESIGN One of the best ways to involve parents in the school counseling program and the educational program overall is to solicit their input. Many authors (Schmidt, 2003; Baker, 2000; Gysbers & Henderson, 2000) have advocated for surveying parents or conducting needs assessments with parents to help with the design of the counseling program. If school counselors do not take parental input into consideration, they are missing information from key players in the education process. When people are asked for their input into a program, they tend to be more committed to that program. Therefore, if parent input or opinion is requested and taken into consideration for program planning, parents will feel more invested in the counseling program and are more likely to be supportive and involved.

Cuthbert (2002) suggested that involving parents in the design of the school counseling program can have several positive effects: greater insight into what parents want and expect for their children in schools, increased likelihood that skills learned through the counseling program will be reinforced at home; increased knowledge about the goals and objectives of the school counseling program; a sense of shared ownership in the school counseling program and greater support for program goals; and greater trust of and respect for school counseling and its purpose in schools (p. 81). Being asked for input and being told that it will be used when designing school counseling programs empowers parents and helps them feel that they are an essential component of the school counseling program. They will be encouraged to be more invested in counseling program goals and services.

ACTIVITIES THAT FOSTER PARENTAL INVOLVEMENT Another way to engage parents in the counseling program is to provide activities that involve parents in their child's academic success. These activities might include parenting programs in the community, information sessions on topics that are relevant to parents and their children (e.g., financial aid, college information), parent coffees or open forums at which relevant issues are discussed, or other activities at which parents might provide information, speak to students or other parents, or volunteer. Some parents do not participate in their children's educations because they feel they are unwelcome in the school. The more opportunities parents have to participate in school events, the higher the level of overall parental involvement. Therefore, school counseling programs should offer programs that are relevant to parents' needs. Another suggestion for engaging parent involvement is to provide transportation to and childcare at school events, or to conduct parent activities in various communities so that parents can attend.

PARENTS' EVALUATION OF THE PROGRAM It is sometimes difficult for a school counselor to ask parents for their opinions because it opens him or her up to criticism. However, parental evaluation of the school counseling program must be a key component of the ongoing evaluation process. If parents are dissatisfied with some component of the counseling program, school counselors should know so that the problem can be addressed. If parents feel that the school counselor considers their opinions and input to be valuable, they will be more likely to look for and support changes that are responsive to their needs.

If school counselors are to focus on systemic change, no part of the system can go unnoticed or unrecognized. Parental involvement can be a great asset to the school counseling program, and support from parents is essential in order to provide truly effective counseling programs in schools.

Conducting a Successful Parent Conference

There may be times when the school counselor will conduct a conference with parents and school personnel. It is essential to be prepared and to help everyone feel comfortable in the conference. Involving the student in the conference, if appropriate, is beneficial, particularly at the secondary level. Our professional practitioners offer sound suggestions for maximizing the success of parent conferences.

Professional Practice

RENEE (ES)

When I conduct a parent conference I try to establish a connection with the parents right away. I begin each conference with a positive comment regarding their child. I try to reflect the parents' feelings and validate their concerns. I may make a statement such as, "I know we're all here to do what is best for Bobby, let's put our heads together and see if we can develop some ideas about how to give him as much support as we can."

BETH (MS)

I always try to start a parent conference on a positive note and with a solution-focused approach. I might say, "I know we've all come here because we're concerned about Joey, and I was hoping that you could help us develop strategies for working with him more effectively." Also, we give the parents the chance to share what they see as their child's strengths and challenges. The parent's response is usually very enlightening because it indicates a great deal about the child's environment.

ESTHER (HS)

When conducting a parent conference, it is always important to establish parameters, goals, and a mutually agreed upon agenda. Once this is done, have everyone agree to the following items.

1. Establish a time frame for the conference, which includes an ending time.
2. Collectively problem solve and structure some kind of follow-up concerning the student's progress and the parent's concerns. Be sure to include the student in the problem solving.
3. Promote a positive, nonthreatening atmosphere. It is very intimidating to a student to have to face parents and teachers when they know they are not doing well.
4. Check with everyone present at the conference to ascertain if you have accomplished what you set out to address.
5. Summarize the key points.

Providing Parent Support

There is an assumption that when a parent makes contact with school personnel, it is to discuss a situation or concern about his or her child. Sometimes parents reach out for help with learning to parent more effectively. The school counselor is in a unique position to provide tremendous support for parents who are looking for ways to be better parents.

There are several ways that school counselors can provide support for parents. First, school counselors can plan and implement parent education programs—weekly or bi-weekly gatherings at which the school counselor leads sessions on parenting issues. Established programs that are often used include Active Parenting (Popkin, 2003) and Systematic Training for Effective Parenting (STEP) (American Guidance Service Publishing, 2003). These parenting curricula provide activities for parents to help them learn more effective parenting skills.

Another source of support for parents might be monthly Parent Nights. Conroy and Mayer (1994) suggested that school counselors provide monthly opportunities for parents to gather to discuss a parenting topic of interest. In their survey, the most popular topics included discipline, dealing with a strong-willed child, and helping the child be successful in school. The school counselors worked with the school's parent-teacher organization to provide materials for the workshops. Free childcare was provided and refreshments were served. Often in these informal, yet structured, meetings, parents become comfortable working with the school counselor on issues involving their children. School counselors can also feel they are providing an important service by helping parents learn how to help their children be more successful in school and at home.

A final way that school counselors can support parents is by developing a parent resource library. The library might offer books and literature on parenting; information on child and adolescent issues; community resources for health, social, or emotional needs; and contact information for mental health agencies and facilities in the community. Establishing a library of resources may take some time and involves gathering pertinent information. In addition, finding space to store these materials may be an issue that has to be addressed. Another important consideration in the development of these resources is to also make sure that teachers know the resources are available to parents. Providing resources is another way that school counselors can collaborate with teachers and parents.

These are just a few of the ways that school counselors can connect with and provide supportive services for parents. When parents feel they are working in a partnership with school personnel and the school counselor is at the forefront of developing positive interactions, effective collaboration has occurred and student needs can be approached in a more systemic manner.

REFLECTION AND DISCUSSION

1. As a new counselor in a school, what specific strategies would you use to connect with parents of students? What factors might you need to consider in your interaction with parents?

2. In some cases, the relationship between a student and his or her parents is a source of the difficulty the student is having. How would you approach parents about attending a meeting to discuss the student? What if the parents become defensive?

3. Providing support to parents is an essential practice for school counselors. As a school counselor, how would you promote this counseling service? What obstacles might arise in your efforts to be supportive to parents? How would you address these?

Working With Families in Schools: The School Counselor's Role

Family systems theory is certainly not a new concept in counseling. In the counseling field, working with families has been popular since the late 1960s. It is only recently that school counseling has focused on interventions that include families, not just individual students. The concept of *triangulation* (Bowen, 1978) described the effect of the family system on the individual. Triangulation occurs when two people in conflict project or deflect their tensions and anxieties onto a third party. The result may be that the third party (a) takes on the characteristics that have been imposed by the other two parties or (b) extends the pattern of interaction into other situations and relationships. For example, if parents are having difficulty in their marriage, it is not unusual to take the frustrations of the marriage out on one or more of the children or to involve a child as a confidante or ally. In turn, the child may exhibit more aggressive behaviors toward other students as a way of dealing with the frustrations at home.

Another caution involving triangulation is that the school counselor might be targeted or triangulated into the family system (Edwards & Foster, 1995). The family members may turn their hostility and frustration toward a classroom teacher, administrator, or school counselor. The school counselor can utilize counseling skills that help the members of the system refrain from blaming and determine the source of the problem. Keeping family members focused on the presenting problem and the development of solutions is one of the school counselor's tasks.

Hinkle and Wells (1995) defined family systems counseling as a theory that ". . . focuses on the structure, hierarchical relationships, and rules within the family" (p. 17). To try to help the individual student without understanding the family system seems to discount an important part of the equation. This is not to say that school counselors should engage in intensive and long-term counseling sessions with families in the school; it does, however, acknowledge that the student's issue should be considered in light of family situations and circumstances. It also suggests that if behavioral change is to be effective over time, the behavior must be practiced and reinforced in all settings (e.g., home, school, recreation, church).

A New Role for School Counselors

School counselors have not traditionally provided family counseling in schools. The current trend is for school counselors to be more directly involved in providing family counseling, with an overall focus on the difficulty the student may be experiencing in school.

One consideration for school counselors is the skills that are critical to effective counseling with families. Feature 9.1 lists several techniques that might be utilized in counseling sessions involving families. The skills described are not unfamiliar in counseling, but the context is different when working with families. Counseling skills should be adapted to the unique circumstances of the family and its members.

Stages in Family Counseling in Schools

Hinkle and Wells (1995) identified a process by which school counselors engage families in a student concern. The first task is making the initial contact to ask that the parent(s) or family members come in for a meeting with the school counselor (p. 59). The meeting may include other school personnel who have insight into the student's situation. If the family agrees to come in, it is important to have all parties define what they feel is the primary concern with the student. The student needs to be active in this process, since he or she knows the nature of the problem best of all. There is the possibility that one parent might not be able to or want to attend, in which case the counselor and participating parent should make a concerted effort to involve the parent who is not present in goal-setting or interventions that might occur.

Professional Perspective

RENEE (ES)

Often parents are feeling isolated and overwhelmed. Using your counseling skills with the parents will help you establish rapport and create an atmosphere of trust. Parenting is an extremely difficult job, and parents are usually doing the best that they know to do at any given time. Empathy and an attitude of collaboration, rather than approaching them like "an expert" who is critical of their parenting skills, will help combat feelings of defensiveness.

In this initial meeting, the school counselor would begin with the *social stage* (Hinkle & Wells, 1995, p. 64), in which developing a relationship with the family members is a priority. Acknowledging and appreciating a family's willingness to work with the school to address the student's issue reinforces the likelihood that they will be willing to meet again. During this stage, the school counselor can get a better sense of the family dynamic, the role of family members, and the problem relationships or interactions that might affect the student's behavior. This stage gives the school counselor insight into the workings of the family and may shed light on issues or dynamics that are related to the student's issue.

The next stage, according to Hinkle and Wells (1995), is the *problem stage*, in which the school counselor helps the student and the family members come

FEATURE 9.1
_____

Family Systems Counseling Skills

Joining

This technique involves basic counseling skills that are used to develop rapport, establish a relationship, and put family members at ease. One way to join all members of the meeting (especially if other school personnel are included) is to continually remind everyone that each member's goal is the same. For example, "I know we all have different concerns today, but it's important that we realize we are in agreement about wanting Devon to be successful in school and in life. I'm sure we all want the best for her." This strategy will be important in the later stages of counseling.

Normalizing and Reframing

For many parents and families, this will be their first counseling experience. They may feel very intimidated or uncomfortable with the counseling session and may perceive the entire situation negatively. This could result in blaming behaviors rather than focusing on a solution. The school counselor can reframe the situation in a positive light. For example, "I think that Luis may be acting out in order to get your attention. It says a great deal about how he feels about you to want to have your attention. Maybe we can focus on ways that the family can spend more time together."

Use of Siblings

Siblings are an important source of information and may have unique insight into a student's problem. They might be able to talk about what they observe at home and if they have noticed a difference between at-home and at-school behavior. Sometimes, though, siblings may try to sabotage each other, so it is important to make sure to hear each member's comments.

Daily Routine Questions

School counselors can learn a great deal about families by simply asking them to describe a normal day. Listening to responses and noting disparities in activities or perception of events may provide important information for the counselor. Discrepancies or disagreements may be the catalyst for change.

Solution-Focused Strategies

Using strategies such as finding exceptions to the problem situation or asking the "Miracle Question" might be appropriate to address the immediate needs of the student.

Encouragement

Constant encouragement and reinforcement to all members will help continue the counseling process. Parents may feel that they have failed at parenting, and the student may feel hopeless or may defiantly refuse to implement change. It is important to thank each member for coming and for the willingness to talk about issues. Even if little progress is made, the school counselor should acknowledge how hard it is to simply agree to meet. Refocusing on the common goal and encouraging members to implement any strategies for change will be helpful in engaging commitment from all members of the group.

Source: Adapted from Mullis, F., and Edwards, D. (2001). Consulting with parents: Applying family systems concepts and techniques, *Professional School Counseling,* 5(2), 116–123.

to some agreement about what the problem is (p. 66). The awareness of the problem may produce anxiety or heighten emotions as different members of the family discuss the problem (Edwards & Foster, 1995). This might involve intense dialogue and disclosure with regard to how the student responds to the family dynamic. In this stage, the school counselor may sense discomfort or dissension among family members. It is important to continue to remind parents and family members that the goal of these meetings is to help the student with the problem that is occurring at school. Any school personnel who have insight into the student's issue should also contribute to the problem definition stage. The school counselor can help the family or school members adjust and proceed to looking for solutions. Nicoll (1992) suggested that the school counselor direct the discussion by asking school personnel to identify specific problems they have observed.

> Beginning the session by focusing on the parents and home can mistakenly suggest that the school's problem is to be blamed on the parents. This will inevitably lead to resistance and defensiveness by the parents, and appropriately so. The counselor must start by obtaining a complete description of the school problem in behavioral terms. (Nicoll, p. 353)

Then, the school counselor can ask the parents what they observe at home. One strategy that can provide useful information is to have the parents describe a typical day at home. Asking specific questions about things such as schedules, sibling interaction, and outside activities may provide insight into other things that may be going on with the student.

The third stage is the *interaction stage* and is the action phase of the process (Hinkle & Wells, 1995, p. 68). This stage involves encouraging dialogue between the student and family members, the student and any involved personnel, and the family and school personnel. The question at this stage is: *Now that we have defined the problem, how will each part of the system address it?* This stage also includes goal setting and developing the steps to address the issue. If it is determined that the problem is most related to issues at home, the school counselor can work with the family to determine what steps need to be taken to address the issue. If the problem seems to be related to school, school personnel can decide how to proceed with the issue. If the problem appears to be affected by a combination or interaction of both, goals may be established for each environment. Deciding on specific steps to achieve behavioral goals is an important component of this stage. The next step is making sure each individual in the system is committed to the steps involved in reaching the established goals.

The final, yet ongoing, stage is *evaluation*. If a plan has been put into place, the family is committed to taking steps toward goals, and the school has committed to complementary action, there should be ongoing evaluation to determine if goals are being reached. Further, a follow-up session should be scheduled with all involved individuals. Nicoll (1992) suggested that the follow-up session occur one or two weeks after the plans are implemented. This commits all parties to the process and also provides impetus for assessment and evaluation to see if the plan is working.

If any person in the system neglects his or her responsibility, it is likely the results will not be positive. The metaphor might be a machine in which all of the parts are not working in sync; therefore, the machine does not work. In order for the student to have the greatest potential for success, all members of the support system must work together toward a common goal. The stages described require that school counselors possess and utilize effective counseling skills, including the ability to facilitate the process. Bemak (2000) made specific recommendations for facilitating cooperation with parents through effective collaboration, including developing family advocacy programs, including families in decision-making processes about their children, and utilizing strategies to make schools more responsive to family needs.

This section has discussed family counseling skills and strategies that might be implemented by a school counselor. While it may be idealistic to believe that school counselors should intervene with each student's family in order to maximize student success, school counselors need to recognize specific situations in which family intervention might be appropriate. Some student issues will be primarily school-related in nature and may not require a systemic approach. Other situations may involve problems within the family that are relevant to the student's problems in school and may be beyond the realm of the school counselor's training. School counselors will need to learn to recognize that any situation that does not improve after a few meetings is probably a situation that needs to be referred for outside family counseling.

REFLECTION AND DISCUSSION

1. As mentioned, some families are intimidated by meetings with school personnel. What could you do, as the school counselor, to help alleviate some of the negative feelings that family members might have toward the school?

2. A member of a family may not want to participate either in counseling or in working on the student's goal. How would you respond to dissension or lack of commitment to work on the student's problem?

3. Identify specific steps you would take when deciding whether to intervene with a family. Include a plan for any situation that might extend beyond your level of expertise.

Connecting With the Community: The School Counselor's Role

Chapter 4 discussed the need for a positive and collaborative relationship with community agencies in terms of referrals, consultation about students, and learning about the role of each agency in the community. Chapter 7 explored how school counselors can work with community-based student assistance personnel. Historically, there is evidence that the collaboration between school counselors and community agency professionals has not been very effective. A study by Hobbs and Collison (1995) suggested that school counselors rethink their role in working with community agencies. They recommended that school counselors understand their role in the context of the community and accept that utilizing outside resources does not undermine the effectiveness of counseling services provided in school (p. 63). Consultation and collaboration with community agencies throughout the counseling process can only enhance the efficacy of school counseling services for the student.

Keys and Lockhart (1999) concurred with this reformed role for school counselors and acknowledged the significance of a collaborative relationship with community agencies through prevention and intervention services that benefit students and families. Thompson (2002) also acknowledged the need to "[i]dentify and integrate resources and services from the community (health, social services, substance abuse, juvenile justice, recreation, service clubs, and organizations) to strengthen school programs, family practice, student learning, and personal development" (p. 174). Further, Bemak (2000) suggested that counselors work with community agencies in three ways: (a) linking students and their families to community resources based on unique needs (i.e., mental health, employment, health care); (b) coordinating with community services to bring them into the school as much as possible (e.g., substance abuse counselors who provide services to students during the school day); and (c) collaborating on the development and implementation of prevention and intervention services that may be provided inside or outside of the educational setting (p. 327). The community can serve as an important partner with schools to provide services for students. For example, many communities have before- and after-school day care opportunities in which the schools have joined with recreational departments in the community. These joint efforts lead to community-wide support for students and their families. Whether services are received inside or outside of school, the partnership is pivotal in the provision of services for students.

School counselors can work collaboratively with community partners to help provide useful services to all students based on their unique needs. For example, the school counselor or counseling office might be involved in disseminating information regarding summer programs, enrichment programs, camps, alternative education, or job opportunities for students. Further, providing information about service-learning projects through partnerships with community organizations or summer internships with local businesses might be another way school counselors promote this connection. Mentoring partnerships with local businesses also provide an opportunity for school counselors to make use of the assets in the community. These connections will enhance the services of the school counseling program, while also benefiting the community.

Many of the projects or relationships that form between schools and communities require proactive initiation of contact with community agencies. As a new school counselor, it will be critical to learn about the agencies, businesses, and opportunities in the community in order to tap into available resources. This connection will be important in a systemic approach to providing counseling services.

REFLECTION AND DISCUSSION

1. There has been a history of "turf" issues between school counselors and community mental health personnel. As a school counselor, how would you break down the barriers that separate the two? What specific actions would you take to try to promote a collaborative relationship with agency professionals?

2. Not every community has a large number of resource personnel. Imagine that you are a school counselor in a rural area with very few local resources available. How would you collaborate with professionals in neighboring schools and communities? What are specific ways that you would reach out for help?

3. What community services do you feel would be helpful in schools? How would partnerships with these agencies benefit students?

School–Family–Community Connections:
The School Counselor's Role

It is obvious that connecting schools, parents, and the community is critical to providing successful and comprehensive services for students. School counselors, as consultants and coordinators in the school, are certainly pivotal players in making this connection.

Much of what has already been said focuses on promoting interaction and collaboration of schools, families, and community agencies/personnel. Keys and Bemak (1997) identified critical tasks for school counselors in the process of linking schools, families, and communities, including developing or being a member of a mental health team. The role of such a team is to assess the needs of the student and the family, identify available community services and resources, and develop plans and goals for providing services to students and families. Taylor and Adelman (2000) asserted that the establishment of a school-based, resource-oriented team will help reduce fragmentation and will be cost-effective in terms of coordination and implementation of services. It will also prevent redundancy and unnecessary overlap in services provided.

School counselors should emphasize prevention rather than reaction (Keys & Bemak, 1997). Involving community agencies and connecting at-risk students and families with services before a situation becomes detrimental should be a major goal for school counselors. An important part of this step is to recognize when students and families are vulnerable and volatile.

School counselors should also seek training and professional development in skills related to short-term counseling and family counseling. Community agencies and mental health professionals should certainly be involved in these training opportunities, particularly if family counseling or short-term therapy is an area of expertise.

School counselors should be aware of the community resources that are available for families, including various cultural and ethnic groups (Keys & Bemak, 1997). Often, schools are a clearinghouse for the exchange of information and families that are new to a country or region may not be aware of the resources available to them. Ultimately, students suffer when basic needs are not met. Therefore, the school counselor is in an important position to help students and families adjust to life in a new country, community, and/or school.

Perhaps the most important task for school counselors is to serve as change agents. Clarifying misunderstandings or misconceptions about the role of schools and community resources will provide a greater and more effective working alliance. Keys and Bemak (1997) stated:

> In this role, the school counselor helps community agency professionals understand school climate, existing norms, policies and procedures, and the different responsibilities of other school personnel. At the same time, counselors can help school personnel and families understand how this new form of service can be of assistance and connect those in need of services with relevant programs. (p. 261)

It makes sense that students and families have more comprehensive and varied services when schools and communities work together. "Counselors should move quickly to play a greater role, a leadership role, in helping schools and communities restructure support programs and services to create comprehensive, multifaceted approaches to ensure all students succeed" (Taylor & Adelman, 2000, p. 306).

CONCLUSION

This chapter has focused on the necessity of collaboration and connection between schools, families, and communities. Students are naturally a part of all three systems—school, family, community. Therefore, counseling services should focus on integrating all three in order to meet the needs of students in a comprehensive program. Strategies for making the connection were offered throughout this chapter. In connecting with parents, school counselors must be willing to work with parents and meet them where they are in terms of how they participate in their children's educations. Further, school counselors must extend themselves to community agencies and professionals to try to integrate services and opportunities into the school program. These support systems are invaluable to the overall success of students. Finally, while the relationship might appear to be a triangle, it is advantageous to imagine it more like a circle, where schools, parents, and community all influence and work together, with the student as the focus. This joint effort ultimately fosters optimum student development, which is hopefully the shared goal of everyone involved.

REFLECTION AND DISCUSSION

1. Consider the collaborative relationship between schools–communities–families. On a sheet of paper, make three columns, with a heading for each (SCHOOL/COMMUNITY/FAMILY). List the unique assets and challenges for each group. Consider how each will help or hinder the other by engaging in a collaborative relationship. Discuss this with classmates.

2. If you are a new counselor coming into a school that seems resistant to utilizing community resources, how might you approach the issue with colleagues and administration? What would be your argument in favor of greater collaborative relationships?

3. What school, parent, family, or community issues do you think might hinder the development of collaborative working relationships? Anticipate the questions, concerns, or issues and discuss how you would respond to each.

CHAPTER 10

The Professional School Counselor as Leader

Contributed by Dr. Paul L. Phillips, State University of West Georgia; Dr. Susan Sears, Ohio State University; Dr. Brent M. Snow and Dr. C. Marie Jackson, State University of West Georgia

*T*his chapter begins the discussion of the transformed roles of school counselors. One of the roles emphasized in many school counselor training programs is leadership, a necessary component of effective school counseling programs. In this chapter, the authors first provide an overview of school counseling leadership and identify leadership skills that should be developed in order to ensure effective school counseling practices. The perspectives and practices of our veteran counselors are included. In addition, school counselors-in-training have the opportunity to assess personal leadership attributes and identify areas where leadership skills should be developed.

What Is Leadership?

A review of school counseling literature reveals that there are as many definitions of leadership as there are authors on the subject; however, most authors agree on some basic themes. The most obvious is that leadership occurs within a social context—an organization and its internal and external key stakeholders. For school counselors, the organization is, of course, the school. The internal stakeholders include students, teachers, administrators, and other support personnel. The external stakeholders include families, social agencies, businesses, government agencies, and others with vested interests. Another theme shared by many researchers is that leaders influence people. The kinds of influence range from authoritarian to inspirational. While an authoritarian leader motivates individuals through compliance with expectations, an inspirational leader motivates individuals through passion.

We offer the following definition of leadership: *the process of influencing others to create a shared commitment to a common purpose.* This definition has been influenced by such authors as Worzbyt and Zook (1992), Cash (1997), Peterson and Deal (1998), Henderson (1999), Schwahn and Spady (1998), and Zigarmi, Blanchard, O'Conner, and Edeburn (2000). Using this definition as a foundation, this chapter reviews the role of the professional school counselor as a leader and places this role in the context of the *Transforming School Counseling Initiative* (Education Trust, 2003), funded through a grant by the Wallace–Reader's Digest Fund and administered by the Education Trust in 1996. The majority of this chapter is dedicated to exploring the knowledge, skills, and values required of effective leaders. It concludes with a message to school counselors-in-training about the critical importance of the professional school counselor's role as a school-wide leader. This chapter provides the framework for chapter 11, which focuses on examples of responsive leadership in school counseling.

Leadership Challenges for School Counselors: A Historical Perspective

Historically, there have been several challenges that school counselors and school counselor training programs faced. The rapid growth of counseling in the 1950s and 1960s, as well as the public's expectations that guidance counselors would take the lead in helping all children meet their educational and career goals, created many challenges for school counselors. The most critical challenge was lack of sufficient training. Wittmer (2000) maintained that counselor education programs were not prepared for the consequences of the 1958 National Defense Education Act (NDEA), and therefore counselors were trained too quickly and insufficiently. Some counselors started their jobs without a clear understanding of their role in schools. Critics would argue that today's counselor education programs are still not preparing counselors to work effectively in the school context.

Another historical challenge emerged from the vague definition of the role and functions of school counselors. Role ambiguity for school counselors has been a problem for some time. As has been reiterated throughout this book, this challenge still presents itself in school counseling today. The role of leadership in school counseling establishes new challenges for practitioners: (a) to understand and advocate for the importance of comprehensive developmental school counseling programs in the overall educational arena, and (b) to assume a leadership role in the development and implementation of educational programs in order to define the roles and responsibilities of school counselors as contributors to student academic success.

Today's educators are hearing many of the same criticisms they heard in the 1970s, 1980s, and 1990s. Politicians and concerned citizens call for accountability in schools and improved student achievement almost daily. One of the American society's most pressing problems is the achievement gap between Black and Hispanic students and non-Hispanic whites. Poverty cannot explain all of the achievement gaps because both grade and test score disparities appear in middle-class communities with diverse schools. This gap has been documented since at least the 1960s. Between 1970, when the National Assessment of Educational Progress (NAEP) first began monitoring national achievement, and 1980, Black and Hispanic students made great strides in narrowing the gap that once separated them from white peers. However, beginning in 1988, African-American and Latino high school seniors on average scored at the same level as non-Hispanic white eighth graders on NAEP math and reading tests (Viadero, 2000). That disparity still exists today. Do counselors have a responsibility to address this issue? One could argue that counselors should be tackling this achievement gap by helping to identify the factors that contribute to the disparity between student groups. Professionally, school counselors should be catalysts for educational change and leaders in educational reform.

The School Counselor's Role as Leader

The new vision for school counselor roles (House & Martin, 1998) has moved beyond the old roles, which were often passive, reactive, and largely clerical in nature. Today's school counselor must accept the role of passionate leader and advocate for change. This new vision has been stated clearly in the Transforming School Counseling Initiative and advocated by The Education Trust (2000):

> Some school counselors might even deny that they are in a leadership role—especially that they are in an educational leadership role. If they have seen their primary domain as a mental health specialist in the school who works with persons who come to them or who are sent to them, then leadership may be an uncomfortable concept. . . . The mental health component remains, but the goal is not to be a counselor in private practice who works in the school. Brent Snow from the State University of West Georgia has stated the goal this way: "The school counselor is the mental health expert in the school. The school counselor is not the mental health counselor in the school." (p. 13)

Counselors impact the mission and the climate of the school through student advocacy efforts, which involve leadership for academic success, staff development, school reform, and institutional decision making (Clark & Stone, 2000). School counselors lead the way in identifying and removing barriers to high academic achievement and increasing learning opportunities for all students (Education Trust, 2003), but a unified approach is clearly needed. Individuals need the ability to succeed in a global society, and pressing issues in our society affect at-risk populations, minorities, and various other populations who have not always been served well in the school environment. The school counselor with strong leadership skills can lead the way to meeting student needs through team building with teachers, parents, administrators, and the community (Jackson, Snow, Phillips, Boes, & Rolle, 1999).

Professional Perspective

RENEE (ES)

I believe the school counselor is a leader in the school. He or she must model appropriate behavior and protocol in a variety of situations, serving as a leader for students, staff, and parents. Whether handling student disagreements, disgruntled parents, or crisis situations, the school counselor must lead by example. The school counselor will also serve as a leader by sponsoring student activities, such as peer mediation, or school-wide initiatives, such as character education. Staff members often view the school counselor as someone who is knowledgeable and capable, someone who has the characteristics and qualities of an effective leader.

School counselors must serve as proactive leaders for the school counseling program and develop the image of this program as central to learning, change, and improvement for all students. The school counselor is a school leader; however, it is critical to note that in this context leadership is not administrative, but refers to the action and impact the school counselor can demonstrate within the school environment. The opportunities for school counselors to be in contact with all those involved in the overall school program may be greater than for any other school personnel. This unique role of school counselors allows the school counseling program to be perceived as the center of school activity. It is important that school counselors be active on various work teams in order to lead in the development of school-wide programs that meet the changing needs of students. Working with various community members, parents, and the school faculty and staff, the counselor can lead in program improvement to increase the academic, social, and emotional growth of students. Further, the professional school counselor is a key leader in school and community collaboration (Jackson, et al., 2001) through sustained efforts to foster effective communication and purposeful interaction.

Research provides several examples of school counseling leadership activities that can be demonstrated through a variety of practices:

- development and presentation of local, regional, and national data to support the need for systemic change to better meet student needs (House & Martin, 1998);
- identification of resources and the implementation of linkages between the school, students, families, and the identified resource agencies (House & Martin, 1998; Jackson, et al., 2001);
- recognition and development of leadership skills in students (Gladding, 2000);
- identification of support systems and various safety nets for students to enhance success and achievement (Hart & Jacobi, 1992);
- overall development of the school counseling program and its implementation, from needs assessment to evaluation (Gysbers & Henderson, 2000);
- staff development programs and in-service programs for teachers and parents that create a shared vision of high expectations and high standards for all students and the perception that the school counselor and the school counseling program are integral parts of the overall school program (Myrick, 2003); and
- maintenance of a professional image by participating in professional, civic, and social organizations, furthering the attainment of the overall mission of meeting the needs of all students (Clark & Stone, 2000).

School counselors have always needed various leadership skills, such as planning, organizing, coordinating, implementing, monitoring, and evaluating.

Today's school counselors need to utilize these leadership skills in a focused manner to better meet the challenges facing 21st century schools. School improvement may seem to be merely a buzzword, but the realities of our rapidly changing global society speak loud and clear to the need for a better way of educating today's youth for success in school and life. School counselors can help all school stakeholders recognize the need for improvement and help develop plans for productive change.

Professional Perspective

ESTHER (HS)

The role of the school counselor encompasses many responsibilities, and changes as the needs of students change. Administering new tests, diversified staffing assignments, staff in-services, counseling groups, department liaison, faculty advisory committee representative, conference presenter, program promoter, publications editor, and program initiator could all be added to the list of leadership responsibilities that a counselor might have. Counselors do not simply "work a job," they "develop" the job. Showing initiative; being sensitive to the needs of students, faculty, and parents; and developing programs in response to these needs are all part of demonstrating effective and responsive leadership.

If students and their future contributions to society are central to the school reform movement, then it follows that school counseling programs are essential to this mission. For many years, the authors of school counseling literature have offered suggestions for planning development-based programs to meet student needs and evaluating student outcomes. School counselors must move beyond "talking a good game" and take action to develop effective programs for all students. Many researchers and authors have called for the design and delivery of uniform programs to ensure quality development and the survival of school counseling (e.g., Dahir, 2000; Gysbers & Henderson, 2000; Sears, 1999). Burnham and Jackson (2000) surveyed school counselors and concluded that the school counselors in their study continued to meet student needs largely through traditional means (i.e., individual counseling, scheduling, and advising). This study supported the need for continued efforts to transform the manner in which today's school counselors deliver effective counseling programs. Developing leadership skills in school counselors is of the utmost importance. Without the ability to use leadership skills at the most opportune time and in an appropriate manner, many opportunities for positive change can be lost. The students, their families, and the community are the recipients of the benefits of school counselors with strong leadership skills. Because of the likelihood that effective leadership in school counseling will perpetuate positive change in students, the remainder of this chapter is dedicated to the knowledge, skills, and values required for effective leadership.

Foundations of Effective School Counseling Program Leadership

A fairly well-defined body of knowledge about leadership has been developed in the last several decades. The knowledge base referred to in this section specifically relates to the definition of leadership provided at the beginning of the chapter: Leadership is the process of influencing others to create a shared commitment to a common purpose. This definition incorporates the following concepts: being mission driven, promoting core values, commitment as opposed to compliance, and shared responsibility. The following discussion of these concepts is provided as a basic foundation of knowledge in the area of leadership.

Mission Driven

To be mission driven is to constantly refer to the mission or organizational purpose when making decisions and taking action. Focusing on a specific purpose and working toward common goals are key elements of a mission-driven program. Whether in education or in other occupational areas, an effective leader knows the importance of a common purpose that is a viable, working dimension of an organization. In the school setting, the common purpose is the mission of the school, expressed in a clear and concise statement (Covey, 1989). A mission statement, developed as an outcome of a shared vision, generates unity, commitment, and focus among all those involved. A clear focus establishes direction for concrete action, to which stakeholders can become vigorously committed.

The process of developing a viable mission statement for the school or school counseling program requires participation of key stakeholders. Participation in developing a mission statement is one aspect of shared commitment. While it is not necessary that every parent and teacher participate in the process, they and other key stakeholders need to be represented on the team that develops a school or counseling program mission statement. An effective method for developing a mission is to establish a leadership or steering team composed of representatives from each group of stakeholders. The leadership team members need to communicate with their respective stakeholders to gather diverse input as the mission is developed. Gysbers and Henderson (2000) discussed the need for a steering committee, under the leadership of the school counselor, to guide school counseling program development. A school–community advisory committee can be an extension of the steering committee and a source of valuable input and support.

Presently, most schools have mission statements, and it is common to see these statements posted on school walls and printed in materials disseminated by schools. It is crucial that a mission statement functions as a working document. Effective leaders use mission statements to frame issues that will lead a mission-driven organization. They explore issues in the context of the mission. They ask questions such as, "How will this proposed program increase the academic achievement of all students, which is a part of our mission?" or "If we hire this new person, will he or she be a good addition to our staff and help us further our mission?" As the mission is used to guide decisions and take action, it becomes more than a statement posted around the school; it becomes a working document that is continuously evaluated for modification. A natural consequence of being mission driven includes functional alignment, which occurs as each function in the school is aligned with the mission. When aligned with the school's mission, developing curriculum, designing instructional activities, selecting faculty, and other functions contribute to a mission-driven school. The school counseling program mission must be considered in light of the overall school mission statement. An effective school counseling steering committee and/or advisory committee will align the program mission with the school mission. Carrying out functions aligned with the mission is evidence of shared responsibility and commitment by those involved.

Core Values

Effective leaders understand the importance of core values. Core values must be clearly stated and generally accepted. They are the values that key stakeholders believe are important. Evidence of core values is typically reflected in behavior. The core values of a school should be developed as mission statements are developed. These values are the shared beliefs that guide an entire school, as well as the school counseling program plan and design. Core values may be influenced by a number of factors, such as the demographics of the school population, geographic location of the school, local financial support for education programs, and availability of resources to address mission goals. With these considerations in mind, it is critical that the school counseling program personnel identify and describe the shared values on which the program is founded. Further, these core values, once identified, should be the basis for the development, implementation, and maintenance of school counseling program goals and services.

Commitment Versus Compliance

As individuals become dedicated to the school mission, they become motivated. Their motivation becomes commitment to the mission and its accomplishment. A commitment is self-initiated from a desire to be a part of the organization and to contribute to the mission of the school. As a result, the school culture becomes one of commitment based on shared values. Motivation through commitment is important, valuable, and useful when making decisions, taking action, and using resources.

In contrast, an organization in which individuals are motivated by compliance requires a different kind of leadership. Leadership of individuals motivated by compliance is different from leadership of individuals motivated by a shared commitment. It is a type of leadership that emphasizes the expectations of the leader and requires the leader to guide individuals toward meeting those expectations. While both commitment and compliance can be mission driven, complying with the expectations of the leader generates motivation, but only in terms of the leader's vision and mission. That is, the group is motivated in compliance with the leader's goals. On the other hand, the leader of a committed organization motivates commitment to the mission through an outgrowth of shared values and beliefs. This requires the development and demonstration of effective leadership skills, such as encouraging teamwork and collaboration as the organization tries to achieve the mission through shared goals and vision.

Effective School Counseling Leadership: Skills, Qualities, and Values

There are essential skills, professional qualities, and personal values that contribute to effective leadership. These factors can be assessed through self-reflection and feedback from others. Based on these assessments by self and others, a leader can increase his or her effectiveness (Bennis & Namus, 1985; Zigarmi et al., 2000). We recommend the Leadership Development Profile (LDP) (Phillips, 2000) as an instrument to be used for leadership development. A copy of the profile is located in Feature 10.1. The LDP identifies and describes 21 key indicators of leadership that comprise the skills, qualities, and values of effective leaders. School counseling and leadership literature support the skills, qualities, and values defined by the LDP (Leithwood, Jantzi, & Steinbach, 1999; Burns, 1978).

The LDP enables a leader to reflect on self and on systematic feedback from others. It offers a rating scale for each of the 21 indicators: (a) extraordinary—so remarkable that few (three or four people) could receive this rating; (b) excellent—outstanding and constant; (c) good—solid and consistent; (d) area to develop—an area that can be improved, but is not necessarily a weakness; (e) not observed—not necessarily applicable.

We encourage school counselors-in-training, as well as practicing school counselors, to carry out a self-assessment. Complete the profile in Feature 10.1 before continuing in this chapter. As you review your responses, read the description of each key indicator in the remainder of the chapter. Then seek a trusted colleague or peer with whom you can share your self-assessment and discuss the accuracy of your assessment. In the following material, the key indicators of leadership used in the self-assessment are discussed.

Indicators of Effective Leadership

As you review your responses to the LDP, refer to the following material, which discusses the key indicators of effective leadership and the implications for school counselors.

FEATURE 10.1

The Leadership Development Profile

Instructions: This Leadership Development Profile (LDP) is designed for self assessment, as well as assessment by others. As you reflect on each key indicator, place a check next to the category that most accurately describes your assessment. If you wish to qualify your assessment, space is provided for comments.

Key Indicators of Leadership

Vision—The capacity to see beyond the current status and formulate other possibilities

___ Extraordinary ___ Excellent ___ Good
___ Area to develop ___ Not observed

_____

_____

Unity—The ability to build unity within an area of responsibility, between areas of responsibility/departments, and throughout the school

___ Extraordinary ___ Excellent ___ Good
___ Area to develop ___ Not observed

_____

_____

Continuous Improvement—The insight to see improvements that can be made, to coordinate resources, to take initiative to make those improvements, and to monitor action in order to assure the effectiveness of the action

___ Extraordinary ___ Excellent ___ Good
___ Area to develop ___ Not observed

_____

_____

Custodial Care—The value of making decisions and taking action as a temporary custodian of the school; to seek in every way to make the school stronger and more effective in a non–self-serving manner

___ Extraordinary ___ Excellent ___ Good
___ Area to develop ___ Not observed

_____

_____

Teamwork—The skill of getting associates to work together toward common goals in a non-blaming, supporting, problem-solving manner

    __ Extraordinary   __ Excellent   __ Good
    __ Area to develop   __ Not observed

_____

_____

Reliability—The skill of meeting commitments on time and responding in a timely manner to requests; to follow through to completion of a task

    __ Extraordinary   __ Excellent   __ Good
    __ Area to develop   __ Not observed

_____

_____

Integrity and Trust—The quality of maintaining the standard of integrity required to gain trust from associates, students, parents, and community stakeholders

    __ Extraordinary   __ Excellent   __ Good
    __ Area to develop   __ Not observed

_____

_____

Commitment—The quality of delivering consistent and dedicated support of the mission and core values of the school

    __ Extraordinary   __ Excellent   __ Good
    __ Area to develop   __ Not observed

_____

_____

Problem Analysis—The ability to recognize interrelationships of problems; to be perceptive; to see the major parameters of a problem; to consider the complexity of the many facets that a problem may have

    __ Extraordinary   __ Excellent   __ Good
    __ Area to develop   __ Not observed

_____

_____

(Continues)

Decisiveness—The ability to choose quickly at times; to decide what to do about an issue and take action; to identify, choose, and balance between needs, alternatives, and actions

__ Extraordinary   __ Excellent   __ Good
__ Area to develop   __ Not observed

_____
_____

Planning and Organizing—The ability to plan an approach before taking action; to organize information and resources; to define tasks and prioritize; to establish objectives and measures; to consider contingencies

__ Extraordinary   __ Excellent   __ Good
__ Area to develop   __ Not observed

_____
_____

Strategic Thinking—The process of analyzing a range of strategies and selecting the most effective strategy for meeting a commitment, accomplishing an objective, and furthering the mission of the school

__ Extraordinary   __ Excellent   __ Good
__ Area to develop   __ Not observed

_____
_____

Judgment—The ability to take into consideration the multitude of possible ramifications of a decision or an action

__ Extraordinary   __ Excellent   __ Good
__ Area to develop   __ Not observed

_____
_____

Communication—The skill of effectively listening, speaking, and writing in order to achieve a clear and accurate mutual understanding between self and others

__ Extraordinary   __ Excellent   __ Good
__ Area to develop   __ Not observed

_____
_____

Resolve Issues—The skill of identifying issues in a straightforward manner, facilitating genuine discussion, and achieving a consensus on how to resolve issues

__ Extraordinary   __ Excellent   __ Good
__ Area to develop   __ Not observed

Shared Responsibility—The ability to lead individuals so that everyone assumes responsibility for the results of their work and the work of others on the team; acknowledges mistakes; takes corrective action; and believes the entire team is responsible for its decisions and actions

__ Extraordinary   __ Excellent   __ Good
__ Area to develop   __ Not observed

Advocacy—The valuing of equity and justice for all students; taking action on behalf of individuals and groups to correct inequitable, unjust situations

__ Extraordinary   __ Excellent   __ Good
__ Area to develop   __ Not observed

People Skills—The insight and emotional capacity to interact with people in a problem-solving (non-blaming), exploring (non-restrictive), creative (non-traditional), challenging, and supporting manner

__ Extraordinary   __ Excellent   __ Good
__ Area to develop   __ Not observed

Compassion—The capacity to recognize, embrace, and support individuals in need

__ Extraordinary   __ Excellent   __ Good
__ Area to develop   __ Not observed

(Continues)

Consensus Building—The ability to listen accurately and effectively so that individuals disclose concerns and raise issues before the group in order to achieve consensus of the group

___ Extraordinary   ___ Excellent   ___ Good
___ Area to develop   ___ Not observed

_____

_____

Initiative—To make recommendations and offer suggestions; to express a position on issues; to offer ideas for consideration

___ Extraordinary   ___ Excellent   ___ Good
___ Area to develop   ___ Not observed

_____

_____

Source: Phillips, P. (2000).

VISION   Vision is the capacity to see beyond the present situation and formulate other possibilities. Visionary leaders employ reflection to consider possibilities. They look at their schools and their key stakeholders and formulate possibilities by seeking answers to questions such as "Could we . . . ?" or "What about the possibility of . . . ?" Visionary leaders are restless because they are not satisfied with the status quo. This restlessness is quieted by a belief in possibilities. The possibilities are an outgrowth of the optimistic nature of visionary leaders. As they talk about their visions, they often excite and inspire others. They believe and have confidence in the capacity of their associates to change. Chapter 8 discussed the development of a shared vision between the school counselor and school administration. Effective leaders continue to work toward a shared vision with all school personnel to build consensus and commitment to the school mission.

UNITY   Unity refers to the ability to build a sense of community or togetherness within an area of responsibility, between departments or groups throughout the school. Effective leaders build unity between people. They understand the power of synergistic energy, or energy that comes from individuals supporting and believing in each other. It is not enough that school counselors build unity within their counseling programs. They must also build unity throughout the entire school; they must champion the theme "Together we can." There is a certain amount of humility required to build unity among individuals. Leaders who are able to give credit to others, even at their own expense, will be more effective in their ability to unify people. The greater the sense of unity in a school, the more focused individuals can be in carrying out their common purpose. Chapters 7, 8, and 9 emphasized the school counselor's role in collaboration with stakeholders in schools. Developing the ability to unify others around a common goal is part of the collaboration process and a necessary skill for school counselors.

CONTINUOUS IMPROVEMENT The capacity to improve requires having the insight necessary to identify improvements that can be made, coordinate resources, take initiative to make those improvements, and to monitor action in order to assure the effectiveness of the action. Continuous improvement is a daily, moment-by-moment awareness of opportunities for improvement. This awareness is of little value unless action is taken to implement improvements. A common roadblock to continuous improvement is the belief that "hitting a home run" is necessary to improve—improvement must be immediate and resolve all issues. This "all or nothing" thinking can be detrimental. Instead, effective leaders believe that any improvement, regardless of how small, is good. Every action that results in making schools better for students is signifi-cant. As improvements are made and then monitored to ensure that the change lasts over time, the school is continually being improved. School counselors must constantly monitor and evaluate the school counseling program to make improvements that will benefit students.

CUSTODIAL CARE Custodial care refers to the value of making decisions and taking action as a temporary custodian of the school. Effective leaders seek ways to make the school stronger and more effective in a non–self-serving manner. Leaders who understand custodial care want their schools to be stronger and better when they leave. They know that for a relatively short period of time, a few years for some and 25 or 30 years for others, they are entrusted with the care of a school. They realize the school is more important than they are as individuals, and their role as leaders is to serve the school and its key stakeholders. This realization is critical for school counselors because caring is a natural quality for most school counselors. Assuming responsibility for the care of others is a huge responsibility and a demonstration of committed leadership.

TEAMWORK The skill of motivating associates to work together toward common goals in a non-blaming, supportive, problem-solving manner is called teamwork. Effective leaders build teams and believe that teams make more sound decisions than do individuals. Team building leaders delegate respon-sibilities, as well as the authority to carry out those responsibilities, to teams. A team leader thwarts blaming and emphasizes problem solving. School coun-selors demonstrate leadership through collaborating with other stakeholders in the educational environment, identifying the roles that each will assume, and deciding how each person contributes to the school mission.

RELIABILITY Reliability refers to the skill of meeting commitments on time and responding in a timely manner to requests, as well as following a task through to completion. Reliable individuals pay attention to detail, make schedules, and meet their schedules. They foresee commitments that cannot be met and notify others in advance. The more leaders are reliable, the more they influence others. This leadership role for school counselors has been addressed in previous chapters, but the need for consistency, reliability, and dependability should be further emphasized.

INTEGRITY AND TRUST School leaders must possess the quality of maintaining a standard of integrity that will engender the trust of associates, students, parents, and community stakeholders. The integrity of leaders is measured to a large extent by the level of trust others place in them. Marginal integrity equals marginal trust, and no integrity equals no trust. Trust between leaders and their associates is developed when leaders place the interests of others above their own. Developing trust takes time, but leaders who make their personal and career goals secondary to the needs of others in the organization are able to develop trust. School counselors must demonstrate the ability to trust and be trusted so that others perceive them as effective leaders.

COMMITMENT Commitment refers to consistent and dedicated support of the mission and core values of the school. When individuals are motivated by commitment to the mission rather than by compliance to expectations of leaders, they share dedication to the common purpose of the school. Effective leaders are skilled in persuasion and inspire others to make a shared commitment. School counselors demonstrate commitment through obvious actions and interactions that promote the school counseling program, as well as the school's mission and goals.

PROBLEM ANALYSIS A leader skilled in problem analysis possesses the ability to recognize the interrelationships of problems, be perceptive, see the major parameters of a problem, and consider the complexity of a problem. Problem analysis is a skill effective leaders use in a multifaceted manner. Recognizing and considering a range of alternatives for solving a problem is fundamental to analyzing and solving problems. Effective problem analysis involves openness and the ability to dialogue with others. School counselors are specifically trained to address problems and seek solutions that benefit all involved individuals.

DECISIVENESS Decisiveness is the ability to quickly identify an issue, choose a course of action, and balance the needs of all those involved. Decisiveness to some extent requires a willingness to be responsible and accountable for a decision. It also requires effective leaders to refrain from allowing their needs to prevent them from making decisions. Decisiveness requires knowledge of the situation, including an awareness of the needs of the students and the school, and an element of wisdom. For school counselors, some decisions are difficult, and others may not agree with a school counselor's decisions. School counselors demonstrate effective leadership when they adhere to a decision that will be most beneficial for students, even when the decision may be unpopular.

PLANNING AND ORGANIZING Leaders must possess the ability to plan an approach before taking action; to organize information and resources, define tasks, and prioritize; to establish objectives and measures; and to consider contingencies. Planning and organizing are skills for focusing time, space, people, money, and other resources on the school's mission. The greater the command of resources, the broader the responsibility and influence will be. The involvement of others in planning and organizing helps develop commitment. The Career Week example in chapter 4 illustrates how school counselors utilize these effective leadership skills.

STRATEGIC THINKING Strategic thinking is the process of analyzing a range of strategies and selecting the most effective strategy for meeting a commitment, accomplishing an objective, and furthering the mission of the school. Leaders who need to be right often miss the concept of effectiveness. An individual may be right and at the same time ineffective. In the arena of strategic thinking, it is important to be both effective and right.

JUDGMENT Leaders must possess the ability to take into consideration all possible ramifications of a decision or an action. Sound judgment requires foresight. The capacity to make reasonable decisions requires discernment— the ability to understand the dynamics between the impact of a decision and the responses of those impacted. While judgment may be an internal attribute, school counselors often develop this leadership skill with time and experience in the school counseling job.

COMMUNICATION Being a skilled communicator means effectively listening, speaking, and writing in order to achieve a clear and accurate mutual understanding between self and others. Effective communication is a means for developing relationships and for building an atmosphere of inclusion. Individuals who are not informed can feel isolated. The skill of accurately listening to others so that they feel understood helps establish solid relationships. Being able to say what you mean when speaking and writing allows others to view you as solid and predictable. Because communication is the crux of a school counselor's interactions with others, this skill must be developed early in one's school counseling training program.

RESOLVING ISSUES The ability to resolve issues requires the skill to identify issues in a straightforward manner, facilitate genuine discussion, and achieve a consensus on how to resolve issues. Leaders demonstrate a noticeable degree of influence as they skillfully resolve issues between disputants. Leaders who are secure are able to place hidden agendas before everyone involved and thereby bring resolution to problematic issues. School counselors can demonstrate problem resolutions through effective intervention and by following through when addressing student issues.

SHARED RESPONSIBILITY   Shared responsibility refers to the ability to lead individuals so that everyone assumes responsibility for the results of their work and the work of others on the team. Each team member acknowledges mistakes, takes corrective action, and believes the entire team is responsible for its decisions and actions. Leaders generally accept responsibility for themselves. Effective leaders also assume responsibility for others. They believe errors in judgment, ineffective programs, and failure are shared problems. They skillfully avoid blaming others and openly acknowledge their responsibility in all issues. The school counselor can emulate shared responsibility through participation in activities such as curriculum development, discipline policy development, and other activities that may not be specific to the school counseling program but are related to the overall educational program and academic success of students.

ADVOCACY   Effective leaders value equity and justice for all students and take action on behalf of individuals and groups to correct inequitable, unjust situations. At the heart of the mission of almost all schools is a dedication to students. It is critical for school leaders to advocate for the removal of impediments to learning. An effective leader will model advocacy and encourage recognition of barriers, including inequitable, unjust policies, procedures, and situations. Further, effective leaders will encourage follow-up action to alter those circumstances. Chapter 12 will further discuss advocacy as a leadership skill.

PEOPLE SKILLS   Possessing the insight and emotional capacity to interact with people in a problem-solving (non-blaming), exploring (non-restrictive), creative (non-traditional), challenging, and supportive manner is essential to effective leadership. Leaders must balance the challenges and support they offer to students. In some instances, too many challenges can generate anxiety and hinder performance. However, too much support and entitlement may also hinder performance. Providing sufficient challenges and sufficient support enhances performance. Of course, performance in this instance means making a contribution that furthers the school mission. Because of the constant interaction with faculty, parents, students, administrators, and community members, the ability to work with and relate to people is a mandatory skill for school counselors.

COMPASSION   Compassion is the capacity to recognize, embrace, and support individuals in need. The value of compassion is especially important in the context of sound judgment. Compassionate leaders earnestly consider individuals as persons and have the foresight to consider the impact of a decision or action on others. To recognize individuals in need and neither embrace nor provide support for them is negligent. The nurturing nature of most school counselors is an obvious example of compassion. School counselors serve as leaders by modeling compassion in their interactions with others.

CONSENSUS BUILDING   Consensus building is the ability to listen accurately and effectively so that individuals disclose concerns and raise issues before the group in order to achieve an agreement that all members of the group are able to accept. Organizations, schools, leadership teams, committees, and other groups with members who are able to establish consensus on issues are more effective. The greater the consensus on important decisions, the greater the individual support for the group goals. A consensus underlies an attitude of "community of mind," which permeates successful schools. School counseling programs that demonstrate high levels of consensus with other stakeholders will have an increased likelihood of student achievement and success.

INITIATIVE   Leaders must be able to make recommendations and offer suggestions, express a position on issues, and offer ideas for consideration. To initiate is to start something rather than respond to something. While being a visionary is a key indicator of leadership, initiative is an important ability of effective visionaries. To merely consider alternatives to the current situation without taking the initiative to realize a new vision will result in ineffective leadership. Without taking the first step toward achievement of an identified goal, the goal will never be accomplished. School counselors who maintain the status quo and do not initiate new and innovative ideas may have difficulty in a leadership role. However, effective leadership can be accomplished when school counselors are willing to take risks and take the lead in new challenges.

These 21 indicators of leadership are the basis of the Leadership Development Profile. This instrument has been used with several groups in leadership development settings and has received positive feedback from individuals who reflected on the various ratings from self, peers, and supervisors. Responses indicated that the LDP enhanced self-understanding and insight regarding strengths and areas in need of development.

CONCLUSION

Counselor educators, as well as practitioners, have generally focused on the specific skills associated with theories and techniques of counseling and psychotherapy. As important as this knowledge base is, leadership skills will be critical in the 21st century work of the professional school counselor. The counseling profession has done an excellent job in providing counseling skills training over the past few decades. In the future, leadership skills, identity, and focus will be required areas of emphasis. The school counselor should assume a leadership role and be identified as the key person in the school who maintains a focus on understanding the needs of all students and advocating for student success. The school counselor should be aware of the "pulse" of the school community and the leadership opportunities in the school counseling and education programs. With the opportunities and responsibilities inherent in the position, the school counselor is, and must be, a leader. Without leadership, the role of the professional school counselor is diminished, and the positive influence of school counselors may be diluted.

This chapter has provided an overview of the professional school counselor as a leader in the school. It is the hope of the authors that the Leadership Development Profile presented in Feature 10.1 will be useful for developing and strengthening leadership skills both for students in school counselor education programs and for practicing school counselors. The next chapter will provide examples of leadership programs and opportunities in which school counselors can be involved and demonstrate effective leadership.

REFLECTION AND DISCUSSION

1. Leadership roles for school counselors may take many forms. Consider the programs and services that are part of a comprehensive counseling program. List as many leadership roles as you can for a school counselor at any school level.

2. Sometimes, leadership can be ineffective. Under what circumstances do you think that a school counselor's attempts at leadership might be negative or ineffective? Identify ways to overcome barriers to effective leadership.

3. There is the misconception that leadership implies being "in charge." In what circumstances or situations should school counselors not take on leadership roles? Think of specific examples in which leadership and being in charge may not work well together.

4. Complete the Leadership Development Profile (LDP) in Feature 10.1. If you are not currently in a school counseling position, project how you might function as a leader in the school as a school counselor. Based on your self-assessment, what key indicators do you find are areas of strength for you? What areas need further development in order to help you become a more effective leader?

CHAPTER 11

The School Counselor as Responsive Leader: School Violence Prevention and Crisis Intervention

*B*ased on the school counselor's specialized training and skill development, he or she may take on various leadership roles in school programs. Chapter 10 discussed a variety of skills that are indicative of effective leadership. School counselors often assume the important leadership role of responding to current issues that are relevant to the school setting. The violent events that have occurred in our schools in the last decade have prompted society and schools to consider why children and adolescents are so angry. Were we paying attention as children were harassed and became more and more frustrated? Why didn't we see the signs or investigate more closely when students acted out or became withdrawn? These are questions that have been asked often in the last few years.

School counselors may assume consultative, collaborative, and/or coordination roles in the implementation of violence prevention and crisis intervention programs. In some schools, counselors may serve as leaders or coordinators for special programs in the school, such as character education or peer mediation. In other schools, counselors may serve as team members or support resources for other school personnel who are implementing schoolwide programs. Regardless, school counselors should be involved, since they are specifically trained in programs that promote a positive and supportive school environment.

This chapter focuses on the school counselor's role as a responsive leader in school violence prevention and crisis intervention. In particular, the chapter will address the school counselor's involvement with bullying and harassment programs and prevention efforts. Further, we will also explore intervention programs, such as the school crisis response team, and the school counselor's potential for involvement with crisis intervention. In general, the school counselor should be at the forefront of efforts to create a school climate that promotes peace in order to facilitate learning.

Research on School Violence

School violence can range from minor incidents to major life-threatening events. Hanke (1996) suggested that school violence behaviors exist on a continuum. On one end are behaviors such as teasing and bullying and on the other end are more severe behaviors, such as homicide and suicide. Regardless of the position on the continuum, all violent behaviors lead to disruption of the educational process and, even worse, trauma for the victims, the perpetrators, and the observers.

In 2001, the National Center for Student Aspirations (NCSA) (2001) conducted a nationwide Web-based survey of nearly 70,000 students in grades 6 through 12 and asked for their perceptions of school climate. Slightly more than half (59%) reported feeling safe at school. However, the Josephson Institute of Ethics (2001) surveyed 15,877 middle and high school students and found that 43% of high school and 37% of middle school boys felt that it is

"OK" to hit or threaten a person who makes them angry. Nearly one in five (19%) of the girls surveyed concurred. Researchers have also sought to identify those people that students turn to for help. Sadly, surveys have indicated that students do not feel they can turn to anyone. A recent survey of 477 teens (The Empower Program, 2002) found that 50% would tell their parents if they were being harassed, yet only 16% of the students would speak with a teacher. School counselors fare only slightly better. The survey indicated that only 22% of students would tell a guidance counselor or school administrator.

Responding to crises or violence in schools is an important role of school counselors. According to Caplan (as cited in Poland & McCormick, 1999), crisis intervention occurs at three levels:

1. *Primary*—the activities devoted to prevention of crisis;
2. *Secondary*—the steps taken in the immediate aftermath of a crisis; and
3. *Tertiary*—follow-up assistance after the crisis.

The next section will discuss examples of *primary* crisis intervention and the role that school counselors play in the prevention of violence at school.

Primary Crisis Intervention: Violence Prevention Programs

Recently, schools have made efforts to implement programs that prevent violence prior to catastrophic events similar to the Columbine massacre. Feature 11.1 outlines the horrific events of that tragic day. Among the reasons that these two young men attacked their fellow classmates and then killed themselves were claims that they had been ignored, teased, and made to feel like outcasts by their peers and the school personnel. No interventions had occurred to help these students deal with the issues that upset them to the point of homicide and suicide. Could prevention programs have been effective? Would a supportive relationship with a school counselor have made a difference? Obviously, we will never know; but an intervention, even at the most primary level, might prevent tragic events. According to Glasser (2000), "What all these violent students share is exactly what the violence-prevention program is designed to address. They lack good relationships with warm, caring, responsible adults. . . . The success of the program will be directly related to how well the counselors can do this" (p. 79).

Research supports the development of a variety of violence prevention programs. Because there does not appear to be a single solution to the problem of violence in schools, Peterson and Skiba (2001) suggested that the implementation of multiple programs that focus on changes in the school climate has a more positive effect on student behavior and learning. They identified five key approaches to improving the school climate and preventing school violence: (a) parent and community involvement (which was discussed in chapter 9), (b) character education, (c) violence prevention and conflict resolution curricula, (d) peer mediation, and (e) bullying prevention. The following discussions

FEATURE 11.1

Student Violence at Columbine High School

It was an ordinary Tuesday morning at Columbine High School on April 20, 1999. The students had gone through their regular routines, attending classes, forgetting assignments, laughing as they walked down the hall. No one knew that the events that would occur later that day would inevitably change their lives forever. The following is a timetable of the events that are to live in infamy as one of the most tragic days in our nation's school history.

11:00 a.m. Several hundred of Columbine's 900 students head to the cafeteria for lunch. Others are in class or have gone to the library.

11:30 a.m. Dylan Klebold and Eric Harris, wearing black trench coats, arrive at school. They pull out weapons and begin firing at students in a student parking lot. They walk into the cafeteria, shooting as they go, and then proceed upstairs to the library, still shooting. Some students later reported they were shouting that they were going to "kill all the jocks"; other students simply remember running for cover or running for their lives. In the library, Klebold and Harris massacre several students while leaving others untouched. One reporter wrote: "Some kids play dead. By the time it is over, 12 aren't playing." Some time after killing their classmates, Klebold and Harris turn their weapons on themselves and fire.

12:00 p.m. While the shooting has been going on inside, small explosions are signs that bombs have been planted throughout the school building. Police SWAT teams are now surrounding the building and are trying to usher more and more students out of the building. Ambulances begin to take the first wounded students to local hospitals, the media begin to arrive, and parents hope that their children will emerge from the building.

12:30 p.m. Since gunshots are no longer being heard, SWAT teams begin entering the building and doing a room-by-room sweep of the high school.

2:30 p.m. SWAT teams continue to free students and teachers who have been in hiding. Everyone exiting the building is told to put their hands behind their heads so that they can be frisked; they are also questioned and offered medical care before being bused to a local elementary school.

> 4:30 p.m.   The school is declared safe and SWAT teams survey the dev-
> astation.
>
> The identity of those killed is uncertain as parents wait for children who
> are not coming out of the building. The bodies will have to remain for
> another day before being sent for formal identification and autopsies. A
> medical examiner pronounces 13 dead—1 teacher, 10 students, and the
> 2 students whose anger consumed them.
> The investigation begins, and the horror of this day never ends.
>
> *Source:* Adapted from Anthony, T. (2002). Reconstructing the Columbine Horror, *The Daily
> Camera*. Retrieved May 9, 2002, from http://www.thedailycamera.com/shooting
> /reconstruction.html.

of these programs emphasize the school counselor's role as school leader in
effectively developing and implementing school violence prevention programs. Although bullying is a form of harassment, we will focus on bullying in
isolation, and then discuss harassment in terms of sexual harassment.

Bullying and Harassment Prevention Programs

One characteristic common to students who exhibit violent behaviors is that
they act out because they "can't take it anymore." According to Hazler and
Carney (2000):

> Violence does not begin with gang warfare, rape, murder, and suicide. That is
> when society becomes afraid of violence. Instead it begins as put downs,
> insults, threats, harassment and bullying, where inappropriate lessons of how
> to deal with others are learned and where frustration, resentment, and anger
> build. (p. 108)

The effects of bullying and harassment on the mental and emotional development of students may be underestimated, and since Columbine, schools have
made a greater effort to intervene before disaster strikes.

BULLYING   Bullying frequently involves overt behaviors, such as physical
attacks, verbal threats, name calling, and rumor spreading. However, some
bullying behaviors are covert, such as exclusion from a group. The covert
behaviors also take a toll on students, but may go unnoticed because they are
not as obvious as the overt actions. Any or all of these may be detrimental to a
student's socio-emotional growth, as well as a deterrent to academic success.

Bullying and harassment occur much more frequently than one might
imagine. In fact, research supports that bullying is commonplace in schools.
A national survey by the American Medical Association (as cited by National
School Safety Center, 2001) questioned 15,000 students in public and private

schools (grades 6 through 10) about bullying behaviors. Responses to the survey indicated that 10% of the students reported being bullied by other students at least once a week. Another 13% acknowledged bullying others, and 6% responded that they were both victims and perpetrators of bullying. Other research supports an even greater instance of bullying. A report by Mulrine (1999) indicated that as many as 25% of schoolchildren endured daily taunting, teasing, pushing, and shoving from schoolyard bullies, and more than 43% of middle- and high-school students avoided using school bathrooms, where harassment and assault are most likely to occur. Another report cited by Smith-Heavenrich (2001) indicated that 3 million bullying incidents are reported each year, and more than 160,000 students miss school each day because of the trauma of being bullied. While this number may seem high, it is probably a low estimate, since many victims of bullying never report that they are bullied out of fear of further torment or retaliation.

Not only should there be concern for victims of bullying, but school counselors must also consider the bullies as well. Roberts and Morotti (2000) supported approaches that address the bullies.

> Bullies must be educated about school and societal rules toward aggressive behaviors as well as held accountable for their actions. However, true accountability can only come when bullies understand the full ramifications of their behaviors on both their futures and those of their victims. (p. 154)

What is it that causes children and adolescents to torment others? Why would students think it is appropriate, even admirable, to instigate negative behaviors toward their peers? A survey by Rodkin (as cited in "Portrait of a Young Tough," 2000) found that 950 students in grades 4 through 6 thought that some of the "coolest" boys were the most violent. Students were asked to rate themselves and each other based on the question "*Who is 'really cool,' friendly, athletic, studious, shy, and who starts fights?*" The results showed that the popular violent boys were bullies and were rated as "cool" by all types of girls and most boys, except the unpopular boys, who were probably the victims of bullying. Interestingly, the violent girls in the study were only considered "cool" by other violent girls, whereas all types of girls considered the violent boys to be popular. This study challenges the assumption that bullies are outcasts or socially ostracized by their peers. In fact, it suggests that bullying behaviors might be reinforced by the popularity or notoriety that accompanies the reputation of being a bully.

Bullying Prevention Strategies In response to national concerns about bullying, the United States Department of Education (DOE) (1998) has developed a resource on bullying entitled *Preventing Bullying: A Manual for Schools and Communities.* This resource defines bullying and provides a comprehensive approach to bully-proofing schools. Intervention strategies and action plans for schools are included in the hope that a comprehensive and collaborative approach will help alleviate this problem. The DOE makes this free brochure available to anyone, and the information included would be valuable material for school counselors to have readily accessible. The brochure also mentions several curricula and classroom resources that are available for school counselors and classroom teachers to use in their efforts to prevent and intervene in bullying situations.

Research has offered strategies for preventing bullying and intervening with victims of bullying (Hanish & Guerra, 2000) and bullies (Roberts & Morotti, 2000). For school counselors, prevention efforts can take many forms. Classroom guidance lessons or school-wide activities that focus on themes of peacefulness and tolerance may foster a climate that deters bullying. Small group counseling might help victims develop skills and behaviors to prevent and deal with bullying. Small groups may also help bullies develop appropriate social skills and empathy for others in an effort to curb the bullying behavior. Individual counseling is a useful tool when students need direct intervention and need to focus on specific strategies and skills for either dealing with the bullying or stopping their bullying behavior. Consultation and collaboration with other school personnel and parents are also integral to a holistic approach to resolving a serious problem in schools. There must be a unified effort to address this recurring problem if change is to occur.

SEXUAL HARASSMENT   Harassment can be defined as an extreme version of bullying; it is a serious issue in our schools. Harassment may be verbal, physical, emotional, or sexual. Most recently, the emphasis has been on the issue of sexual harassment in schools. While many of our students do not recall the scandal of the Clarence Thomas/Anita Hill case, there has been an increased awareness of sexual harassment activities since the early 1990s. It is obvious to school personnel that teacher–teacher and teacher–student harassment is blatantly against school rules and against the law. Most students understand that sexual harassment from a teacher is wrong and punishable. The line becomes a little less clear when considering student-to-student sexual harassment.

As mentioned previously, schools tend to mirror society, and the increase in awareness of sexual harassment in the workplace has trickled down to an increased awareness of sexual harassment in schools. Schools became aware of the need to address student-to-student harassment when the Supreme Court decided on *Davis v. Monroe County School Board* in 1999. In this case, a fifth grader in Monroe County, Georgia, was repeatedly sexually harassed by one of her fellow classmates. The harassment went on for months, despite the girl's reports to school personnel and the mother's report to school administration and the school board. Because no intervention occurred, the mother sued the school district. The case had conflicting verdicts in the circuit and district courts and ended up in the United States Supreme Court (Chaves, 2000).

A synthesis of the Supreme Court ruling by Yell and Katsiyannis (2000) indicated that on May 24, 1999, the Supreme Court, in a 5–4 vote, ruled that schools may be held liable for student-on-student sexual harassment under Title IX of the Educational Amendments of 1972, which prohibits sexual discrimination.

Harassment under Title IX includes hostile environment sexual harassment, which occurs when the sexual harassment of another person is so pervasive and severe that it creates an abusive or hostile learning/educational environment. Based on the longevity of Ms. Davis's experience and the fact that the harassment was reported and not addressed, the Court decided that Monroe County was allowing her learning environment to be hostile. The Court also indicated that school districts are in violation of Title IX if they remain unresponsive to reports of sexual harassment (Yell & Katsiyannis). As a result of this ruling, school districts began to pay more attention to peer harassment and many implemented programs to address it.

There are several issues school personnel should consider when deciding how to address sexual harassment in schools. First, sexual harassment is not gender-specific. It is incorrect to make the assumption that victims of harassment are always female. Second, schools should not be forums for sexual harassment; yet there are incidences of sexual harassment in schools (Kopels & Dupper, 1999). Finally, the impact of harassment on self-concept may be long lasting and detrimental. For these reasons, school systems and school personnel must take action, and school counselors should lead the way in implementing services and programs that help eliminate sexual harassment and related problems.

Sexual Harassment Prevention Strategies   It appears that schools are responding to the need to reduce the incidence of sexual harassment among students. Most schools now have programs in place that provide at least brief sessions with students to inform them about sexual harassment law. Further, students are becoming aware of the consequences of sexual harassment, both at the school level and in the legal system. Kopels and Dupper (1999) recommended that schools be proactive and comprehensive in their efforts to minimize and/or prevent sexual harassment. Specific suggestions included (a) prompt and appropriate response in situations involving peer sexual harassment, (b) assistance for victims of sexual harassment, and (c) increased knowledge about and sensitivity to peer sexual harassment. Although Kopels and Dupper suggested that middle school might be a good time for intervention, sexual harassment prevention should probably begin earlier. Since some children seem to physically mature earlier than others, incidents of harassment and teasing in a sexual way may begin even earlier than once believed. Education and prevention efforts may be effective as early as upper elementary grades (fourth or fifth grade). While it may vary from school district to school district, in many instances the person responsible for leading prevention efforts is the school counselor.

Effective Prevention and Intervention: The School Counselor's Role

While prevention efforts are critical, schools must also establish specific intervention strategies and consequences for bullying and harassment in schools.

These efforts should occur at state and local government levels, as well as in schools. Colorado has set a precedent for prevention and intervention measures (*Safe Communities, Safe Schools*, 2001). In July 2001, the Colorado legislature passed Senate Bill 01-080, which mandated that school districts create specific policies on bullying, including discipline codes to be followed when bullying occurs. School districts in Colorado must submit annual reports with information about bullying prevention and education efforts. Similar ideas have been implemented in other states, and most school districts now have policies addressing bullying and harassment.

While these global efforts are essential and valid, bullying and harassment must be handled at the school level; in fact, school counselors must deal with such incidents on an individual or case-by-case basis. School counselors can play an integral role in helping not only the victims of harassment, but the perpetrators as well. Whether the counselor is the leader of the prevention program or participates in a school-wide effort to address this problem, it is absolutely necessary for him or her to be a catalyst for improving relationships between students.

Professional Perspective

ESTHER (HS)

Counselors play an important role in the school's violence prevention program. They organize an active conflict resolution program. At each grade level, counselors carry out a sexual harassment prevention program. They offer counseling and group guidance strategies.

Specific tasks of school counselors to address bullying or harassment might include:

- classroom or large group presentations about the protocol or process for reporting bullying and harassment;
- classroom instruction about behaviors that constitute bullying and harassment and how to respond as a bystander;
- small group counseling sessions for either victims of harassment or students who harass that focus on issues that are relevant to each group;
- individual counseling sessions with victims and perpetrators that explore the effects of bullying and harassment on self and others;
- consultation with parents and teachers to address the impact of bullying and harassment on students;
- coordination of student-led programs on bullying and school-wide efforts to enforce a "no tolerance" position on bullying and harassment;

- coordination of or participation on a team of administrators, teachers, parents, and students who continually monitor and seek to improve the school's prevention programs;
- collaboration with outside agencies and organizations that focus on bullying and harassment prevention and that might provide support or services to the school;
- assuring that policies and procedures are being followed when bullying or harassment is reported and supporting students who are going through this process; and
- proactive efforts to update and improve school or school board policy on bullying and harassment so that students feel safe, secure, and unthreatened when they are in the school environment.

School counselors are trained to help students work through the trauma of harassment and teasing. Only within the last few years have schools been proactive in addressing these issues. By providing education about and increasing awareness of bullying and harassment—defining bullying and harassment, identifying strategies for victims and bullies, and publicizing procedures for reporting occurrences of bullying and harassment—schools hope to thwart the occurrence of harassment.

Professional Perspective and Practice

RENEE (ES)

My job is to help students develop skills and coping strategies that will help them in life. My school system provides a set of prescribed lessons on bullying and sexual harassment that must be taught to all kindergarten through sixth grade students in the fall of the school year. I follow this up with more lessons on conflict resolution and tolerance/acceptance. We role-play and try to give the students as much practice as possible in dealing with difficult situations. In addition, I coordinate character education activities, which are designed to promote a positive atmosphere. I also coordinate a school-wide positive reinforcement program in which a staff member can recognize any student for a good deed. I also sponsor peer mediators who undergo intensive training in conflict resolution, and conflict resolution skills are taught school-wide through classroom guidance lessons. We start helping students develop the skills to resolve conflict peacefully in kindergarten. All of the hard work shows; we have very few major discipline problems or referrals to the office.

In order to make school an environment in which maximum learning can be achieved, school counselors must confront the situations and conditions that interfere with the learning process. Bullying and harassment can be devastating for the victims, the perpetrators, and the bystanders, and create the antithesis of a positive environment and peaceful climate that fosters learning. School counselors should take a leadership role in working with students, teachers, administrators, and parents to combat the issues of subtle yet harmful attacks that, if not confronted and dealt with, can have catastrophic results.

Zero Tolerance Policies: Have We Gone Too Far?

The good news is that most schools have now instituted programs focused on prevention of violence. Even though acts of bullying, harassment, and violence do occur, they are being addressed, and consequences are being implemented in most circumstances. However, it seems that school systems may have gone to the opposite extreme. Due to the implementation of *zero tolerance policies* for violent behavior, there have been several incidents in which students were suspended for actions that previously would have been considered play or part of normal developmental curiosity.

Zero tolerance means that there are no warnings and no second chances for violent or aggressive behaviors, whether they are verbal, written, or physical. Consequences are imposed regardless of the circumstances in which a behavior occurred. Arguments for and against zero tolerance policies have begun to surface. Proponents insist that in order to maintain school safety, zero tolerance policies must be followed without exception, and punishment must be swift and consistent. Critics rely on research that indicates that zero tolerance policies do not curb acts of violence, but in fact may perpetuate them. According to *The Washington Times* (Richardson, 2002), zero tolerance policies are starting to have a deleterious effect on otherwise good students. The article described an elementary school in Centennial, Colorado, (20 miles from Columbine) where seven fourth grade boys were suspended for making "finger" guns while playing a game called "Army and Aliens" during recess. The students were suspended for the rest of the day, but parents said the effects of the punishment have been long lasting. The boys were given in-school lunch detention for a week following the incident, which turned into a week of "public humiliation" (p. A14). Other children stared and laughed at the boys as they passed them in the hallway. As a result, the boys reported not wanting to attend school and developed symptoms such as headaches and stomach problems to avoid being placed in the public detention area. The school district maintained that the incident was handled properly and in accordance with the zero tolerance policies of the school system. Some would say that being ridiculed or ostracized are natural consequences of the choices these boys made; others might argue that students suffer enough public punishment and should be given second chances.

Similar incidents have been reported nationwide. The arguments for and against zero tolerance are varied, but the consensus seems to be that each case must be considered in isolation. Do the students pose threats at other times, or is this an isolated incident? Should students be punished regardless, since it only takes one incident to produce tragic results? What types of programs support both the victims and the perpetrators, and how can we meet the needs of both?

The issue of zero tolerance is a true dilemma. Should students be allowed to break school rules and create hostile and/or violent environments for other students? Most would agree not. But should we suspend students for engaging in developmentally understandable, although not appropriate, behavior, such as using their fingers as pretend guns? Do students deserve second chances or the benefit of the doubt? Or will the one time the behavior is excused result in a later incident that is devastatingly tragic? There are no easy answers to any of these questions. As a school counselor, you may feel strongly one way or the other, but your role in these issues is to help students deal with the consequences of their own actions and the effect of those actions on other students. If students are suspended for behaviors that violate zero tolerance policies, they may eventually return to school, depending on the severity of their punishments. The school counselor is a person who can help with the transition back into the school. There could be social and even physical repercussions from peers, who may ignore or ridicule the students. These students could also feel animosity from teachers and administrators. When a student is expelled, it is appropriate for the school counselor to support the student and the family as much as possible when he or she is making the transition into another school or an alternative education program.

As a school counselor, you may have strong personal feelings about an incident or behavior, and it is important to be aware of your feelings so that you can be an effective advocate for the student. If your feelings are negative or intolerant of the student, seek out other school personnel (other counselors, if available) to assist you in this process. It is critical to be involved in order to advocate for the student and the family, but you must professionally and ethically consider your personal reactions to the student and seek appropriate assistance.

Secondary and Tertiary Prevention: Conflict Resolution and Crisis Intervention

Preventive measures are critical to deescalating the emotions that often provoke school violence. But the reality is that, despite best efforts in schools, bullying and harassment behaviors still occur, and the school counselor must be a leader in developing and implementing appropriate interventions. Whether the school counselor is the person to whom these incidents are reported or a liaison to and resource for school administrators who take disciplinary action, the school counselor, because of his or her training, is an important link in the chain of intervention.

One aspect of the effectiveness of the prevention programs discussed earlier is the students' realization that there are serious consequences to violent or harassing behaviors. For example, students should be informed of the policies for bullying and harassment, as well as the seriousness of the infraction. In addition, schools must develop very specific guidelines for the consequences of rule violation. Finally, schools must establish boundaries for potentially violent behaviors and decide if first-time offenders should be granted second chances.

It is difficult for students to report incidents of sexual harassment or teasing, even though they might know it is the appropriate procedure. As mentioned previously, research indicates that students typically do not come forward due to fear of retaliation and further harassment. Students must believe that something will be done, and that consequences will be consistently enforced, or they may not bother to report these incidents. For this reason, school personnel must make sure that the consequences associated with unacceptable behaviors are enforced.

While the school is responsible for responding quickly and justly to incidences of violence or harassment, the school counselor can be a leader in promoting intervention programs that focus on deterring potentially violent behavior. An intervention strategy that promotes a more peaceful school environment and better relationships among students is the conflict resolution program.

Effective Intervention: Conflict Resolution Programs

Conflict resolution programs are an important piece of the overall goal of preventing school violence. Cromwell (1999) summarized research that indicated that there has been a reduction in suspensions, fights, discipline referrals, and administrator time spent on discipline, as well as an overall positive change in classroom and school climate due to the implementation of conflict resolution programs. According to Cromwell, there are four basic approaches to creating conflict resolution programs in schools: (a) process curriculum—teaching conflict resolution in isolation outside the curriculum, (b) mediation programs—training selected students in the principles of conflict resolution so they can mediate disputes between other students, (c) peaceable classrooms—integrating conflict resolution principles into the curriculum and classroom management, and (d) peaceable schools—using conflict resolution principles as a system for managing the school as well as the classroom by involving all members of the school community. We will explore each of these areas in order to understand how they work collectively to create direct interventions that avert further crisis among students.

One way to implement conflict resolution programs is to provide curricula that focus on problem solving and decision making in situations outside the classroom setting. Role-playing or creating scenarios that involve dealing with conflict in real-life situations is one way to instill conflict resolution behaviors in students. For example, the school counselor might present the scenario of a student who is teasing another student in the hallway between classes. One student could play the harasser, one could play the victim, and other students could be bystanders. The students could discuss the situation from each of the players' perspectives. How does it feel to be the teaser? The victim? Should the bystanders intervene or stay out of the situation? What are the consequences of each role? The role-play can initiate effective dialogue about how to handle difficult situations involving harassment. It was my experience that children of all levels enjoyed playing roles and acting out situations that were relevant to everyday experience. Through participation and observing how others react to difficult situations, students are able to develop plans for responding to similar situations.

The most obvious setting in which to foster conflict resolution is the setting in which students spend most of the school day—the classroom. Teachers are the most obvious leaders to implement activities that create peaceable classrooms. The school counselor can serve as a consultant for these activities and can participate as needed. Examples of activities that create a peaceable classroom follow:

- Developing and implementing class rules with student input— students should be involved in this process so that they are invested in maintaining these rules.

- Establishing a protocol for what will happen if there is a conflict— students know the steps to be taken in the event that a conflict occurs (e.g., try to resolve it yourself, and if that doesn't work, involve an adult).

- Acknowledgement and agreement that peace is a necessity for the classroom to be a place of learning—students may develop a pact or sign an agreement that they will abide by the rules of peacemaking in order to promote learning.

Regardless of the level (elementary, middle, high school), students should be aware that the ultimate goal in every classroom is to create a peaceful environment in which everyone has a right to conflict-free learning.

It follows that if all classrooms are peaceable, the school as a whole will be more peaceful. However, students are not in classrooms every minute of the school day. Bullying and harassment often occur at times when there is less structure, such as in between classes in the hallways, during lunchtime, and on the playground during recess. Therefore, school-wide programs, such as character education, create an overall climate of peacekeeping throughout the school. Another way to promote peace throughout the school environment is through the development and implementation of peer mediation programs.

The School Counselor's Role in Peer Mediation

In most schools, school counselors or counseling departments are directly involved with, if not in charge of, peer mediation programs. This seems natural because school counselors have had training in the skills needed for successful mediation. As the leader in the program, the school counselor or counseling team becomes responsible for the recruitment, selection, and training of students who will serve as peer mediators. In addition, the school counselor typically implements the program, which includes developing a mediator schedule, determining where mediations will take place, maintaining records of mediation that occur, and continually monitoring the mediations and the program in general. Therefore, in a peer mediation program, the school counselor may serve as counselor, trainer, consultant, and/or coordinator.

When peer mediation programs first became popular, school counselors seemed to be an obvious resource to involve in the recruitment, training, and implementation of the program. Now, other school personnel (i.e., teachers, school social workers) may become more involved. In many schools, especially secondary schools, student assistance personnel might oversee peer mediation and/or peer helper programs. Leadership skills, such as shared responsibility, can be useful to school counselors when defining roles and responsibilities in the peer mediation program. Regardless of the extent of their involvement in the peer mediation program, school counselors should promote the program as an intervention that is intended to reduce incidents of conflict and violence.

If the school counselor is the leader in the peer mediation program, there are steps that should be taken to develop the program. These tasks are recruitment, training, and implementation.

STEP 1: RECRUITMENT Most peer mediation programs begin with the recruitment of students to serve as mediators. The number of students needed will depend on several factors: (a) the size of the student body, (b) the schedule of the school day in terms of students missing class, and (c) the criteria by which students are selected. In many situations, students are nominated by their peers, a process that makes sense because the students will be helping to resolve disputes among their peers. Elementary schools typically recruit fifth or sixth graders, since the students should be developmentally capable of understanding and implementing the mediation steps. In middle and high schools, mediators might be selected from each of the grade levels in the school. A technique for recruitment at the middle school level is to make contact with the

My Story

The first time I recruited mediators, I was sure that it would be a popularity contest and that the most appropriate students might not be selected. Surprisingly, the students chose mediators who they felt were trustworthy, honest, and could help them in a time of conflict. Some of the chosen students had strong personalities, others were quiet. I found that the students who were chosen by their peers were often the best choices to carry out the responsibilities of the program.

students at each grade level at the end of the school year and ask them to nominate a number of girls and boys from their classes who they could talk to about problems and trust to help them solve their problems.

After accepting nominations, students will vote on the list of recommended mediators. Females and males with the most votes would be selected. The number selected will depend on the number of students in the grade level and the number of conflicts that have historically been reported. Once mediators are selected, permission slips should be sent home to acquire parent permission for participation as mediators in the program.

Recruitment at the middle school and high school levels may vary from the elementary selection process. Often, students who are selected at the elementary level are encouraged to continue as mediators in middle school and high school. It is beneficial to have trained students available the first day of school in middle and high school. In addition, recruitment of new mediators might be solicited through advertisement, teacher recommendation, or offering a class in conflict resolution and allowing students who register to become mediators. As new mediators are selected, the training process is repeated. Often, experienced mediators, as well as the counselors or teachers who coordinate the program, conduct the training of new mediators. This provides a great deal of lateral support as students progress through the school ranks.

STEP 2: TRAINING   The conflict mediation training process is the ultimate determinant of the success of the program. Participants must understand the basic concepts and process of conflict mediation programs in order to carry out the steps that will make the program work. In general, training includes a variety of exercises and role-plays that help participants understand conflict and how to resolve it. The training focuses on teaching participants the steps in the process. In general, there are six steps:

1. The disputants (students involved in the conflict) agree to meet, and mediators set the ground rules.
2. Mediators gather information about the conflict from each disputant.
3. Mediators identify what the dispute is about through reflective listening and clarifying information.
4. Disputants identify possible options for resolution of the dispute.
5. Disputants select one or more workable options.
6. Disputants reach consensus on an agreement and mediators document the decision.

When two or more people are in conflict, these basic steps move the disputants toward an agreeable resolution. Peer mediators are trained to monitor and guide the students through this process and peacefully resolve the issue.

STEP 3: IMPLEMENTATION   Peer mediation programs are school-wide programs that need support from administrators, teachers, parents, and students in order to be successful. It will be futile for a conflict mediation program to be

My Story

At the elementary level, I always sat in on mediations. I was never directly involved (unless there was an escalation in emotion), but I was usually at my desk or sitting elsewhere in the room. I did this for liability reasons and so that I could evaluate the mediators and give them feedback for future mediations. The mediations could take as little as 10 minutes, but there were a few that took an hour or more. Only once did we actually have to come back the next day to resolve a dispute.

The number of mediations conducted also varied. Some days there were no disputes, and on other days there were two or three. Certain times of the year also seemed busier than others in terms of the need for mediation; for example, it seemed that there was a notable increase in the number of student conflicts in the spring.

established unless the population for which it is intended is invested in the process. For that reason, it is necessary to publicize the program and educate members of the school community about the goals, purpose, and potential benefits of the program. The school counselor's level of involvement with the mediations may vary. See the "My Story" box for further discussion of this issue.

At the middle and secondary levels, two or more persons typically sponsor peer mediation programs. In addition, mediators may only be available during a certain block of the day or before and after school. Because the number of mediators is typically large, it is usually not as difficult to have mediators available. In fact, there may be mediators assigned to every period/block so that the entire day is covered. Further, if there are many sponsors, supervision of mediation sessions becomes less of an issue.

There are several key elements of successful implementation and maintenance of the peer mediations, including:

- providing a process for referrals;
- making teachers and students aware of that process;
- securing space for mediations to occur;
- making sure mediators have all necessary materials to conduct mediation (e.g., contracts, rules, steps in the process);
- reminders (e.g., P.A. announcements, posters, bulletins) that the mediation program is available when conflict arises;
- scheduled meetings (monthly or bi-monthly) with the mediators to discuss issues, concerns, successes, challenges, and ideas for improvement; and
- ongoing evaluation of the program both internally (the mediators and coordinators of the program) and externally (teachers and students).

The largest source of referrals will probably be teachers and administrators, but students should be encouraged to use the peer mediation program as an option when dealing with conflict.

Conflict resolution programs are an integral and necessary part of our schools today. Whether the school counselor is the leader or part of a team of leaders, it is an important program for the overall good of the school. Being involved in conflict resolution programs is an important leadership and advocacy role for school counselors, as the programs are essential to teaching students important life skills, such as working through problems and settling disputes. Successful intervention in the personal and social struggles of students will help resolve some of the situations that might interfere with effective learning.

While peer mediation is an example of a planned intervention that promotes peace, there are times when unexpected events occur. When a crisis occurs in a school, school counselors should be leaders in responding immediately and effectively.

Crisis Response Team: The School Counselor's Role

> *You are a high school counselor, sitting at home on a Sunday evening, preparing for the coming week at school. The phone rings.*
>
> *You hear your principal's voice on the other end, and by his tone, you know that something bad has happened. He informs you that the high school football coach and two student athletes were killed in a car accident on Saturday. They were coming back from a scouting trip in a nearby school district. The two athletes were seniors, both popular, good students. Both had college football scholarship offers. The coach had been at the school for 12 years. Not only was he a beloved coach, but also was a popular and respected history teacher who taught 10th grade geography and 11th grade U.S. history.*
>
> *You sit stunned as your principal asks you to come in early to help inform the faculty of the news and carry out the Crisis Response plan. While you have been the Crisis Response Team Leader for a year, you realize you have not been called into action until now. What do you do? Where do you begin?*

Another important program that school counselors are typically part of, if not in charge of, is the crisis response/intervention team. This team responds to crises that occur (a) in the school environment, such as the example above; (b) in the school community, such as a youth kidnapping or murder; or (c) on a national level, such as the terrorist attacks on the World Trade Center and the Pentagon on September 11, 2001.

Because school counselors are trained in promoting a peaceful school environment, empathic response, and dealing with volatile emotions, they are appropriate members or leaders of a school's crisis response team. Counselors are often notified immediately when a local, state, or national crisis has occurred, and the crisis plan is implemented. The level of crisis, as well as which situations are deemed school crises, may vary. As in this example, crisis can be local, such as the death of a student or staff member. If the crisis is local, it is appropriate to invite extra counselors from other schools or from the community to be available in the event that students are struggling with the loss. When crisis occurs close to home, it is particularly critical for the school counselor to take a leadership role in organizing and implementing the support services needed throughout the crisis.

Poland and McCormick (1999) focused on how school personnel, parents, and communities must come together in times of crisis and outlined specific behaviors that should be incorporated into a school plan. They also provided important considerations regarding counseling after a school crisis. These points are summarized in Feature 11.2. While this is not an exhaustive list (see Poland & McCormick), it provides a foundation and basic strategies for school counselors who must respond to a crisis that occurs within or near the school community.

When the World Changes: Responding to National Crisis

On a larger scale, crisis response teams also respond to national crises, such as the terrorist attacks of the World Trade Center and Pentagon on September 11, 2001. Schools across the country implemented full or partial lock-down as school personnel responded to the needs of students. In some situations, students were unaware of the events; in others, students watched on TV as the towers crumbled, killing thousands. School counselors responded in a variety of ways. Some helped retrieve students as parents flooded schools to pick up their children in the midst of the crisis. Others roamed the halls looking for students who had become distraught or panicked as a result of the attacks and making sure that students stayed in classrooms inside school buildings that were, for safety's sake, locked. Our veteran counselors had varied experiences during this event.

Professional Practice

RENEE (ES)

On September 11th, 2001, our administrators made the decision not to tell our students about the terrorist attacks. Because of our proximity to Washington, D.C., we knew we had students whose parents worked in the Pentagon and other government buildings that may have been targeted. We believed that any kind of announcement would have just created panic and distress. The teachers were notified individually and privately and were asked to view televisions only in areas that were not accessible to students. We attempted to maintain a normal school day. The teachers and staff were provided with a respite room

FEATURE 11.2

Responding to Crisis

- If the crisis has occurred at school when students are present, assist in getting everyone back to their classrooms where they will be safe and accounted for after the crisis.

- Cancel all scheduled appointments and counseling activities not related to the crisis in order to respond to the crisis itself.

- Target the following five groups for counseling assistance, in this order: (a) those who were injured in the crisis event, (b) those who witnessed the event, (c) those emotionally close to the victims of the crisis (e.g., family members, close friends), (d) those known to be at risk or to have suffered recent loss, and (e) those known to have had a previous suicide attempt or other students/faculty members at risk for irrational responses.

- Provide counseling services for those who self-refer or are teacher-referred.

- Provide a forum for students to express their feelings about the crisis; writing, artwork, and small-group discussions are all important ways to help students process what has happened.

- Given the immediacy of the need for counseling services, suspend the requirement of parental consent for counseling services; most parents will understand that the response must be immediate.

- Communicate with parents of affected students as soon as possible. Provide support both emotionally and physically by having materials available, such as contact numbers for outside agencies that specialize in pertinent services, and assisting families in accessing these resources.

- Debrief the faculty immediately following the crisis and in the days (possibly weeks or months) to follow. Maintain an open door policy to deal with individual concerns and issues.

- Remain "in tune" with the individual reactions in a group situation. While some may recuperate quickly, others may struggle. Approach them privately and offer support.

- If students or faculty members have perished, follow the school schedule of the deceased and process with all persons who had contact with these persons.

- Review the daily attendance lists to identify students who may be out of school due to the crisis. Follow up with students and their families to offer support in helping these students make the transition back to school.

- Be a presence in the building and observe emotions and behaviors. Be present in the hallways, at the bus drop-off, in the cafeteria, and in other locations where students gather.
- Offer to stay for extended hours or to arrive early to provide assistance to students and their families.
- Communicate with the counselors throughout the school district and either (a) ask for their help if the caseload is overwhelming or (b) offer to go to their schools if the crisis has had a greater impact on them.
- Designate areas that are available throughout the school day where students, staff, and parents can access counseling services.
- Utilize local resources to help provide coverage. In addition to the on-site personnel (i.e., school psychologist, school social worker), contact local agencies and practitioners to see if they can be available to help.
- Provide bilingual services for students whose primary language is not English.

Source: Reprinted by permission of the author from *Coping with crisis: Lessons learned (A resource for schools, parents, and communities)* by Dr. Scott Poland.

and someone to cover their classes if they were feeling too overwhelmed and needed to take a break. Ten percent of our students were signed out early that day. There seemed to be a need for families to gather their loved ones together.

BETH (MS)

We had parents coming in droves to pick up their children, so there was no way to contain the information. I encouraged my principal, saying, "You've got to tell the children something." I think I acted as a consultant because of my training in crisis management. As a group, we went into each classroom and said, "This is what we know." We only gave them the facts. We told them that if their parents came to pick them up, we would release them. We also said that we didn't know what might happen with school the next day. Then we answered questions. For the students who were visibly upset, we took them to another room and provided support as necessary.

After a tragedy of the magnitude of that horrific day, school counselors had to be prepared for the nightmares, fears, and emotions that came with the scenes that will forever play in the minds of our youth, while also dealing with their own emotional responses to the events of that day. In the aftermath of the events of September 11, students had to struggle with fear of war, biological warfare, and further terrorism.

Professional Perspective

ESTHER (HS)

The sense of loss from September 11, 2001 would manifest itself long after the events of that day. The counselor's role was to provide support, address crises, and facilitate communication. Maintaining normalcy provided continuity for students. Counselors offered student counseling groups on loss, stress management, and made referrals to outside grief groups for families who lost relatives that day.

Professional Practice

RENEE (ES)

For me, the day we returned to school after the attacks was much more difficult than the day of the attacks. Many of the staff and the students seemed to be in shock. Teachers needed support for talking to their students about it. I was available to work with any students or teachers who needed counseling that day. I also disseminated information to teachers and parents on how to help their youngsters cope with the tragic events. I definitely saw an increase in anxious behavior and somatic complaints after 9/11. On the anniversary of 9/11, I again distributed information to staff members and parents to help them deal with their students and any issues that might surface.

In uncertain times, it is important for school counselors to be in the forefront of efforts to reduce the anxiety and tension surrounding the events occurring in our communities and in our nation. One key characteristic and role of school counselors is reacting calmly in times of crisis. While the natural response may be panic, distress, or fear, school counselors are given the paramount task of being stable (emotionally and physically) and practical (able to keep a clear head). In addition, this role includes a responsibility to soothe students and help them feel secure during times of crisis. Even if events are uncertain and information is obscure, school counselors should reassure students that everyone in the school and community is working to maintain their safety and security. While administrators and community personnel must keep their fingers on the pulse of the events, school counselors should be aware of the emotional effects of the events on students and staff, while also keeping personal emotions in check. This is an awesome task, but one that must be considered in order to provide effective counseling services.

CONCLUSION

In general, recent news about school violence and the efficacy of prevention programs has been good. The U.S. Departments of Education and Justice (2000) found that school crime rates have decreased significantly in the last decade. This, coupled with initiatives and grants focused on safe schools and students, indicates that prevention and intervention efforts might be making a difference. While certainly encouraging, this information has to be regarded cautiously. The number of violent acts in schools is decreasing, but the degree of violence seems to be increasing. School counselors are leaders in violence prevention and intervention efforts and must ask: *How can we prevent such heinous acts in our schools?* There is no clear answer, but there must be an effort by school personnel, specifically school counselors, to deter and diffuse potentially violent situations. Task forces on school violence are recognizing that school counselors are logical persons to be leaders and consultants in formulating and implementing prevention and intervention programs. Further, in unfortunate times of crisis, school counselors are also key resource personnel to help regain and maintain a sense of peace and security in the school environment. School counselors must come forward as leaders in efforts to protect students and to maintain peaceful learning environments that foster academic and personal success.

REFLECTION AND DISCUSSION

1. Although the majority of students help maintain peaceful schools, other students defy the structure of schools and the authority of school officials. As a school counselor and leader, how might you engage students in peace-promoting efforts?

2. Sometimes it is difficult to identify students who have the potential to become suddenly violent. What signs and symptoms might you look for when trying to prevent violent acts by students? As a school counselor, how would you intervene?

3. This chapter discussed prevention and intervention services to address school violence and school crisis. Are there additional issues that should be explored? List other types of violence-related or crisis-related issues that might occur in schools and discuss how the school counselor might address these issues.

CHAPTER 12

The School Counselor and Advocacy: Taking a Stand

*A*dvocacy is one of the primary responsibilities and a professional practice of school counselors. It is such a critical role for school counselors that one of the themes of the ASCA National Model for School Counseling Programs (ASCA, 2003a) is advocacy.

> As educational leaders, school counselors are ideally situated to serve as advocates for every student in meeting high standards. Advocating for the academic success of every student is the key role of school counselors and places them as leaders in promoting school reform. (p. 22)

The role of advocacy, however, is not limited to serving students, although student advocacy is a priority for school counselors. School counselors are constantly being asked to advocate for the job, for the profession, for parents, and for educational programs. Whether representing a humanistic point of view in a heated discussion among school personnel or making sure a student's point of view is considered when making decisions about his or her future, school counselors must assume the essential role of advocacy in the 21st century.

The notion of advocacy is not new. It is not unusual to advocate for the underdog, pull for the "little guy," become passionate and committed to changing conditions that require social action. "The social advocacy approach is based on the belief that individual or collective action must be taken to improve conditions for the benefit of an individual or group" (House & Martin, 1998, p. 284). It also involves informing and educating interested parties about the services and opportunities available to make a student's educational experience as successful as possible. Focusing specifically on advocacy in schools, it is evident that school counselors may be called upon to advocate more than any other school personnel. School counselors can exhibit their commitment to advocacy in several ways. Myers, Sweeney, and White (2002) identified the essential issues in professional advocacy—professional identity, the public's image of and access to counseling and counselors, collaboration and coalitions, professional pride, and accountability. In order to provide services for current and future generations of students, school counselors must make advocacy a priority. School counselors are, and should continue to be, advocates for pupils, as well as personnel, programs, policies, and procedures that positively impact the planning and implementation of effective school counseling programs.

Dr. Marie Jackson of the State University of West Georgia, along with her departmental colleagues, has participated for 6 years in the Transforming School Counseling Initiative with the Education Trust (2003). The State University of West Georgia is one of the six universities across the nation that received a competitive grant to transform the curriculum for training school counselors. She has firsthand experience practicing and providing training on the school counselor's advocacy role. She is a former school counselor and a current counselor educator who understands the importance of school counselor advocacy. The following section is her professional contribution to the topic of school counseling and advocacy.

Professional Perspective: The School Counselor as Advocate

The following material, to the heading "Action + Advocacy = Effective Services for Students," was contributed by Dr. Marie Jackson, State University of West Georgia

> Counselors trained or retrained for the new vision must be proactive advocates for system change, knowledgeable about schools, and equipped to assist students in meeting their educational and personal goals. (House & Martin, 1998, p. 290)

Those in the school counseling profession have "talked a good game" for many years, contending that school counselors are leaders of change. We began presenting the school counselor as change agent in the 1960s and alluded to the necessity of the school counselor being in the forefront of change. However, when speaking of change, school counselors' focus was primarily on change in the school counseling program, developing the school counselor's role description, and increasing the number of counselors in the schools. All of these issues are worthy arenas for advocating change and growth. Yet today's society cries out for a different type of advocacy role for school counselors. The new vision for today's school counselors is as advocates for the academic success of all students in an equitable environment. Becoming an advocate for students and their families requires developing a new set of skills and often a new attitude.

Advocacy for children has been considered the domain of various community agencies outside of the school. Even though advocacy is a service often provided by community agencies, it is also an important role for today's school counselor. Who better than the school counselor to recognize existing barriers to educational opportunities and glaring inequities, especially those impacting various ethnic, minority, and lower socioeconomic groups? In our global society, with rapidly increasing diverse student populations, school counselors cannot assume that the services and curricula that met the needs of white, middle-class America in the past will meet the needs of all students today.

Advocacy is sorely needed, but is a skill that must be acquired and practiced. Simply having the desire to be a caring and concerned counselor who believes in the development and success of *all* students is not enough. In fact, having a mindset focused on the beliefs that support advocacy without possessing the advocacy skills to support change can be detrimental to school counseling and to school counselors. A school counselor who attempts an advocacy action without an informed and carefully planned approach may damage the cause of the individual, the group, or maybe even his or her own career.

It is critical to explore the history of advocacy in relation to school counseling, the definition of advocacy, types of advocacy, advocacy actions, the role of the school counselor as advocate, and strategies appropriate for use by the school counselor.

What Is Advocacy?

Advocacy has been defined in a variety of ways in counseling literature. Hepworth and Larsen (1986, as cited in Ezell, 2001) provided a working definition of advocacy:

> [T]he process of working with/or on behalf of clients (1) to obtain services or resources for clients that would not otherwise be provided, (2) to modify extant policies, procedures, or practices that adversely impact clients, or (3) to promote new legislation or policies that will result in the provision of needed resources or services. (p. 22)

For the purposes of this discussion, the definition of advocacy adapts Hepworth and Larsen's points to relate to schools and includes ideas from Toporek (1999). In the school counseling setting, advocacy is an action taken by the professional school counselor "to facilitate the removal of external and institutional barriers to the students' well-being" (Toporek & Liu, as cited in Toporek, p. 34). Advocacy in the school setting serves two primary goals for students and their families: (a) increasing a sense of personal power and (b) fostering environmental changes that reflect greater responsiveness to the personal needs of those the school counselor serves (Lewis, Lewis, Daniels, & D'Andrea, 1998).

Bradley and Lewis (2000) referred to advocacy as taking action to make environmental changes on behalf of clients. Lee (1998) used stronger words, saying, "When counselors work as advocates they plead on behalf of the client or some social cause" (p. 387). Advocating for a social cause requires a focus on social justice and social action. Many debate the extent of the school counselor's involvement in social justice.

According to Kiselica and Robinson (2001), *advocacy counseling* involves social action, social justice, social activism, and "cuts across the disciplines of counseling, psychology, social work, sociology, and religion" (p. 388). Advocacy counseling has a long history and has targeted domestic and professional issues. For the purposes of this text, advocacy refers to an arena in which the school counselor operates in order to serve the needs of all students, both directly and indirectly. This arena cuts across all program domains or components. In some way, advocacy actions may be needed in all counseling roles.

Advocacy as an Arena for School Counselors

The movement for transformative change in the role of the school counselor was ushered in with the advent of the new millennium. A study of recent school counseling literature uncovers numerous books, articles, and reports related to the school counselor in the 21st century (e.g., Baker, 2000; Baker, 2001; Green & Keys, 2001; Schmidt, 2003). These all indicate a need for transformation of the counselor role or for new skills in a new age. One might ask why or even if the school counselor in the 21st century is portrayed differently than in recent past. Considering the critical changes and the tragic events that have occurred in schools in recent years, it is easy to recognize the need for evolving roles and responsibilities. Some of the major changes affecting schools are increasing violence, globalization, terrorist actions, and family dysfunction. Globalization requires students to complete the academic process having attained high-level skills, preparing them for success in an increasingly competitive worldwide marketplace. Without major adjustments via school and social reform efforts, it will not be possible for all students to leave school prepared to find a place in this complex society. Where does the school counselor's role as student advocate begin?

School counselors are in a position to be on the first line of defense against barriers to student success and achievement. School counselors can help empower students and families to make a difference in their own lives and to initiate social action for groups that have been collectively prohibited from attaining success through no fault of their own. This sounds like an overwhelming task, but it is not solely the responsibility of the school counselor. The school counselor, however, must be a leader in this regard, armed with an understanding of advocacy actions and strategies that bring about change for the betterment of all students.

Advocacy Roles of the School Counselor

The advocacy roles of the school counselor are at the forefront of what school counselors do. The emphasis on advocacy in the *Transforming School Counseling Initiative* (Education Trust, 2003) and the ASCA National Model (ASCA, 2003a) are indicative of the necessary role that school counselors must assume as advocates. Bradley and Lewis (2000) indicated that advocacy roles might occur in two areas of counseling: *client advocacy* and *political advocacy* (p. 3). The first area refers to responding to the individual needs of clients or, in the case of the school counselor, the student. It should also be noted that the "client" might also be a teacher or parent who is in need of support or help in an educational circumstance. Political advocacy addresses a more global perspective in which counselors respond to the greater economic and political forces that are often present in society (Bradley & Lewis). This is especially true for school counselors who are sometimes considered dispensable when school budgets are being cut or when the political arena regarding support services for students becomes vulnerable.

This section focuses on a variety of advocacy roles that may be assumed by school counselors. The initial area explored will be *student advocacy*, followed by *educational advocacy, program advocacy,* and *political advocacy.*

STUDENT ADVOCACY   Throughout this book, one of the more prominent themes has been that the primary role of the school counselor is to advocate for students. This is the central task and focus of effective school counseling programs. Student advocacy roles may involve a variety of tasks:

- defending the need for more comprehensive student services;
- educating students about their personal and educational rights;
- representing students in administrative hearings or meetings;
- testifying in court on behalf of a student or their family; and
- representing the best interests of students in meetings or forums that impact educational programs.

It is sometimes challenging to take a stand or assert a position in situations where others are supporting a different position. The appropriate school counselor advocacy role is to consistently and constantly consider the impact of decisions and actions on the student. Whether supporting a group of students or the individual needs of one student, school counselors may find themselves in a position that does not concur with the thoughts or actions of others. It becomes imperative that school counselors serve as a catalyst to remind all constituents that the best interests of the student are a priority.

Many of the daily actions of a school counselor can be considered student advocacy. When a counselor consults with classroom teachers about curricula or the proper placement of a student, the counselor is advocating for student success in learning. Participating on a student support team that investigates individual students in need of further assistance and identifies resources and programs to meets those needs is also an advocacy action. Advocacy may also be as simple as securing an interpreter to explain policies and procedures to the non–English-speaking parents of a new student enrolling in school. It is important for school counselors to remember that student advocacy tasks do not have to be blatant in order to be effective. Any intervention on a student's behalf is an example of appropriate student advocacy.

PROGRAM ADVOCACY   School counselors have the critical task of promoting the school counseling program. While most school-counselors-in-training may not think of public relations as an important task for school counselors, demonstrating that the school counseling program is effective is a primary advocacy role for school counselors. "Regardless of setting, type of clientele, or types of intervention, an essential question for all counselors is whether or not our methods 'work' to help persons in need" (Myers, Sweeney, & White, 2003, p. 398). Program advocacy includes demonstrating accountability and being able to show how the school counseling program contributes to the success of the overall education program. Accountability in school counseling programs will be discussed in detail in the next chapter.

What actions constitute school counseling program advocacy? The following are tasks that school counselors can perform to advocate for their program:

- distributing newletters or brochures that include current and future programs and services in the school counseling program;

- creating bulletin boards or public address announcements that keep students, faculty, and administration aware of current events in the counseling program;
- developing accountability reports on a monthly or bi-monthly basis that demonstrate the efficacy of school counseling programs and sharing them with key stakeholders; and
- inviting the media to publicize programs or events that highlight the activities that are sponsored by the school counseling program.

These are only a few of the many ways that school counselors advocate for their program. Some might feel that school counselors should not have to sell their program or prove that counseling services are effective. However, it is important to recognize that program advocacy is not solely for the benefit of promoting the school counseling program. It is also an affirmation to the school counselor that the program is meeting the needs of the students and the educational program, which is a crucial goal of effective school counseling programs.

Program advocacy requires that the school counselor remain open to new ideas and opportunities to enhance school counseling services. It is often easier to maintain the status quo. This, however, defies the action-oriented focus of effective advocacy. Effective school counselors are constantly assessing and revising the services and activities that comprise the school counseling program. Another advocacy role is to seek new and relevant programs to meet the needs of students. Program advocacy involves being able to assert that the school counseling program is developed around the success and achievement goals of students, which requires being actively engaged in professional opportunities to explore new programs and alternative ways to provide services. It is much easier to advocate for a school counseling program that is successfully meeting the needs of students than to explain why counseling services are ineffective.

EDUCATIONAL ADVOCACY It is important for the school counselor to understand the educational environment and academic programs that influence the school counseling program. While program advocacy asks the question: "How does the school counseling program support the educational program?" educational advocacy asks: "How does the educational program benefit students?" Since school counselors are student advocates, it makes sense that they must also understand and advocate for educational programs and services that promote student success.

While school counseling is a specific program that contributes to the educational program, it is imperative that school counselors understand how the overall education system works in order to work more effectively within that system. Specific tasks might include:

- learning how the school and school system work;
- knowing the chain of command;
- becoming familiar with who is the best and most credible person to present a concern and what is the process for reporting the concern;

- identifying what types of situations should be brought to the attention of school leaders; and

- supporting curricular or program changes in the school or school district.

It is not enough to simply be aware of issues or situations that will ultimately affect the education process. If school counselors are to be effective advocates, action is a necessary part of the plan. In addition to remaining informed, school counselors can be actively involved in educating others about the issues, decisions, and actions that impact educational programs. Further, school counselors can be catalysts for helping others advocate their positions about issues and actions that influence school programs. School counselors can teach advocacy skills to students, parents, and others in order to help them have a voice or constructively address situations that influence student academic success. For example, if the local school board is considering a change in curriculum and a group of students and parents believe this change will negatively influence their educational success, school counselors can help the group develop a plan for approaching the administration in a constructive way about their concerns. While the school counselor may or may not agree with the position of the concerned group, it is important to help others, particularly students, develop skills to advocate for themselves and the cause they feel is important. Because school counselors are members of the education community and employees of the educational institution, they can provide valuable insight and appropriate guidance for those who wish to address a situation or issue that has implications for the education program.

POLITICAL ADVOCACY   Bradley and Lewis (2000) defined political advocacy as counseling actions that focus on "influencing the political, economic, and social systems that oppress a whole population of clients" (p. 3). Some of the situations discussed in the *educational advocacy* section might also fall into the political category. However, this section will discuss opportunities to engage in activities that affect school counseling in a more global sense, such as issues discussed at the state or national level. Advocacy activities in this area might include:

- monitoring legislative actions that influence school counseling programs on a state and national level;

- talking to political and/or legislative decision makers on behalf of students;

- lobbying policy makers;

- networking with community resources outside of school to provide more comprehensive services for students; and

- organizing coalition groups to address issues that affect students and/or the school counseling program.

In general, when one thinks of political advocacy, the mental image might include protestors carrying signs or making verbal attacks on government decisions. However, political advocacy in school counseling does not have to be militant or excessively overt, but school counselors should be proactive. It is important that school counselors remain informed of the social and political issues that affect educational programs in general and, more specifically, school counseling programs. Being aware of relevant decisions and how they impact students, reading reports of local and state school board actions, and keeping abreast of legislative actions are a few of the ways that school counselors can become more effective political advocates.

The advocacy roles of school counselors are too numerous to mention. In many cases, school counselors are engaged in advocacy roles without even realizing it. Yet the significance of these roles cannot be ignored. Whether the school counselor advocates specifically for one student or for the profession of school counseling in general, the advocacy role is critical to the efficacy of school counseling programs. The next section will discuss a process for becoming an effective advocate.

Becoming an Advocate: A Personal and Professional Process

Becoming an advocate as a school counselor is a challenging process. School counselors moving toward advocacy begin by looking at who they are both personally and professionally. Personal exploration begins with the following questions: Do I have the attributes and the skills to be a student advocate, a self advocate, and an advocate for the profession? Am I knowledgeable about the costs, the hazards, and the ethical issues involved as I pursue an advocacy role? It is essential to carefully assess personal beliefs and values regarding equity for all students, and determine personal strengths and weaknesses in relation to performing advocacy duties. Then, after becoming more self-aware, a school counselor will begin to develop a personal advocacy style.

As you begin to assess your beliefs, values, strengths, and weaknesses on your journey to self-awareness, you might ask yourself, "Where on the advocacy action continuum am I?" Toporek (1999) discussed advocacy in counseling as ranging from empowerment to social action. Empowerment is a process whereby the counselor focuses the interaction on facilitating the student's self-efficacy. Empowerment involves increasing a student's ability to bring about change in self or his or her environment to make a difference regarding a problem or issue. In this way, the school counselor helps the student recognize, understand, and address the barriers that are prohibiting his or her success or attainment of a goal. In social action—the other end of the continuum—the school counselor becomes involved in the larger socio-political environment to affect removal of barriers to student academic success. Differences of opinion exist regarding the extent to which a school counselor should become involved in politics in order to facilitate student growth. However, there are a variety of legitimate ways to involve oneself ethically and professionally to make a difference in students' lives.

One way to effectively advocate is to work through professional organizations and other community groups to indirectly impact students' lives, as these groups potentially influence local school and public policies both at the state and federal level. Choosing where one stands on the advocacy continuum between empowerment and social action, and then developing the skills for that level of advocacy, is indeed a demanding task for today's school counselor.

Effective Advocacy: Necessary Attributes and Skills

Kiselica and Robinson (2001) outlined six attributes important for advocacy counselors:

- the capacity for commitment and an appreciation for human suffering;
- nonverbal and verbal communication skills;
- maintaining a multi-systems perspective;
- being adept at individual, group, and organizational interventions;
- knowledge and use of media, technology, and the Internet; and
- assessment and research skills (pp. 391–393).

While these seem to have a global focus, there are specific attributes and skills that facilitate effective advocacy.

INTEGRATING ATTRIBUTES AND SKILLS Kiselica and Robinson (2001) suggested that advocacy counselors need to exhibit compassion and empathy for their clients, as well as possess a desire to enhance the growth of their clients. They also noted, "complicated social problems, such as teen parenthood, homophobia, and domestic violence, are the result of a complex interaction of forces originating from the many different systems influencing a client's life" (p. 392). These problems increase the need for school counselors to understand how each of these systems work. It is important to be aware of the impact of social systems on students and to develop interventions with this in mind. Being skilled in the delivery of individual, group, and organizational/environmental interventions, as well as being knowledgeable of the various interacting systems, can also facilitate client access to information and enable the counselor to provide mediation for clients during advocacy actions (Kiselica & Robinson).

ADVOCACY THROUGH TECHNOLOGY According to Kiselica and Robinson (2001), the use of media, technology, and the Internet can be powerful instruments for advocates. Stone and Turba (1999) reminded school counselors that supporting student achievement is more than a philosophical orientation in that it requires a set of specific skills. These authors also focused on the skilled use of technology as an effective tool for advocacy practice. Others have also discussed the value of technological skills in advocacy. For example, House and Martin (1998) supported the use of technology when performing such actions as monitoring student progress, helping students with career planning, and acquiring and accessing data in order to make effective and informed decisions about individual students or the entire school. School counselors need to be trained and understand how technology can help them advocate successfully for students and for their profession.

ASSESSMENT AND RESEARCH   Assessment and research skills are often cited as being among the tools least preferred by school counselors. However, in order to perform advocacy actions, these skills are needed to evaluate the outcomes of advocacy initiatives, to determine needs, and to identify successful strategies for intervention (Kiselica & Robinson, 2001). Assessment and research can raise awareness of inequities and other advocacy needs. Awareness is the starting point for all advocacy actions. As a research tool, the case study is valuable and often overlooked. The development or presentation of a case study can serve a variety of purposes related to advocacy. Case studies of students dealing with specific concerns can be used with students to provide ideas for handling their current problems. A case study can also be used in legislative advocacy to support a request for increased services. When involved in advocating for the school counseling program, program evaluation and assessment data can provide justification for the provision of better counseling services. Chapter 13 will focus on specific ways that school counselors can use evaluation and assessments as advocacy tools.

Becoming an effective advocate is an important task for school counselors today. In order to be an effective advocate for students and their families, school counselors need to assess their personal level of motivation for pursuing advocacy as a strategy. It is also important to consider one's capacity for commitment, the desire to alleviate human suffering, and the ability to follow through. Advocacy is not a simple procedure that can be implemented in a routine step-by-step fashion. It requires much reflective and analytical thought throughout the process. Before attempting advocacy actions, school counselors must develop a working knowledge of advocacy, including an understanding of the various types, strategies, and tactics involved in each category. It is also critical to consider the reasons for using advocacy actions, and the surrounding ethical issues that are sometimes inherent to situations that might require advocacy actions.

Effective Advocacy: The Choice Is Yours

Because existing barriers sometimes seem to block advocacy actions, some counselors choose the path of least resistance, avoiding their advocacy role. School counselors sometimes give varied reasons or excuses as to why they stop short of acting on behalf of a student. School counselors often say they have neither the time nor the know-how to be an effective advocate. Others may believe that advocacy is not in their job description or even a part of their role. Examining the job description and assigned duties is critical. Some of these reasons may be valid and need to be considered. However, reviewing the American School Counselor Association's Ethical Standards for School Counselors (ASCA, 1998; also see the Appendix) and the ASCA National Model (ASCA, 2003a) should remind school counselors of the professional obligation school counselors have in advocacy. Ezell (2001) stated that "lack of time, energy, resources, and training are real barriers . . . to advocacy" (p. 12). Yet the constraints in place in a particular job setting can be overcome in varying degrees by focusing on self-empowerment and empowerment of students and their families. According to Ezell, those who advocate in spite of obstacles identify a need, believe in the efficacy of advocacy, understand when advocacy is needed and how to effectively advocate, and embrace the challenges that are often inherent to advocacy.

How will you know when advocacy actions are necessary? Through your own observations of student clients, noting the quality of their educational experiences and the various services provided and not provided. Hart and Jacobi (1992) encouraged counselors to become proactive in meeting student needs. One of the approaches suggested was to implement outreach programs to inform students of opportunities to further their education or develop a talent or skill. Correcting any myths or misconceptions about what it takes to succeed and designing motivational activities to encourage school success can lay the groundwork for student advocacy. Continually assessing the barriers to education that exist for students will identify necessary advocacy actions. It is not always easy to become aware of inequities and injustices toward others without heightened self-awareness regarding the various ways that individuals and groups are overlooked (i.e., gender, ethnicity, race, socioeconomic status). Even if being aware of inequalities comes easily, it is much more difficult to know what to do and to actually have confidence in your ability to make a difference. Recognition of the usefulness of advocacy skills and the desire for the know-how often appear when a need for action arises. Then it is much too late. Prior recognition and acknowledgement of the power of advocacy is a proactive way to approach advocacy situations.

Ideally, school counselors are prepared for advocacy actions in their counselor training programs. Coursework on advocacy has been included during the recent school improvement and school counseling transformation work in the last decade. Yet having advocacy skills and seeing a need for them is often not enough. Fear and uncertainty may cause hesitation. Being afraid that employers and community members will not appreciate your actions can interfere with the motivation to pursue advocacy actions. These fears, hesitations, and feelings of being overwhelmed are legitimate concerns. One way to overcome such barriers is to work with fellow counselors, supportive community action groups, and professional organizations. There is safety and support in teamwork. Working with others is often more productive than working alone. However, keep in mind that there are many things you can do as "just one counselor" to empower students and their families to act on their own behalf, especially if you have the support of school leaders.

An essential ingredient to successful advocacy by the school counselor is the degree to which the school and school system support advocacy actions on behalf of students. The level of support provided by school leadership is likely to be linked to the system's identified beliefs and values in regard to equitable education for all students. Bailey, Getch, and Chen-Hayes (2003) included working as a team, educating principals and staff, building effective relationships, and making sure the administration is onboard as essential actions before taking advocacy risks. The concept of teamwork and collaboration continue to emerge as essential practices for school counselors, and this is nonetheless true when talking about the school counselor's advocacy role.

There is an old adage that states, "Be sure you are right and then go ahead." This phrase means that the first step in taking action is to make sure there is a need for action, that there is no other solution than an advocacy action, and that you have the knowledge and skills to take the action. It is essential to possess the motivation and stamina to pursue the action and, most of all, recognize when it is time to stop or put an issue to rest. Knowing when to move forward and when to slow or cease the pursuit of change is critical to the success of an advocacy action. Without this knowledge and awareness of timing, it is possible to do more harm than good for students and their families.

House and Martin (1998) indicated that school counselors must become advocates for helping all students gain access to rigorous academic preparation and support for success in these programs. These authors provided a list of practices for school counselors in order to advocate for students and to become recognized as a viable and integral part of a school. These items were divided into categories of (a) when working with students, (b) when working with the school system, and (c) when working with the community. Following are some examples.

- Teach students how to help themselves (e.g., organizational skills, study skills, test-taking skills).
- Teach students and their families how to access support systems for academic success.
- Use local, regional, and national data to promote systemic change.
- Work as a resource broker within the community to identify all available resources to help all students achieve (p. 289).

Advocacy actions of school counselors are a necessary part of educational reform. It makes sense that the school counselor may be the best person to develop greater opportunities for students to achieve and succeed in the future. In this regard, House and Martin (1998) stated:

> [School counselors] have access to critical data about student placements, academic success and failure of all students, and course-taking patterns. They know which teachers are seen as ineffective by students and administrators and are in a position to provide consultation and staff development for teachers in need of assistance. They are in touch with parents and they can easily access community resources. (p. 285)

These proponents of advocacy challenged school counselors to embrace the responsibility that comes with advocacy and utilize this empowering tool as a way to address barriers that may prevent students—all students—from reaching their maximum potential.

The time has come for school counselors to further develop their role as change agents. With proper training in leadership skills, focusing upon the change effort, and with proper training in the skills of advocacy, better understanding of the counselor's role as an advocate will evolve. Today's school counselor must assume an integrated role within the entire academic community and skillfully communicate and demonstrate this role to all the various stakeholders.

Action + Advocacy = Effective Services for Students

When considering the wide range of social issues and conditions that accompany students, parents, teachers, and community members into our schools, it is clear that school counselors must rise to the challenge of being effective advocates. Whether advocating for the school counseling program or for a specific student, there are common themes that should permeate the actions of school counselors: *putting student needs first, demonstrating passion and commitment, doing what is right,* and *staying the course.*

Putting Student Needs First

The school counselor's first commitment is to the students. This is nonnegotiable. Any program changes, policy changes, decisions, or alterations should always be considered in light of the effect they will have on *all* students.

Professional Perspective

RENEE (ES)

The school counselor should, above all else, be an advocate for students. Parents or teachers may become caught in power struggles or emotionally entrenched in a situation. The school counselor must always step back and say, "What is in the best interest of the student?" This may not always be the easiest stance to take, but it is the school counselor's responsibility to advocate for the child and mediate between the adults involved, if necessary.

Demonstrating Passion and Commitment

It is difficult to advocate for something that does not seem beneficial to students. If a school counselor has feelings of discomfort or is hesitant to participate in or lead activities toward or for a cause, he or she should really explore the reasons for hesitancy. Examination of the personal and professional level of commitment and emotional response should either affirm the school counselor's next steps in the advocacy process or allow the school counselor to decide not to pursue advocacy actions. If a school counselor feels strongly about a decision or action, he or she must have the passion and commitment to take a stand and be prepared to defend the position. Balancing passion and commitment with the ability to communicate valid reasons for taking a stand is a skill that often takes time to develop and certainly takes time to finesse.

Professional Practice

BETH (MS)

I try to acknowledge the parents, teachers, or other persons involved with the child in order to normalize their feelings of frustration. For example, I might say, "It must be very challenging to have this student in your class when you've got 24 other students," or, "I know it must be difficult to be a single parent of a child that has so many needs." The other aspect is to acknowledge that this child does have needs and to try to engage others in the solution. I try to make it clear that I am not trying to give the child an easy way out, but that someone needs to support him or her. Most of the time, if you acknowledge that it is not easy to be involved with or responsible for the child, but that the child needs help, the involved parties will almost always be supportive.

School counselors have a wonderful opportunity to advocate for a unified approach to issues and situations. The concept of *unity* was also discussed as a necessary element of effective leadership. It is crucial that school counselors use passion and commitment as a means of advocacy and unification. For example, if the school board does not have a clear understanding of what the school program is doing and the difference that it makes with students, then the school counselor needs to educate and inform the board of the necessity of the program in the school. This could be accomplished by a presentation of the effective outcome results of school counseling interventions or a demonstration of how school counselors are committed to working as a support service for students, parents, and school personnel. Another example would be if parents are unhappy with a teacher's policy or procedures, the school counselor can be an important facilitator in helping the parents and teacher arrive at a greater understanding of each other's positions. Advocacy for collaboration is a key role for school counselors.

Doing What Is Right

One of the most valuable lessons to remember in your school counseling career is that appropriate and ethical decisions are not always popular. However, in order to be an advocate for a student or a cause, school counselors may have to take a stand on what they feel is in the best interest of the involved parties. As a school counselor-in-training, you will hopefully develop skills to facilitate dialogue, explore issues, and respond effectively to conflict or disagreement.

One skill that is as instinctual as it is teachable is the belief that what you do or say is the right thing. As long as the students are the highest priority, acting appropriately should come very naturally. Further, it is beneficial to consult with colleagues and peers to consider different perspectives before acting on a situation or making a decision. Doing the right thing professionally also means being informed and having a basis for a position on an issue. Most importantly, the "right" thing involves considering what is best based on overall circumstances and the implications of advocacy actions in any given situation.

Staying the Course

Advocacy may be as simple as providing information about the school counseling program so that parents are aware of the counseling services available. It may also be long-term and intensive, such as trying to convince state legislatures that school counselors at all levels are necessary to the overall effectiveness of a school program, and not ancillary services that can be cut from the budget. It may be personally and emotionally draining, for instance, advocating for a student who is struggling so that parents, teachers, and administrators give him or her another chance. These long battles can sometimes be frustrating and discouraging. However, school counselors must persevere in their advocacy role by doing what it takes to address students' needs as effectively as possible.

Professional Perspective

ESTHER (HS)

Counselors are first and foremost student advocates. They have the opportunity to make a difference in a child's life everyday. Counselors advocate for students as they apply for college, apply for jobs, and interact with parents, teachers, and administrators. Counselors must keep students' needs as their primary focus.

CONCLUSION

This chapter has examined how school counselors can participate in advocacy. At this point, you may find yourself asking, "How can I begin to advocate for myself, the program, the students, and families, especially as a new school counselor?" Kuranz (2002) offered some suggestions of where to begin:

> We advocate by understanding our voices make a difference. School counselors have the skills to be effective advocates. A good advocate listens, communicates, embraces different points of view, sets goals, develops strategies, provides feedback, works with people no matter who is in charge, thinks on his or her feet, coordinates, mediates, juggles more than one job at a time, identifies resources, and sticks with a task until a solution is found. (p. 178)

Effective advocacy is a skill that can be acquired early, developed over time, and utilized throughout a school counselor's career. Sometimes, school counselors engage in advocacy roles out of necessity or immediacy, such as pleading a student's case to teachers and administrators or responding to the school board's consideration to eliminate a counseling service. Other times, advocacy is organized and planned, such as participating in state-level activities related to school counseling legislation or approaching a community organization about supporting the counseling program. Whatever the situation, an important guideline is to honor your commitment to being a professional school counselor and be ready to advocate for the programs and practices that you know will sustain the students and the profession. Hopefully, your training will prepare you to face the challenges and opportunities that might present themselves as you begin your school counseling career. Practicum and internship experiences will shed light on how school counselors integrate advocacy into their roles. If advocacy stops, effective counseling programs may become ineffective. Therefore, advocacy skills and practices should be integrated into all facets of a school counseling program.

REFLECTION AND DISCUSSION

1. Advocacy is a role that school counselors fulfill in order to meet the needs of all students. Are there any student populations that you think might require greater advocacy than others? What are the unique issues of these groups of students, and how do school counselors provide support?

2. Dr. Jackson discussed different types of advocacy. In terms of school counseling, how do you think the categories should be prioritized? Which type of advocacy seems to be the most critical to promoting student success and effective counseling programs?

3. What specific behaviors do you expect to perform in your advocacy role? Imagine the following and then identify how you would advocate in each situation:

    a. There has been some discussion by the School Board to cut the budget by increasing the student-to-counselor ratio in the district's schools, thereby eliminating some school counseling positions.

    b. Parents are vocally upset about a new program that the counseling program is trying to implement with students.

    c. A 17-year-old student has indicated to you that he would like to drop out of high school and pursue his GED. You know that this student has accumulated very few credits toward his diploma and that truancy and completion of assignments are two major issues. You are about to attend a meeting of administrators, the student's teachers, the student's parents, and the student to determine the best plan of action for the student. What will you say in the meeting?

CHAPTER 13

The School Counselor and Results-Based Accountability

*F*or school counselors, the concept of *accountability* seems to conjure up images of research and statistics that require intense number crunching and hours of data analysis. With the current emphasis on school reform and results-based evaluation, it is important to examine the school counselor's role in accountability. According to Otwell and Mullis (1997):

> Many children come to school with personal problems that interfere with learning, and the counselor who can help to limit or prevent these obstacles is a valuable member of the educational team. However, counselors can no longer assume that people outside the counseling profession understand and accept the idea that students need this type of assistance and that the assistance provided is effective. School counselors, therefore, face the daunting task of providing empirical data to bolster support for their unique contribution to the school's instructional team. (p. 344)

Assessment and evaluation provide an opportunity to demonstrate the contributions that school counselors make to the educational success of students. The age of accountability is upon us, and school counselors will need to embrace accountability, using results to secure their position as an integral part of the education team.

There are several scholarly sources that offer extensive coverage of evaluation and accountability in school counseling programs (Baker, 2000; Gysbers & Henderson, 2000; Schmidt, 2003). Whiston and Sexton (1998) provided a summary of school counseling outcome research that had been conducted and published between 1988 and 1995. While the research provided useful results for school counseling, the summary described an increasing need for data that supports the efficacy of school counseling programs. Thus, accountability has emerged as one aspect of the transformed role of school counselors. School counselors are being asked to reframe traditional notions about evaluation. This chapter will focus on the new accountability—what can be measured, how it can be assessed, and how data can be presented. As you enter the profession of school counseling, it is important that you understand the importance of accountability, as well as the process in which it can occur.

We will begin by exploring evaluation—the *process* in which results are measured. Dr. Pamelia Brott, a counselor educator at Virginia Polytechnic Institute and State University and editor of *Professional School Counseling*, contributes a practical perspective on how accountability and evaluation are natural outcomes of effective school counseling services. It is not enough to say that, as school counselors, we help students feel better. The question is, *"How are students more effective learners because of the school counseling program?"* Finally, we will discuss *school counselor performance evaluation* as a process that develops effective counseling skills.

Evaluation: Reasons for Resistance

Historically, data collection in school counseling has consisted of "head counting," or calculating the number of lessons or amount of time spent in specific counseling activities. For example, "Thirty-two students participated in four small group counseling units on anger management" or "I spent 25% of my time providing classroom guidance lessons this week and 10% conducting individual counseling sessions." In the past, quantity has defined quality in many school counseling programs. The demand for results-based reform in education has led to a demand for results-based counseling programs in schools. Rather than waiting for change, school counselors must now be focused on making change happen through documentation and reporting of results.

Professional Practice

ESTHER (HS)

In the past, we have not effectively used results-based evaluation. Counselors fill out a time survey, which details how much time is given to counseling and noncounseling activities. This came about as a result of state legislation requiring that 60% of counselors' time be spent in counseling activities.

Researchers and professionals have offered several reasons for school counselors' resistance to evaluation. Kuranz (2002) offered the following reasons:

- no time to add another responsibility,
- lack of resources,
- lack of confidence in the ability to conduct research or collect data,
- lack of models or samples of what others have done,
- no opportunities to collaborate with other professionals, and
- new and unfamiliar frameworks to help counselors conduct research (p. 177).

Maybe the most understated excuse is that school counselors sometimes fear that they will find shortcomings in their programs (Dahir & Tyra, 2002). School counselors feel fear and uncertainty related to the risks of evaluating their programs and themselves. School counselors might ask, *"What if we evaluate the program and find that what we're doing isn't working?"* Otwell and Mullis (1997) stated, "Being accountable does not always mean being successful" (p. 346). However, discovering that a program is not successful or effective is useful information. If a school counselor is implementing a curriculum that is not making a marked improvement in students' lives or educational achievements, it may be time for the counselor to rethink the use of the curriculum. Counselors should approach the evaluation process positively. Rather than thinking, "We don't want to perform an evaluation because what we're doing may not be working," counselors should be thinking, "If what we're doing isn't working, then maybe we need to revisit what we're doing." Evaluation, whether the results are positive or negative, provides valuable information that should guide the development and maintenance of comprehensive school counseling programs.

Another reason for the lack of research on accountability measures in school counseling is that counselor education programs may not prepare school counselors-in-training to conduct results-based evaluation. Trevisan (2000) found that only 19 states and Washington, D.C. require skills in program evaluation as part of the state certification for school counselors. This suggests that school counselors are not proficient in evaluation skills, which could be a reason that they avoid or are intimidated by research and are resistant to data collection and evaluation.

At present, the concepts of accountability and evaluation are sweeping through school counseling programs across the country. The Transforming School Counseling Initiative (The Education Trust, 2003) devoted an entire segment of its school counselor training programs to teaching school counselors to use accountability to connect counseling programs to the missions of schools and involve school counselors in standards-based reform. School counselors must assert their positions on plans for reform and provide results that reveal how the counseling program supports the academic program.

Perhaps the greatest challenge for school counselors is to change the negative thinking that emerges when considering evaluation. According to Allen (1992), "School counselor efficacy is enhanced by action-oriented research which documents the value, effectiveness, and necessity of school counseling programs. . . . Research is a proactive professional activity which will contribute to the accountability, advocacy, and advancement of school counseling" (p. 1). If school counselors reframe evaluation and accountability by considering the benefits for the counseling program, the positive implications of evaluation will be evident. Evaluation does not have to be all-encompassing and may be very specific at first. Taking "baby steps" toward evaluation is a good rule of thumb because any evaluation, even if only of one aspect of the school counseling program, is a good start.

Professional Practice

BETH (MS)

In group counseling and classroom guidance lessons, I usually do pre- and post-tests. The test might be as simple as a small questionnaire, for example, on decision making: "What do you know about decision making? How do you make decisions?" You can really find out how much the students are actually gaining from sessions by conducting very simple evaluations.

The following contribution by Dr. Pamelia Brott will be useful for veteran counselors, as well as counselors entering the profession. With the emphasis on accountability in the Transforming School Counseling Initiative (The Education Trust, 2003) and the National Model for School Counseling Programs (ASCA, 2003a), it is critical that school counselors are prepared to produce data that demonstrate the impact of school counseling programs on student development and achievement. The next section describes specific ways that data can be gathered and utilized in practical and efficient ways that are meaningful to schools and their constituents. This information will be invaluable to you as you begin your school counseling career.

Making It Count: Accountability for School Counselors

This section (to the heading "School Counselor Performance Evaluation: Professional Accountability") was contributed by Dr. Pamelia Brott, Assistant Professor, Virginia Polytechnic Institute and State University. Recognition is given to Judy Bowers and Trish Hatch for their presentation, "ASCA Intensive Training Workshop: The ASCA National Model," at the 2002 ASCA National Conference in Miami, Florida, and for being catalysts for accountability practice in comprehensive developmental school counseling programs.

Professional school counselors are continually challenged to demonstrate the effectiveness of the programs and services provided to the school community—students, teachers, parents, principals, superintendents, and school board members. Evaluation and accountability are the measurable means used to demonstrate the effectiveness of school counseling programs and services (Nystul, 2003). In other words, the question school counselors should be attempting to answer is, "How are students different as a result of the school counseling program?" (ASCA, 2003a, p. 59). One element of the ASCA National Model is the accountability system, which is composed of results reports, school counselor performance standards, and the program audit. The focus of this section will be on the accountability system that professional school counselors can use to demonstrate the effectiveness of the school counseling program and of the services provided by school counselors to the school community.

Data-driven decisions in comprehensive school counseling and guidance programs (CSCGP) provide a systematic approach for aligning the school counseling program with the school's academic mission (ASCA, 2003a; Hatch and Holland, 2001; Bowers & Hatch, 2002). Data are used to identify services provided (process data), what others know as a result of the services (perception data), and the impact of the services (results data). The collection and analysis of data provides a measure of program effectiveness, which in turn becomes an advocacy tool for the school counseling program. Therefore, measures of accountability are used to ensure that the program is carried out, every student is served, the program is analyzed to improve services and to advocate for systemic change, and the information is shared with stakeholders (e.g., teachers, principals, parents, school board).

Professional school counselors must be competent in collecting, analyzing, interpreting, and sharing data. Data can document the immediate, intermediate, and long-range impact of the school counseling program (ASCA, 2003a). Through the use of data, professional school counselors can identify what is working and ways for closing the gap in student achievement.

Student success is supported through the activities included in the delivery system—school guidance curriculum, individual student planning, responsive services, and system support (ASCA, 2003a). The delivery system focuses on student progress in such areas as attendance, discipline, transitions, post-secondary plans, and standardized measures of academic achievement. Therefore, the accountability system provides an indicator of the impact of the delivery system (i.e., school counseling program) on student success over time. Accountability indicators can be identified for activities that address such issues as:

- academic failure notices,
- school dropout percentages,
- retention rate,
- discipline referrals,
- attendance rate/truancy,
- standardized achievement test scores,
- number and diversity of students involved in recognition programs,
- parental involvement,
- high school graduation rate,
- course enrollments (honors, AP, IB, college-level courses),
- individual academic and career plans,
- successful completion of curriculum in courses for credit,
- GPA,
- individual portfolios with 4-year/6-year plans,
- postsecondary plans,
- participation in support services (e.g., tutoring, mentoring),
- school transitions (e.g., new building, transferring to another school, moving),
- school safety, and
- positive school climate.

Foundation

What is the foundation of the school counseling program? Building from the ASCA National Model (ASCA, 2003a), a professional school counselor should be able to articulate the following: (a) the beliefs and philosophy that direct the program; (b) a mission statement that communicates the vision of the program; (c) how the professional school counselor facilitates student development and learning in three broad domains—academic, career, and personal/social; and (d) the "standards and competencies [that] define the knowledge, attitudes, or skills that students should obtain or demonstrate as a result of participating in a school counseling program" (p. 22). The foundation provides professional school counselors with the ways and means to identify goals for the school counseling program and to determine if the goals have been accomplished.

	School Events	Goal: Academic	Goal: Career Development	Goal: Personal/ Social
August				
September				
October				
November				
December				
January				
February				
March				
April				
May				
June				

Figure 13.1 Aligning the school counseling program with the school calendar

Management

Once goals for the school counseling program have been identified, the implementation of the program needs to be aligned with the school calendar. Is the program making the most of the time available? Developing an action plan for the delivery system will ensure that conflicts with other school activities (e.g., parent-teacher conferences, exams, athletics), deadlines (e.g., reports, applications), and holidays (e.g., spring break) are avoided. Figure 13.1 is an example of a table that can be used to align a school counseling program with a school calendar.

Professional school counselors should begin to think in terms of what data will be of use in planning and delivering an effective school counseling program. The use of data enables the professional school counselor to monitor the program and identify activities that can be developed to close the gap between where the program is and where it should be.

A starting point is crosswalking current practices to accountability measures, reports, and calendars. Crosswalking involves making sure that the school counseling program goals and objectives integrate and support the overall mission of the school. Professional school counselors can find ways in which the school counseling program supports and enhances student learning by crosswalking the guidance and counseling delivery system (e.g., classroom guidance, individual and group counseling, coordination, consultation) with the school's mission and curriculum. Figure 13.2 is an adaptation of the "ASCA National Standards: Developmental Crosswalking Tool" (ASCA, 2003a,

ASCA National Standards and Competencies
Crosswalking Tool

Symbol	Activity or Classroom Guidance Unit	Grade Level
*	Career Day	K, 5, 6–8, 9, 11
–	Career as Life	K–5, 6–8, 9–12
+	Be a Good Worker	4, 5
o	School Transitions	K, 5, 6, 8, 9–12

CAREER DEVELOPMENT DOMAIN

STANDARD A: Students will acquire the skills to investigate the world of work in relation to knowledge of self and to make informed career decisions.

Competency A:1 Develop Career Awareness

		K–2	3–5	6–8	9–12
C:A1.1	Develop skills to locate, evaluate and interpret career information	*	* +	*	*
C:A1.2	Learn about the variety of traditional and nontraditional occupations	*	*	*	*
C:A1.3	Develop an awareness of personal abilities, skills, interests and motivations		+		
C:A1.4	Learn how to interact and work cooperatively in teams		+		
C:A1.5	Learn to make decisions	o	+ o	o	o
C:A1.6	Learn how to set goals	o	+ o	o	o
C:A1.7	Understand the importance of planning	o	+ o	o	o
C:A1.8	Pursue and develop competency in areas of interest				
C:A1.9	Develop hobbies and vocational interests		+		
C:A1.10	Balance between work and leisure time				

Competency A:2 Develop Employment Readiness

		K–2	3–5	6–8	9–12
C:A2.1	Acquire employability skills such as working on a team, problem-solving and organizational skills		+		
C:A2.2	Apply job readiness skills to seek employment opportunities				o
C:A2.3	Demonstrate knowledge about the changing workplace				o

Figure 13.2 Crosswalking school counseling program with school curriculum

Source: Adapted from ASCA. (2003a). *The ASCA national model: A framework for school counseling programs.* Alexandria, VA: Author, pp. 87–92.

pp. 87–92) that provides an example of crosswalking activities and units in the school counseling program to reflect a comprehensive program addressing the career development domain.

School counselors should develop reports that describe what is being offered by the CSCGP to support student learning. Data will succinctly organize the information so that it can be visually displayed in charts that support impact statements about the school counseling program and activities. Figure 13.3a (adapted from ASCA, 2003a, p. 108) is an example of a results report compiling program activities that have addressed a specific standard—Career Development Standard C. Figure 13.3b presents examples of impact statements based on the results report.

Assessment

Professional school counselors should seize the opportunity to use data as a means to be proactive in their roles, priorities, and activities. Data-based decision making and ongoing program assessment can be used to clarify school counselors' roles and functions by encouraging others to focus on school counselors' special skills (Nystul, 2003). Data can be used to describe problems, plan interventions, provide advocacy for all students, and target systemic changes (Hatch & Holland, 2001). Further, data can be used to demonstrate the effectiveness of interventions and programs and to increase accountability by evaluating how students are different as a result of the school counseling program. Data can be used to communicate information about the effectiveness of both the school counselor and the school counseling program.

Data can be categorized into four foci: process data, perception data, results data, and data over time (ASCA, 2003a; Hatch & Holland, 2001). Process data tell the story of what you did for whom; gathering process data is a "method of evaluation using figures to show the activities, such as numbers of students served, groups and classroom visits rather than the results from the activities" (ASCA, p. 131). Perception data indicate what others think, know, or demonstrate, measuring "what students and others observe or perceive, knowledge gained, attitudes and beliefs held or competencies achieved" (ASCA, p. 130). Results data are outcome data that demonstrate "how students are measurably different as a result of the program" (ASCA, p. 131). Data over time provide year-to-year information about the effectiveness of the school counseling program and activities. Data can be collected immediately, intermediately, or longitudinally (i.e., long-range) (ASCA; Hatch & Holland, 2001).

PROCESS DATA: "WHAT YOU DID"   Process data are descriptive in nature and indicate if the planned program was conducted (ASCA, 2003a). Examples of process data include the following:

- Forty-nine parents attended the "Kindergarten for Parents" program.
- One hundred twenty-six fifth graders participated in "Be a Good Worker" career education unit.

Career Development Standard C: Students will understand the relationship between personal qualities, education, training, and the world of work

Counselor	Target Group	Curriculum and Materials	Type of Service Delivered	Start Date / End Date	Process Data (# students impacted)	Perception Data (pre-/post-test or activity)	Results Data (how did the students change as a result of the lesson?)	Implications
Mr. C.U. Good	9th Grade—296 students	Self Directed Search (SDS)	Classroom guidance and career counseling groups	October 2002 / December 2002	296 / 100% participation	Three months following SDS activity, 100% of the students could name at least three personal abilities, three personal skills, and three personal interests	100% of the students listed personal abilities, skills, and interests on personal portfolio (4-year plan)	Excellent effect on career development in relation to knowledge of self and ability to make informed career decisions
Ms. R.T. Juan	10th Grade—305 students	Differential Aptitude Test (DAT)	Classroom guidance	October 2002 / October 2002	305 / 100% participation	One month following DAT, 100% of the students identified areas of measured strengths	100% of the students completed the DAT and recorded strength areas on personal portfolio (4-year plan)	Reevaluate follow-up activities cross-discipline (e.g., English essays about personal interests, math graphs of strengths for portfolio)

Mrs. I.C. Yu	11th Grade—287 students	Career Day—non-traditional careers	Career Day using non-traditional career speakers	November 2002 November 2002	281 98% participation	100% of the students completed questionnaire regarding jobs from Career Day that fit abilities, skills, and interests	100% of the students who attended the Career Day could identify at least three non-traditional careers that fit their abilities, skills, and interests, which were recorded on personal portfolio (4-year plan)	Participants in the career counseling groups may need additional resources to support exploration of self-awareness: mentors, extracurricular activities
Mr. M.T. Nest	12th Grade—262 students	Exit interviews	Individual counseling sessions	March 2002 May 2002	262 100% participation	100% of the students completed an exit interview	100% of the students identified a post-secondary plan and recorded the plan on personal portfolio (4-year plan)	

Figure 13.3a School counseling program: activities

Source: Adapted from ASCA. (2003a). *The ASCA national model: A framework for school counseling programs.* Alexandria, VA: Author, p. 108.

Impact Statements

98% or better participation of grades 9 through 12 in career guidance units focused on students' understanding of the relationship between personal qualities, education, and training and the world of work.

100% of the students grades 9 through 12 who participated in career guidance units demonstrated knowledge about personal qualities, education, and training.

100% of the 9th graders listed personal abilities, skills, and interests on their personal portfolio (4-year plan).

100% of the 10th graders completed the Differential Aptitude Test (DAT) and recorded strength areas on their personal portfolio (4-year plan).

100% of the 11th graders who attended the Career Day could identify at least three non-traditional careers that fit their abilities, skills, and interests.

100% of the 12th graders identified a post-secondary plan and recorded the plan on their personal portfolio (4-year plan).

Implications

The planned activities related to the career guidance units in grades 9 through 12 have had an excellent effect on students' career development in relation to knowledge of self and to making informed career decisions.

- The Self-Directed Search, Differential Aptitude Test, Non-traditional Career Day, and exit interviews will be continued at the respective grade levels to reach 100% of the students in grades 9 through 12 in the upcoming school year.

- Additional resources will be identified to strengthen students' acquisition of skills necessary to make a successful transition from school to their post-secondary plans. Resources may include involving academic teachers in cross-curricular student assignments, establishing a mentoring program, and expanding extracurricular opportunities.

Figure 13.3b Examples of impact statements

- One hundred percent of the students in ninth grade participated in sexual harassment prevention classroom guidance lessons.
- Three counseling groups, with five students in each group, were conducted during the fall semester.

PERCEPTION DATA: "WHAT OTHERS THINK, KNOW, OR DEMONSTRATE"
Perception data measure competencies achieved, knowledge gained, or attitudes and beliefs of students, parents, and staff and can be gathered through the use of pre- and post-tests, documented competency achievement, questionnaires, or evaluation instruments (ASCA, 2003a). Results from the

evaluation demonstrate what knowledge participants are perceived to have gained from the activity. The easiest way to collect perception data is by using an existing evaluation tool the school counselor has used to assess an activity. By asking students to complete the assessment before the activity (i.e., pre-test, pre-session) and then again after completion of the activity (i.e., post-test, post-session), the school counselor can gather perception data—what a student knows after completing the activity. Statements using perception data include the following:

- One hundred percent of the first graders named three jobs found in our school at the conclusion of the spring classroom guidance unit, "Our School Workers."
- Ninety-three percent of the sixth grade students can accurately calculate a grade point average (GPA).
- Fifty-four percent of the eighth grade students can identify at least three Advanced Placement (AP) subjects offered in high school.
- Twenty-nine percent of the 11th grade students report an understanding of the relationship between their SAT scores and college admissions.

RESULTS DATA: "SO WHAT"   Results data indicate the effect or impact of school counseling programs and services on students' skills, knowledge, attitudes, and behavior (ASCA, 2003a). Results data demonstrate behavior change in attendance, behavior, participation, academic achievement, and school climate (Hatch & Holland, 2001). They also indicate identified improvements (i.e., decrease in target area, increase in target area). Examples of results data include the following:

- Attendance rates on the scheduled testing days for the state standardized assessment program increased from 90% last year to 99% this year.
- Eighty percent of the sixth grade students on the retention list avoided retention and were promoted to the seventh grade.
- Discipline referrals have decreased by 67%.

DATA OVER TIME: "WHAT HAS CHANGED OVER TIME"   Data over time can be collected and presented based on different time frames: immediate, intermediate, and longitudinal (Hatch & Holland, 2001). Immediate data reflect the impact of an activity on participants (i.e., acquiring information or skills). Immediate data can be gathered through the use of pre- or post-tests for a classroom guidance activity. This data will measure the *immediate* impact on the knowledge, skills, and/or attitudes of the participants. "There was a 100% gain in knowledge about graduation requirements by the ninth graders who participated in the 'I Will Succeed' classroom guidance activity," is an example of immediate data.

Intermediate data reflect participants' application of information or skills from an activity (ASCA, 2003a; Hatch & Holland, 2001). Intermediate data can be gathered by using a questionnaire to follow-up on a classroom guidance activity after a certain period of time (e.g., the next marking period, at the end of the semester). "Eighty-seven percent of the fourth graders described at least three positive ways to deal with bullies one marking period following the classroom guidance unit 'Taking a Stand,'" is an example of intermediate results.

Longitudinal data reflect impact over time (e.g., year-to-year) (Hatch & Holland, 2001). Existing data from activities offered on a recurring basis can be compiled as data over time. Reporting an increase or decrease in attendance at parent education programs, at counseling sessions on standardized test-taking strategies, and at orientation meetings for grade transitions (e.g., elementary to middle school) can indicate use of programs over time, as well as a need for additional activities to close the gap. Longitudinal data can provide valuable information for developing, planning, and implementing effective school counseling services.

Descriptive Statistics

Statistical procedures are methods for handling quantitative data in such a way that the information is meaningful (LaFountain & Bartos, 2002). Descriptive statistics enable us to describe and summarize the data we have collected. Two basic descriptive statistics that can be valuable tools for the school counselor are percent and percent change. Percent is a convenient way to handle large and small numbers and to standardize the numbers with a common base of 100. A percent is a ratio or proportion based on 100 (e.g., 85% indicates 85 out of 100). Percent change is the ratio or proportion of change from a beginning number to a final number (e.g., 91% increase, 12% decrease). Figure 13.4 (adapted from Hatch & Holland, 2001) demonstrates the calculation of percent, and Figure 13.5 (adapted from Hatch & Holland) demonstrates the calculation of percent change.

Communicating Information

Once the identified goals of the counseling and guidance program have been crosswalked to the school curriculum, planned to complement the school calendar, and supported with data collected to demonstrate effectiveness, the information needs to be communicated to the school community. Basically, the CSCGP report can be a series of formative and summative evaluations presented to communication targets (e.g., parents, principals).

FORMATIVE EVALUATIONS The formative evaluation consists of a summary for each activity completed or for a series of activities within a grade level or student group (e.g., at-risk students, special education students, students performing below grade level, gifted and talented students, second graders).

Percent—rate or portion of 100

Number (a) divided by the total (b) then multiplied by 100 (i.e., moving decimal two places to the right) = %

$$a/b \times 100 = \%$$

Example: 194 of 200 seventh graders completed the classroom guidance unit "Be the Best You Can Be."

$$194/200 = .97 \times 100 = 97\%$$

Stated as a percent: 97% of the seventh graders completed the classroom guidance unit "Be the Best You Can Be."

Example: 486 of 521 of our elementary students have participated in at least one school counseling activity this marking period.

$$486/521 = .93 \times 100 = 93\%$$

Stated as a percent: 93% of our elementary students have participated in at least one school counseling activity this marking period.

Figure 13.4   Descriptive statistics—percent

Source: Adapted from Hatch, T., & Holland, L. (2001). *Moreno Valley Unified School District School Counselor Academy Handbook.* Moreno Valley, CA: Author.

The formative report should identify the goal (standard) and objectives (competencies) established by the school counselor, the target group, inclusive dates of the activity or activities, and the data (i.e., process data, perception data, results data). Spreadsheets or tables of information can quickly organize and present formative evaluations. Figure 13.6 is an example of a formative evaluation based on the ASCA National Model (2003a, p. 107).

Once a formative evaluation has been completed, impact statements can be written regarding the effectiveness of the school counseling program.

- One hundred percent of the 11th grade students reported using at least two strategies they had learned in the test taking workshops when they completed the PSAT.
- There has been a 30% decrease in student-reported bullying since instituting the goal of responsible behavior for the sixth graders.
- There has been a 478% increase in parent attendance at evening parent education programs.

SUMMATIVE EVALUATIONS   Summative evaluations constitute a final evaluation of the impact of the school counseling program and activities on the academic achievement of all students in a school over a set period of time (i.e., school year). The summative evaluation summarizes the information from all formative evaluations, highlights the impact of the school counseling program, and identifies goals for the next year. The goals for the next year will include the continuation of proven effective programming, as well as proposed program changes or additions to address discrepancies in program services. Figure 13.7 is an example of a summative evaluation.

Percent change—change from beginning number to final number expressed as a percent

Final # (b) minus beginning # (a) = change (c)

Change (c) divided by beginning # (a) gives a decimal (d) multiplied by 100 (i.e., moving decimal two places to the right) = % change

$$b - a = c$$
$$c/a = d \times 100 = \% \text{ change}$$

Example: There were 42 correct responses on the pre-test; there were 79 correct responses on the post-test.

$$79 - 42 = 37 \text{ (more correct responses)}$$
$$37/42 = .88 \times 100 = 88\%$$

Stated as a percent: There was an 88% improvement in correct answers for identifying Advanced Placement high school courses as a result of the classroom guidance activity, "Movin' Up."

Example: 12 people answered all questions correctly on the pre-test; 36 people answered all questions correctly on post-test.

$$36 - 12 = 24$$
$$24/12 = 2.00 \times 100 = 200\%$$

Stated as a percent change: There was a 200% improvement.

Figure 13.5 Descriptive statistics—percent change

Source: Adapted from Hatch, T., & Holland, L. (2001). *Moreno Valley Unified School District School Counselor Academy Handbook.* Moreno Valley, CA: Author.

USING GRAPHS Data can be presented in a graph to provide a visual representation of information. Graphs are figures that show relations, comparisons, and distributions (LaFountain & Bartos, 2002). Types of graphs include bar graphs (i.e., histograms), circle graphs (i.e., pie charts), line graphs (i.e., frequency polygons), and scatter graphs (i.e., scattergrams). The data that are to be presented will determine the type of graph that should be used.

Bar graphs are appropriate representations of pre-test and post-test data using score means (i.e., averages) as the data to be presented. Line graphs effectively display the relationship between two sets of data (e.g., individual items or scores). Scatter graphs display every data point (e.g., SAT scores, GPAs) so that trends can be noted. If you have compiled the data, a graph can be created.

A number of computer programs have been created to assist in presenting data in graphical presentations. One such program is Microsoft® Excel. Once data are entered into a spreadsheet, the Chart Wizard provides step-by-step assistance in designing a graph. Figure 13.8 provides instructions for entering data into an Excel spreadsheet, and Figure 13.9 provides instructions for creating a graph using the Chart Wizard.

Graphs can be combined with perception data, results data, and implication statements to create a report of formative and summative evaluations. Figure 13.10 is an example of a one-page summary that includes a goal, perception data, results data, and implication statements. A summary report

XYZ SCHOOL DISTRICT

Grade Level	Standard and Competencies	Guidance Lesson Content	Curriculum and Materials	Number of Guidance Lessons Delivered / What Class/Subject	Start Date / End Date	Process Data (# students impacted)	Perception Data (pre-/post-test or activity)	Results Data (how did the students change as a result of the lesson?)	Who Implemented the Lesson?
9	C:A. Students will acquire the skills to investigate the world of work in relation to knowledge of self and to make informed career decisions. C:A1.3 Develop an awareness of personal abilities, skills, interests, and motivations.	Self awareness of personal abilities, skills, and interests	Self-Directed Search	10 lessons in English language classes	October 2002 October 2002	296 100% participation	Targeted areas showed positive growth: Name three personal abilities: Pre-test = 22% Post-test = 45% Name three personal skills: Pre-test = 33% Post-test = 95% Name three personal interests: Pre-test = 15% Post-test = 80%	Increase awareness of personal abilities, skills, and interests among all ninth grade students 105% increase in awareness of personal abilities 188% increase in awareness of personal skills 433% increase in awareness of personal interests	Mr. C.U. Good, Ninth Grade School Counselor

Impact Statement

100% of the ninth graders demonstrated increased awareness of personal abilities (105% increase), skills (188% increase), and interests (433% increase) as a result of the "Self Directed Search" guidance lesson.

Figure 13.6 Formative evaluation

Source: Adapted from ASCA. (2003a). *The ASCA national model: A framework for school counseling programs.* Alexandria, VA: Author, p. 107.

ABC High School
2002–2003 School Year
School Counseling Program

School's Mission Statement: Our mission is to provide a high quality, comprehensive, meaningful education for all students. Students will experience success and will be expected to succeed within the bounds of their abilities and chosen educational goals. Each student will be treated as an individual, given the tools to be a life-long learner, and taught to be an effective and productive member of society.

School Counseling Program at ABC High School: Through individual and group counseling, coordination of activities, consultation with teachers and parents, and classroom guidance activities, the school counseling program contributes to the meaningful education of all students by assisting students with identifying their abilities and chosen educational goals. Each student is treated as an individual, given the tools to be a life-long learner, and taught to be an effective and productive member of society through the school counseling and guidance program.

Goal 2002–2003: 100% of the students at ABC High School will utilize a student portfolio (4-year plan).

Objective 1: Grade 9 will focus on identifying personal abilities, skills, and interests.

Objective 2: Grade 10 will focus on measured strengths (i.e., abilities, skills, interests).

Objective 3: Grade 11 will focus on connecting personal abilities, skills, and interests to careers.

Objective 4: Grade 12 will focus on post-secondary plans.

Accomplishments 2002–2003

100% of the students at ABC High School utilized a student portfolio (4-year plan) during 2002–2003 school year.

Objective 1: 100% of the 9th graders listed personal abilities, skills, and interests on their personal portfolio (4-year plan).

Objective 2: 100% of the 10th graders completed the Differential Aptitude Test (DAT) and recorded strength areas on their personal portfolio (4-year plan).

Objective 3: 100% of the 11th graders who attended the Career Day could identify at least three non-traditional careers that fit their abilities, skills, and interests.

Objective 4: 100% of the 12th graders identified a post-secondary plan and recorded the plan on their personal portfolio (4-year plan).

Goals for 2003–2004

- The Self-Directed Search, Differential Aptitude Test, Non-traditional Career Day, and exit interviews will be continued at the respective grade levels to reach 100% of the students in grades 9 through 12 in the upcoming school year. Resources needed include the following:

    ❑ 300 copies of the Self-Directed Search
    ❑ expanded number of speakers and careers represented for non-traditional career day
    ❑ schedule DAT for 10th grade during October
    ❑ review grade 12 student portfolios (4-year plan) before school begins to be sure all portfolios are up to date

- Additional resources will be identified to strengthen the students' acquisition of skills to make a successful transition from school to their post-secondary plans. Resources may include the following:

    ❑ involve academic teachers in cross-curricular student assignments
    ❑ establish a mentoring program
    ❑ expand extracurricular opportunities

Figure 13.7   Summative evaluation

Entering Data

1. Open Excel.

2. A blank spreadsheet opens. The horizontal rows are numbered; the vertical columns are lettered. Each cell is referenced by column (letter) and row (number); cell C3 would be in column C (i.e., third column) and in row 3 (i.e., third row).

3. To enter data, first name (i.e., label) each data set in row 1 by selecting
   a. cell A1 and labeling the column "Item".
   b. cell B1 and labeling the column "Pre-Test".
   c. cell C1 and labeling the column "Post-Test".

4. In Row 2, select
   a. cell A2 and enter "Interests" for the item label.
   b. cell B2 and enter "15%" as the pre-test score.
   c. cell C2 and enter "80%" as the post-test score.

5. In Row 3, select
   a. cell A3 and enter "Abilities" for the item label.
   b. cell B3 and enter "22%" as the pre-test score.
   c. cell C3 and enter "45%" as the post-test score.

6. In Row 4, select
   a. cell A4 and enter "Skills" for the item label.
   b. cell B4 and enter "33%" as the pre-test score.
   c. cell C4 and enter "95%" as the post-test score.

	A	**B**	**C**
1	Item	Pre-Test	Post-Test
2	Interests	15%	80%
3	Abilities	22%	45%
4	Skills	33%	95%

7. Save the file.

Figure 13.8 Microsoft® Excel instructions for entering data

is a powerful tool for communicating the impact of school counseling practices on student development.

Communication Targets: Who Needs to Know

The information compiled by the school counselor in formative and summative evaluations needs to be shared with the school community—the communication targets. The communication targets are the stakeholders who need to know about the effectiveness of the school counseling program and specific activities. Professional school counselors should begin with personnel within the school who will support effective programs. Information shared with students, teachers, administration, and parents will communicate the effectiveness of the

Creating a Graph

1. Go to the data table (or open the saved file).
2. Using your mouse, select cell A1.
3. Hold down the left button of your mouse and drag your cursor over to cell C1, and then down to C4. Your data should now be highlighted.
4. Click on the "Chart Wizard" icon (small bar-graph icon) on the toolbar. The Chart Wizard window will open.
5. Select your Chart Type (e.g., Bar, Line, Pie, Scatter) by clicking on the type in the left-hand column.
6. Select your Chart Sub-Type by clicking on the sample in the right-hand column. *Note: You can sample chart types with your data by clicking and holding the "Click and Hold to View Sample" button.*
7. Click on "Next" in the Chart Wizard window.
8. You will see a sample of your graph. If the data range is correct, click on "Next." If the data range is not correct, enter a new data range by moving the window and highlighting the correct data.
9. Type in the title of your chart and the titles of your axes. Click on "Next" when done.
10. Select "As new sheet."
11. Click on "Finish" to complete your graph. If you selected "As new sheet", your graph will appear on a separate sheet labeled as "Chart 1" on the tab. Your data can be viewed/edited by selecting the "Sheet 1" tab at the bottom of the screen.

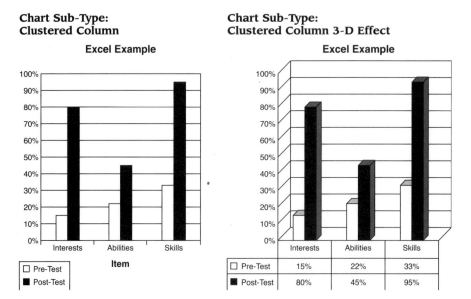

Figure 13.9   Microsoft® Excel instructions for creating a graph

Summary Report
9th Grade Career Development

The goal of the program was to increase 9th grade student knowledge of individual interests, abilities, and skills.

100% of the 9th grade students participated in the pre-test and post-test. Based on pre- and post-test evaluations, 9th grade students increased their knowledge in all three areas.

- **433%** increase in knowledge of interests.
- **105%** increase in knowledge of abilities.
- **188%** increase in knowledge of skills.

Evaluation Questions
List at least three examples of your interests, three examples of your abilities, and three examples of your skills.

	Knowledge of Interests	**Knowledge of Abilities**	**Knowledge of Skills**
Pre-test (n = 296)	15%	22%	33%
Post-test (n = 296)	80%	45%	95%

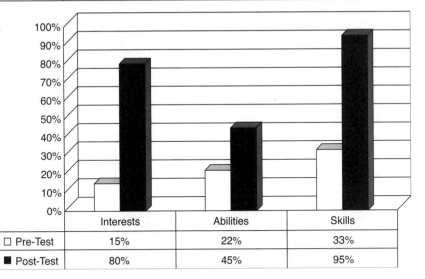

	Interests	Abilities	Skills
☐ Pre-Test	15%	22%	33%
■ Post-Test	80%	45%	95%

Implications

- Additional resources will be identified to strengthen 9th grade student knowledge of individual interests, abilities, and skills.
- Involve teachers in cross-curricular student assignments focused on identifying and using individual interests, abilities, and skills. Initial targets will be English and physical education teachers.
- Expand extracurricular opportunities for 9th graders with focus on matching interests, abilities, and skills with extracurricular activities.

Figure 13.10 Summary report for specific program

program and will garner support for future school counseling endeavors. The next level of communication targets is other school counselors in the district. Sharing information and creating a coordinated plan will ensure that a comprehensive (i.e., kindergarten through 12th grade) school counseling program is made available to the entire school community. Summative evaluations can be compiled into a school counseling program district report that provides information and data that demonstrate that all students are receiving services. The district report should be shared with central administration (e.g., superintendent, associate superintendents, directors) and members of the school board.

Reports should be tailored to the communication targets. The activities, services, and demonstrated effectiveness of the program can be reported through a school profile, yearbook page, newsletter items, newspaper articles, Microsoft® PowerPoint presentations, and written reports. A school profile can be punctuated with significant data reporting student successes based on the school counseling program offerings. A yearbook page can highlight a variety of activities included in the school counseling program with pictures of students, teachers, and school counselors working together. Newsletter items can be brief and provide specific information about school counseling services. Subsequent articles can report the results of the services. Newspaper articles highlight specific activities (e.g., career day, college day, classroom speakers) and recognize the contributions that are made by community members in the school. PowerPoint presentations that are succinct and provide pertinent data on school counseling programs serve to inform parent groups and members of the school board. Written reports can be shared on a yearly basis with principals and superintendents. The written report is a compilation of the process, perception, and results data from summative evaluations, including charts and impact statements on the effectiveness of the school counseling program.

Summary

Accountability provides a vehicle for school counselors to be active leaders in ensuring academic success for every student and provides a method for communicating the effectiveness of the comprehensive school couseling and guidance program. Further, accountability provides an advocacy role for the school counselor, advocating that the specialized skills of the school counselor are used in delivering a planned program of services to the school community.

Professional school counselors demonstrate the effectiveness of the school counseling program and the services provided to the school community through a system of evaluation and accountability. The use of data to demonstrate the effectiveness of the school counseling program will ensure that professional school counselors are providing appropriate and meaningful program services, documenting the impact of the services, planning for future program services, and identifying ways of closing the gap. The goal of the comprehensive school counseling and guidance program must be to ensure academic achievement for every student.

The ASCA National Model (ASCA, 2003a) provides guidelines for the appropriate use of accountability in the school counseling program. Identifying a program philosophy, a mission statement, student competencies within the three domains (academic, career, personal/social), and a planned program of service delivery is the foundation of accountability. Using data—process, perception, results, over time—and communicating information are the building blocks for verifying the effectiveness of the school counseling program and of the services provided by the professional school counselor.

Professional school counselors should embrace the use of data as a means to be proactive in their roles, priorities, and activities. Appropriate use of process data, perception data, results data, and data over time in both formative and summative evaluations communicates the effectiveness of the school counseling program. Communication targets with whom the professional school counselor shares the evaluations include students, teachers, principals, parents, superintendents, and school board members. Reports tailored to the communication targets include the school profile, yearbook page, newsletter items, newspaper articles, PowerPoint presentations, and written reports.

Professional school counselors who establish effective accountability practices for school counseling programs will have the tools to provide leadership, advocacy, collaboration and teaming, and systemic change through an effective comprehensive school counseling and guidance program. Rather than being reactive to the requests of others, professional school counselors will be proactive in ensuring academic success for every student. In other words, students will benefit from the school counseling program.

School Counselor Performance Evaluation: Professional Accountability

As a beginning school counselor, you may be hired with a *provisional* or temporary license until you have gained experience in your school district. School counselors have a professional responsibility to be actively engaged in their performance evaluations. The ASCA (2003c) position statement on evaluation indicates that professional school counselors are proactive in the evaluation process by keeping administrators and supervisors informed about the standards and competencies that school counselors are to demonstrate. Providing current information about the roles and responsibilities of effective counselors is an important component of evaluation. Although the process may vary in each state, evaluation of your performance as a school counselor will be part of the process of achieving a professional license with tenure. Evaluation of the school counselor may occur in one of several ways; for example, checklists, tapes, or portfolios may be used as tools for evaluation (Studer & Sommers,

My Story

In many school districts nationwide, school counselors are evaluated through the use of teacher evaluation forms. This was my experience as an elementary school counselor. Unfortunately, there were several areas on the evaluation form where my principal had to put "not applicable" because so many areas to be evaluated were not related to the types of things I was doing as a school counselor. We had to rewrite and add categories so that the evaluation would reflect at least some of what I *was* doing. When I moved to the high school level, the guidance director had developed his own evaluation instrument that dealt specifically with the goals and objectives of the high school counselor. It was easy for him to use this form, and it provided very specific and relevant information for me in terms of my strengths and challenges.

2000). However, the most common type of evaluation is direct observation by school district personnel with some authority over school counselors, such as the guidance director, the person who supervises counselors in the school district, or a building administrator. The evaluation typically entails one to three observations of the counselor's performance of school counseling responsibilities throughout the school year.

Performance evaluation for school counselors can be unique because the observation may have to be scheduled at a time when the counselor is aware that he or she is being observed. For example, the building administrator may ask for a weekly classroom guidance schedule and arrange to observe during one of those sessions. The confidentiality inherent to small group and individual counseling prohibits outside personnel from sitting in on sessions without participant and parent permission. Therefore, it is easiest for the evaluator to observe a large group counseling session. Observation may also be informal, such as during a parent conference, a large group information presentation, or other counseling services. Because school counselors are not evaluated exactly as teachers are evaluated, there is some flexibility in the type of evaluation that occurs.

The ASCA National Model (2003a) provides a list of professional school counselor performance standards that encompass the myriad skills and practices that professional school counselors should demonstrate.

- Standard 1: Program organization
- Standard 2: School guidance curriculum delivered to all students
- Standard 3: Individual student planning
- Standard 4: Responsive services

- Standard 5: Systems support
- Standard 6: School counselor and administrator agreement
- Standard 7: Advisory council
- Standard 8: Use of data
- Standard 9: Student monitoring
- Standard 10: Use of time and calendar
- Standard 11: Results evaluation
- Standard 12: Program audit
- Standard 13: Infusing themes (p. 63)

It is hoped that school districts will recognize the specialty areas of school counseling and will develop evaluation instruments that are specific to school counselor performance. Other elements, behaviors, or skills that may be evaluated when observing school counselors may include:

- developmentally appropriate materials,
- presentation and instructional style,
- professional behavior and appearance,
- classroom management skills,
- individual counseling performance,
- group counseling performance,
- participation in school-wide programs,
- professional development activities,
- adherence to ethical standards,
- contributions to school climate,
- work ethic and attitude,
- cooperation with other staff members, and
- collaboration with community resources.

One of the most challenging things to remember, especially as a beginning counselor, is that feedback from these evaluations is meant to be constructive and counselors should not expect to be "outstanding" in every area, especially during the first year of employment. In fact, it is personally and professionally advantageous to participate in a performance evaluation process that includes constructive feedback and provides challenges for improvement. Keep in mind that constructive criticism offers opportunity for growth and development.

School counselor performance may also be assessed through surveys or questionnaires to students, teachers, and parents. While this may not be the sole method for evaluation, the perspectives and opinions of constituents is often an influential factor in the performance evaluation of a school counselor.

Professional Perspective

BETH (MS)

Our school district uses a questionnaire that is sent to the whole school. It has a section on the counseling department, and we always receive the feedback. One of the questions is, "How well do you think your counselors are doing?" Besides central office personnel, the counselors get to see the results of these surveys, and we pay attention. I think that the personal touch is as important as the data. Developing a rapport with all of the people in the school helps them trust you. This comes through in the surveys.

It is not correct to assume that *program* evaluation and *performance* evaluation are separate entities. In fact, they are and should be complementary. If a school counselor provides evidence that a program or service is having a positive effect on student behavior or achievement, it also positively reflects on the counselor's performance. Ongoing assessment, rather than "snapshot" observations, might be a more valid evaluation technique for school counselor effectiveness.

Where to Begin: The Beginning School Counselor's Role in Accountability

As you think about a career in school counseling, it is critical to understand the importance of accountability and understand the significance of results-based evaluation in your school counseling program. Your first job as a school counselor will be exhilarating, overwhelming, frightening, exciting, and awesome. Accountability must be a priority when conducting an effective school counseling program that focuses on effective practices and services to meet the academic, personal/social, and career needs of students. Developing successful and accountable programs will require demonstration of the important skills we have explored in this book, such as advocacy and leadership. Beginning the accountability process will require some obvious thought and action.

One way to prevent becoming overwhelmed with the accountability process is to start with small but precise goals. It is unrealistic to believe that you will be able to alter an entire program in your first year. Initially, goals must be simple, measurable, and hopefully attainable. To set huge, lofty goals in the first year of employment may be unrealistic. Change should occur gradually and deliberately. Following is an example of a realistic accountability plan for your first year as a school counselor.

Step 1: Within the first month of school, conduct a needs assessment of parents, teachers, and students.

There are several examples of these types of formal assessments in other scholarly sources (Baker, 2000; Gysbers & Henderson, 2000; Hughey & Gysbers, 1993; Wittmer, 2000). A simple, one-page survey might include the following open-ended questions:

- What types of services do you think are needed from the school counseling program?
- How can the school counseling program best meet the needs of students?
- Please circle any of the services listed that you think are needed. (Possible services to include in the list are individual counseling, group counseling, classroom guidance, parenting programs, career and college information.)
- How can the school counselor(s) in your building be most helpful to you?

Keep the survey simple and easy to read. Consider publishing it in other languages, depending on the diversity of your school population. Ask for a quick response (a week or less). You might also consider including questions that utilize a Likert scale (1 to 5), asking respondents to circle a number indicating their feelings about the school counseling program in order to quantify the results.

Step 2: Based on the assessment responses, identify three goals for the school counseling program and develop a timeline for each goal.

An example of an appropriate goal is, "The school counseling program will conduct six study skills small group counseling experiences (2 at each middle school level) between October and April. A new group will begin every other month and sessions will last 8 weeks." Following is a timeline for this goal:

- September—Solicit group referrals from teachers, students, and parents; check last year's standardized test scores for potential participants.
- October—Conduct sixth grade study skills groups.
- December—Conduct seventh grade study skills groups.
- February—Conduct eighth grade study skills groups.

Step 3: Identify three results you want to achieve in alignment with your goals. Some possible results for the groups might include:

1. Group participants will improve their report card grades during the grading period they are involved in the group. (Results can be gathered from reviewing report cards.)
2. Group participants will acquire at least three new study skills as a result of participating in the group. (Results can be assessed through pre-test/post-test measures.)

3. Group participants' standardized test scores will improve from last year's scores. (Results can be gathered by comparing test scores.)

Step 4: Implement your counseling intervention/service and document progress of the group and its members.

Step 5: Assess results and adjust the program as necessary.
    Any problems or concerns that result from the implementation of the first group should be considered and resolved in order to achieve better results in subsequent groups.

Step 6: Reevaluate the goals at the end of the year to see if they were achieved.
    If the goals were not achieved, consider the reasons and decide whether to keep the goal for the following year. Communicate accountability results to key stakeholders.

These steps are simple and can be implemented in your first year as a school counselor. However, the process will require a commitment to ongoing evaluation and monitoring of the counseling services, in addition to other roles and responsibilities. This commitment will pay off in the long run, as you begin to accumulate evidence that your program is contributing to the overall good of students. This information will be personally and professionally rewarding for you as well as vital to the success of students.

CONCLUSION

This chapter has focused on the evaluation and accountability practices of school counselors. Historically, school counselors have been resistant to accountability measures for a variety of reasons. Currently, the call for results-based evaluation and school-based reform requires that school counselors provide evidence that their programs and services are leading to improved student academic, personal/social, and career performance. The process of evaluation does not have to be complex; in fact, deciding to evaluate just one area of the counseling program is a viable way to begin to demonstrate program efficacy. Program evaluation can also enhance performance evaluation for school counselors. Ongoing assessment and producing results are the best ways to prove that one's performance is effective; however, school personnel who directly supervise school counselors may also conduct observations.
    Finally, accountability and evaluation should be an integral component of the school counseling program. Focusing on specific goals, implementing effective services, and documenting student improvement is the best way to establish oneself as a professional who contributes to the school's mission and educational program.

REFLECTION AND DISCUSSION

1. As a beginning school counselor, develop an accountability plan for your school counseling program. What might be one practice you would evaluate? Give an example of a program goal that is measurable.

2. As a new counselor, you might encounter veteran counselors who are not aware of or supportive of the new accountability role of school counselors. How would you work with these counselors? What types of things might you say or do to get others involved?

3. One of the most important things a school counselor can do is share results data with key stakeholders. What are some creative ways to do this? Who are the key players who need to know that the school counseling program contributes to the overall education program?

CHAPTER 14

Becoming a School Counselor: Your Professional and Personal Journey

*T*his book has a slightly different purpose from that of other textbooks in school counseling. When I considered writing a book in school counseling, it was my intention to provide a practical text about the real-life experiences of school counselors. In my doctoral training, I often found that the things I read about school counseling were different from the things I experienced as a practitioner. I believed that it would be beneficial to talk about the everyday practices of school counselors who were "out in the trenches." In this book, you have read not only about my experiences, but also about the practices and perspectives of veteran practitioners in the field and the scholarly contributions of professionals who have dedicated themselves to the profession of school counseling. As you embark on your journey, please consider the content of this final chapter as a personal and professional challenge to contribute to this worthwhile profession.

The truth is, this book is the proverbial tip of the iceberg. No volume of books could contain all of the things you will learn, need to know, or encounter as a professional school counselor. Therein lies the beauty of the job. Every day is different, unpredictable, and challenging. Therefore, self-exploration is necessary to make sure that school counseling is a good fit for you. Consider carefully what brings you to this field, and make sure that the reasons are valid and appropriate.

This final chapter will provide an overview of the school counselor as a professional and as a person. Because the emphasis is on you, the school counselor-in-training, the second person—"you"—is used more frequently than in previous chapters to promote personal consideration of the concepts. The first section will discuss professional development, including activities that you can begin now in your school counseling training program. The chapter will then explore circumstances that often cause school counselors to burn out and will provide strategies for personal and professional stress management. Finally, the chapter offers admonitions or "words of wisdom" from our veteran counselors, as well as speculation about the future of school counseling. This chapter concludes the book but begins your journey.

Developing as a Professional School Counselor

A major responsibility of a graduate program in school counseling is to emphasize professional development. As you begin to think about your role as a professional school counselor, it is important to consider the many facets of the word *professional;* one aspect of professional school counselor development is development of a *professional identity.*

Developing a Professional Identity

According to Brott and Myers (1999), "It appears as if the development of a professional identity does contribute to defining the role of school counselors, which in turn shapes the counseling programs and services provided to students" (p. 345). It is important to understand that professional identity is not a static event, but a process that continues long after one finishes a graduate program in school counseling. Brott and Myers defined professional identity as ". . . a frame of reference from which one carries out a professional role, makes significant professional decisions, and develops as a professional" (p. 339). Your professional identity is already being formed as a result of your school counseling training program. The courses that you take and training that you receive will influence the professional you become. In order to maximize your professional development, consider the following activities to enhance your educational experience and develop your professional identity:

- Take extra courses or attend conferences, workshops, and in-services in areas that may not be extensively covered in your graduate program.

- If your training program is accredited by the Council for Accreditation of Counseling and Related Educational Programs (CACREP), understand what that means and how this accreditation contributes to the professionalism of the counseling field.

- Join your local and state school counseling associations and the American School Counselor Association. The resources that you will receive as a member of these organizations will be useful to you as a counselor-in-training and when you become a practitioner.

- Consider publishing or co-publishing an article with a counselor educator. If you have an idea for research or a concept to explore, talk with your professors to see if anyone is interested in collaborating on a project.

- Volunteer at school and community functions to gain a general knowledge of the school setting and a better understanding of the types of events and activities in which school counselors participate. If you are already working in the school setting, talk to the school counselors to gain insight into how they contribute to the school program.

- Establish support groups with other graduate students from your program and other graduate programs in the area to discuss the issues that are relevant to school counselors-in-training, personally and professionally.

- Join honor societies through your university program (e.g., Chi Sigma Iota, which is an Honors Society specifically for counseling students).

- Go to the Web site of the Department of Education in your state and read about current events in education, including any updates or changes in licensure requirements for school counselors.

- Attend local school board meetings in order to understand the political and social issues in educational systems.

- Investigate the position of your state government on school counseling issues. If possible, attend legislative sessions or town meetings that address topics relevant to school counseling.
- Advocate, advocate, advocate. Regardless of the group or circumstance with which you are working, publicize the important contributions of school counselors to school programs.

These professional behaviors will carry over into your career as a school counselor. There are no specific guidelines or strategies for how to develop a professional identity, but we can explore a number of ways to cultivate and enhance your professional identity over time.

Professional Perspective

RENEE (ES)

Professional development is a fundamental part of being an effective school counselor. Attending conferences or seminars helps me keep my skills sharp and allows me to grow as a counselor. It would be painfully boring to do the same thing over and over again, year after year. Professional development provides me with an opportunity to explore new techniques and theories. Or it may just serve to remind me of best practices. There is a saying, "If you do what you have always done, you will get what you have always gotten." Professional development allows you to stretch yourself and broaden your repertoire.

BETH (MS)

I truly believe that you need to be a member of professional organizations. I have been a member of local, state, and national organizations for most of my professional life. The state- and national-level memberships provide opportunities to communicate collaboratively with people around the state and nation. I really enjoy the publications and have received lots of good ideas from them. I think it is good to study what counselors are doing nationwide; you can use that information to support your own program.

Spruill and Benshoff (1996) broadly claimed, "Professional development roles for practicing counselors include active participation in professional organizations, obtaining professional credentials, and involvement in continuing education, research and publishing" (p. 469). More recently, Johnson (2000) identified a three-phase plan to promote the identity of the professional school counseling program:

1. Find a way to get all stakeholders to agree on the counseling services needed by students.
2. Develop a plan of action, including identifying ways to promote and conduct the program.

3.   Engage others in the school counseling program by providing infor-
     mation and promoting the program.

Johnson provided several strategies for promoting the school counseling program while demonstrating professional advocacy, such as utilizing technology
when making presentations to constituents, becoming a member of and participant in school- and community-related committees to represent the needs
of students, and publishing a quarterly newsletter for parents, students, and
community members that highlights the counseling program and services
available.

This book has provided many strategies and suggestions for promoting a
school program, which in turn projects a professional identity. In particular, the
discussions on leadership and advocacy offered several suggestions that also
support the development of a professional identity. Leadership and advocacy
require school counselors to be on committees and represent the counseling
needs of students (Johnson, 2000). In addition, being a leader and advocating
for one's profession involves continued education and training in order to
foster professional growth and development.

Professional Practice

ESTHER (HS)

I try to advocate for school counseling by doing presentations at the state, local,
and national level. I try to motivate school counselors to be counseling whenever possible and to fight the sometimes overwhelming administrative tasks. I
have worked with principals to help them understand that we are highly trained
professionals who can offer so much in schools. I have held various offices in
local organizations that advocate for counselors, and I have tried to advocate
in the community by doing presentations for PTOs or churches. I have also presented to counselors-in-training at various universities to offer insight into the
job and help them make a difference in their students' lives. Most of all, I have
tried to continually learn new ways of working with people so that I can offer
the best services to my students.

Professional school counselors seek to promote counseling programs,
advocate for students, collaborate with stakeholders, and provide effective
services. You will not master all of these skills and behaviors by the time you
finish your graduate program, or even after your first year as a school counselor. It is the *process* of development that establishes a professional identity and
the need for continuous change and progress that makes the school counselor's
job both challenging and rewarding.

Two important ways to develop professional identity as a counselor-in-
training are *defining a philosophy of school counseling* and *creating a professional
portfolio*. It is never too early to begin thinking about the type of professional
image you wish to project.

DEFINING A PHILOSOPHY OF SCHOOL COUNSELING When developing a philosophy of school counseling, one of the essential issues to consider is one's theoretical orientation. It is important for counselors-in-training to consider the theory that will serve as the framework within which they will work with students. Typically, a course on counseling theory is required in counselor education programs. This course provides an overview of the major counseling theories that have been developed over time and challenges students to begin to identify with theoretical orientations that they may utilize in their own counseling practices. One issue for school counseling students is that many of the dominant theories are not necessarily applicable to counseling in the school setting. Solution-focused counseling, presented in chapter 3, may be a viable option for use in the school setting. Other theories that may be useful in school counseling include Adlerian Theory, Choice Theory, and behavioral theory and techniques. With the current emphasis on working with families in schools, family systems theory may also be an appropriate choice. More than likely, you will integrate various aspects of different theories into your counseling practices. School counselors typically need a repertoire of techniques and strategies in order to meet the diverse and changing needs of students.

The benefit of a course in counseling theory is that every counselor-in-training, regardless of specialty, can appreciate what each theory contributes to the field of counseling in general. While psychoanalysis may not be ideal for school counseling, one can respect the contributions of Sigmund Freud to the field. Further, the therapeutic conditions identified by Carl Rogers in his Person-Centered Theory provide a foundation for developing rapport with clients and students, regardless of the presenting problem. Knowledge of these theories is integral to the development of one's counseling philosophy.

In order to begin developing a theoretical orientation, you may want to consider two important questions:

- Which theory(ies) reflects my personal view of human nature?
- Am I more comfortable with the techniques of any specific theory?

Developing a theoretical orientation to school counseling is necessary for school counselors to effectively address student, parent, and faculty concerns. The best advice for deciding on a theoretical orientation or technique is to

My Story

It was my experience that the nature of the problem often dictated my choice of theory and technique. Because many cases dealt with student behavior, I found that behavioral techniques, such as behavior contracting, were useful with students. When student issues were more personal/social in nature, I used person-centered techniques to explore the issue, and then moved to more action-oriented techniques, such as solution-focused counseling.

try to match the theory/technique to the presenting problem. Many school counselors are *integrative* in their orientations, which offers greater flexibility when deciding which techniques might be most effective in specific situations. It is a good idea to ask yourself, "What theory or technique will best address this issue?" Effective counseling can occur when counseling practices are based on (a) the nature of the problem, (b) the student's openness to the theory or technique, and (c) your level of confidence in using a specific theory or technique. If the theory or technique doesn't seem to work, change it!

Another aspect of developing a philosophy of school counseling is to determine your perception of the role of counselors in schools. Questions to ask yourself might include:

- What is the school counselor's role in the educational mission of the school?

- What educational/developmental areas should the school counselor support?

- How should the school counselor work with the faculty?

- How does the school counselor contribute to the overall school environment?

It is important to consider the documents and models of our professional organization. The ASCA National Standards (Campbell & Dahir, 1997), ASCA Ethical Standards (ASCA, 1998a, see also the Appendix in the back of this book), ASCA National Model (ASCA, 2003a), and the Transforming School Counseling Initiative (The Education Trust, 2003) will influence your philosophy. In addition, the No Child Left Behind Act of 2001 (U.S. Department of Education, 2002) is an important factor, and school counselors must identify their role in supporting the implementation of this important legislation. Some counselors-in-training include copies of these documents in their portfolios to emphasize that these professional documents affect how they will practice as school counselors. Finally, it would behoove counselors-in-training to sum up in one or two sentences their reasons for becoming school counselors. It is advantageous to be aware of the important current documents and trends in the field, but a personal philosophy must also include one's own motivation for pursuing this career. Perhaps you remember the question, "Why school counseling?" posed in chapter 1. As you have read this book, you may have had experiences in schools that have allowed you to develop your own perspective on the practices of school counselors. Take some time to reflect on this question again, and incorporate your perspective into your philosophy statement.

BUILDING A PROFESSIONAL PORTFOLIO   According to Rhyne-Winkler and Wooten (1996), "The goal of developing portfolios for school counselors is enhanced professional and personal development. The process of portfolio development requires personal reflection, which can initiate changes in counseling skill, personal identity, professional identity, competence, and relationships" (p. 147). In recent years, the counselor portfolio has become a critical element in the school counselor job search and, in some cases, a part of ongoing evaluation once a job is secured. According to Boes, VanZile-Tamsen, and Jackson (2001):

> The portfolio as an employment tool is a brief but powerful visual device to sell the applicant's abilities. Items included should be one's best work and replaced as skills improve. The goal is to present a view of personal and professional growth for the purpose of self-presentation in a job interview and for reflective self-evaluation throughout its development. (p. 230)

There are several different approaches to school counseling portfolios. Rhyne-Winkler and Wooten (1996) provided an outline of the components they feel are necessary, which include documentation of program planning, counseling, consultation, coordination, student appraisal, and educational and professional development. Boes, VanZile-Tamsen, and Jackson (2001) suggested a portfolio format that focuses on the transformed school counselor roles of leadership, advocacy, teaming and collaboration, counseling and coordination, and assessment and use of data. The element that is common to both recommendations is the development of the personal philosophy of school counseling.

I have developed the following recommendations for portfolio composition from my professional and personal experience. The first document that should be visible in the portfolio is a professional resume. The resume should include a professional objective (one sentence describing your employment goal), education background (including your projected graduation date from your school counseling program), work experience (especially internship and practicum experience), professional development activities and projects, professional memberships and affiliations, and references (usually described as available upon request). It is a good idea to have a resume that is limited to one page, front and back. The resume should be a snapshot of relevant information

My Story

My counseling students develop their school counseling portfolios in every course. As students progress through the program, they constantly consider the elements they want to include in their professional portfolios and begin to piece together their professional journeys in school counseling, beginning with coursework and projects in their training programs. I constantly comment: "This should be included in your portfolio." By the time students reach their school counseling internships, they have almost completed their portfolios and are ready to share their information with prospective employers.

for the potential employer, not a detailed recollection of your life history. Also, tailor the resume, particularly the professional objective, to fit the description of the job for which you are applying. For example, if the job opening is for a middle school counselor with expertise in working with at-risk populations, it would be wise to emphasize any experience or training related to working with at-risk populations. While a standard resume is certainly acceptable, the person who is reviewing resumes or portfolios may be searching for someone who has expertise in a specific area.

The philosophy statement, as mentioned previously, is a paragraph that describes your theoretical approach to counseling students, as well as your philosophy of school counseling. It is critical to indicate how you believe school counseling supports the overall education program. This reveals your understanding of the unique nature of school counseling, as well as the team aspects of working in a school.

Other elements in the portfolio may vary. Some students have created their portfolios based on the traditional roles of school counselors (counseling, classroom guidance, consultation, coordination) and included examples in each section. You should include documentation of projects that you develop for your courses, such as examples of counseling curricula (e.g., classroom guidance lessons and small group lessons). In terms of consultation, it is a good idea to include an example of any written correspondence you have had with parents, teachers, or community members. For example, if as a school counseling practicum student you help solicit speakers for Career Day, include a copy of the letter inviting people to participate as Career Day speakers. It is important for potential employers to see examples of your writing ability and proof that you have experience communicating with others about the counseling program.

In a professional development section, include copies of any certifications you may have; certificates of attendance or presentation at in-services, workshops, and conferences; certificates of membership in professional organizations; and proof of your professional liability insurance. You may also want to include any awards or recognition you may have received during your graduate program or as a practicum or internship student. Other important information in this section might include evaluations from your practicum and/or internship experience. It is good for potential employers to know that you are familiar with the evaluation process, and it allows them to see your skill development and progression throughout the school counselor training program.

A final section to include is letters of reference and recommendation. Some students choose to place these near the front of the portfolio, perhaps after the philosophy statement. Others prefer to place the letters at the end as the culminating piece of the portfolio. Regardless, make sure the letters are representative of your training as a school counselor. Letters from your practicum supervisor, your internship on-site supervisor, and your internship university supervisor are critical, since these are the persons who have observed your development as a school counselor. You may also wish to include letters from parents, administrators, or teachers with whom you worked as a counselor-in-training. These letters should speak to your strengths as a potential school counselor and will hopefully identify all of the good qualities that you will bring to a school setting. It may also be appropriate to include letters or notes from students.

The traditional method for presenting a portfolio is with the use of a one-inch, three-ring binder. Remember that the portfolio is to be representative of your training and abilities, not the entire contents of your program. It is wise to make several copies of the portfolio for two reasons: (a) You may interview with more than one person (i.e., a panel), and (b) potential employers may ask to keep your portfolio for more extensive review at a later time.

An innovative approach that some school counseling applicants are using is to provide portfolios on compact discs. The CD portfolio is much easier to send with a resume to prospective employers, and it demonstrates that the school counselor is technologically savvy. Administrators have actually called me to comment that they were very impressed with graduate students who submitted their portfolios on CD because it gave the administrators an opportunity to peruse the documents at their leisure. With the current emphasis on technology, the CD portfolio is certainly worth consideration.

This section has focused specifically on developing the professional portfolio of beginning school counselors. It is important to emphasize that portfolio development does not end when one is employed as a school counselor. James and Greenwalt (2001) emphasized the importance of counselors using a *working portfolio* to document success and achievement. "The working portfolio is a continuous collection of unabridged artifacts one may eventually use as evidence of professional competence" (p. 162). The working portfolio would include such components as professional presentations and publications and professional service to the school or community. Practicing school counselors should maintain documentation of their professional activities and experiences so that they have records of their progress for future potential job searches. In particular, Rhyne-Winkler and Wooten (1996) recommended that practicing school counselors routinely document and evaluate their effectiveness. "A portfolio provides a vehicle for school counselors to take personal responsibility and become proactive rather than reactive in the evaluation process" (p. 147). The portfolio is a critical part of the school counselor's growth and professional development, and it begins on day one of the school counselor training program.

This section has dealt specifically with the school counselor's role and responsibility in professional development. From developing a professional portfolio to becoming active in state and national school counseling organizations, this role is critical to your development as a professional school counselor. The next section is more personal and will provide you with suggestions for self-exploration and self-preservation.

The School Counselor as a Person: Taking Care of Yourself

Why School Counselors Leave

The research on school counselor burnout is limited, but there seems to be some consensus regarding the reasons that school counselors leave the profession. Kendrick, Chandler, and Hather (1994, as cited in Studer & Allton, 1996) listed two significant stressors school counselors identified: (a) lack of role definition and (b) the demands of noncounseling tasks for which they had not been trained. Studer and Allton noted that lack of administrative support for and understanding of the role of the school counselor is also a stressor that takes its toll on school counselors. These issues have all been discussed and addressed in this book.

In my experience, other reasons for school counselor stress and burnout might include:

- excessive caseload;
- lack of support from school board or a misunderstanding about the role of school counselors;
- lack of support from faculty;
- lack of parental support for the school counseling program;
- excessive "administrivia" tasks requiring paperwork;
- lack of time to provide counseling to students;
- pressure to focus only on academic achievement (no emphasis on personal/social counseling);

My Story

When I began my first year as a school counselor, a colleague commented to me, "I'll bet you won't last longer than five years." When I asked why, she responded, "You'll burn out by then. All of them do." She had formerly been a school counselor, and went back to teaching after two years. I have given a great deal of thought to that comment over the years, and also to the fact that I spent nine years as a practicing counselor and would have continued had other professional opportunities not presented themselves. Even though there were days when I questioned why I was doing it, those thoughts were fleeting. Most days, I felt that being a school counselor was the best career I could ever have chosen. However, the tendency to burn out is a reality that should be addressed in order to prevent effective practitioners from leaving the profession.

- lack of respect for counseling time (e.g., being pulled for noncounseling duties); and
- lack of materials, funding, space, and resources to provide effective
  counseling services.

Although these issues can contribute to stress and burnout, they are also areas that can be addressed proactively in order to foster positive change. For example, if lack of school funding results in the cancellation or postponement of a counselor-sponsored event, the school counselor might seek outside grant funding or community support for the program. This would be a professional reaction to an unpredictable stressor. Effective school counselors may need to be resourceful in addressing some of these issues.

A major focus for school counselors that may help avoid stress and burnout is engaging the support of building administrators, faculty, parents, and students in the school. A helpful piece of advice was offered in chapter 4 by our middle school counseling veteran, Beth. She emphasized that one way she prevents being overloaded with noncounseling tasks that might lead to burnout is to make her administrator aware that performing those tasks is not a cost-effective use of her time. Studer and Allton (1996) reminded administrators that using school counselors for administrative or clerical tasks does not promote the educational mission of the school. This can be addressed through the school counselor's professional advocacy role, as well as the leadership positions he or she may fill in the school. Though it may take time, it is worthwhile for school counselors to increase awareness and educate others about the work that school counselors do and the significant contributions that they make to the educational success of students.

Dealing With Stress as a Professional School Counselor

Stress and burnout among school counselors may not always be the result of institutional barriers or misconceptions about role definition. One of the hardest aspects of the school counselor's job is that it is difficult to leave student problems and issues at the school door when it is time to go home. This was discussed as a challenge of school counseling in chapter 1. A key characteristic that school counselors will need to develop, if not already present, is *caregiver resiliency.* According to Siebert (2002):

> As a school counselor, a big part of your job is that of caregiver. You pro-
> vide people in need with a shoulder to cry on, someone to listen to their
> concerns and advice on how to deal with adversity. However, it can be a
> fine line to walk between helping others with their problems and letting
> others' problems have a negative impact on your own mental health. You
> not only owe it to yourself but to your students to be a role model for
> resiliency. (p. 11)

As a practicing school counselor, some of the students' situations and circumstances that you learn of will affect you emotionally. Sometimes, the inability to provide help or relief from the pain and trauma the students are experiencing is enough to discourage even the most optimistic and hopeful counselor. There may be situations so horrific that if you did not know they were true, you would not believe them. The key to dealing with and bouncing back from these types of issues is to understand that they will happen and to decide how you, as a school counselor, can best provide for the student. This may mean simply being a listener and a support system to help a student get through the school day. It may mean going above and beyond the call of duty to make sure that a student has a good meal or has a safe place to go if a situation becomes out of control. This is what school counselors do—we support, we take action, and we give hope.

Because of the emotional toll on school counselors, developing resiliency is an essential skill. Siebert (2002) offered the following steps for improving caregiver resiliency:

1. Enjoy solid self-esteem and self-confidence.
2. Talk with friends.
3. Expect things to work out well.
4. Develop open-minded empathy.
5. Question authority (defend yourself and fight back if necessary).
6. Develop a talent for serendipity (seeing the positive in the seemingly negative). (pp. 12–13)

Professional Perspective

RENEE (ES)

You have to learn to separate yourself from the job while still being an involved and caring person who is invested in your students. It can be overwhelming to be the person that everyone looks to for help. Principals, teachers, parents, and students all seek out the counselor for help. Sometimes, you feel like you don't have the answer, but everyone is counting on you. It is challenging to frame your thinking so that you see your job as supportive of a process (education) rather than a panacea.

Resilience, the ability to bounce back and to succeed in spite of adversity, is a quality that will help you through much of your professional career, and it is a valuable life skill as well. Some people have naturally resilient personalities, while others must develop resilience. Recognizing personal strengths, maintaining an attitude of hope, and working for the good of all are skills that effective school counselors possess.

Daughhetee and Grant (2002) recommended utilizing solution-focused techniques for personal stress management. Rating your stress level on a scale of 1 to 10 and setting goals to de-stress are examples of these solution-focused strategies. Daughhetee and Grant emphasized that stress management plans must be appropriate for the individual, because solution-focused strategies are not a "one size fits all" solution (p. 19). In order to take care of themselves, school counselors should be aware of their stressors, the things that push personal buttons, and the boundaries of their emotions. Awareness is the first step in effectively dealing with stress. Once you become aware of the sources of stress, it is easier to focus on strategies that specifically address each stressor.

> By exploring and intentionally activating the stress buffers you have used in the past, visualizing a less stressful future and identifying action goals, you can construct a unique stress-management plan—one that meets your needs specifically. School counselors have a professional responsibility to be self-caring and to model self-care to the school community. (Daughhetee & Grant, p. 19)

TAKING CARE OF THE CAREGIVER—PERSONAL RESOURCES One source of strength that emerged as a common theme from our veteran counselors is the support of family, friends, and colleagues.

Professional Perspective and Personal Practice

RENEE (ES)

My family and friends are my greatest source of support. I am very fortunate to have a terrific network of friends and a very understanding family. I try very hard to give 110% while I am at work and to leave work at work as much as possible. I also use the other counselors who I work with as a sounding board. We coordinate monthly meetings and use the time to support each other. It takes some effort to coordinate the meetings, but it is well worth it. I take care of myself by making sure that I have time for my family and friends and for myself. I find that exercise is a tremendous stress reliever for me. If you don't replenish yourself, you won't have anything to give to your students.

BETH (MS)

Part of the reason that I am not burned out on counseling is that I love counseling. I do at times get burned out with other tasks, such as testing. That is the part I find stressful. One way I deal with stress is humor. Having other people in your building that you can joke with about what it is about your job that drives you crazy is a good way to deal with stress. Keeping everything in perspective is important. It is also important to remember that even though you might not see it on a day-to-day basis, school counselors make a difference. Sometimes it's small and sometimes it's big, but for me, that's enough to prevent burnout.

What I do personally is spend time with my family. It is important to understand that my role as a school counselor is a big part of my life, but when I go home, I need to focus on other aspects of my life.

ESTHER (HS)

Your family, friends, and colleagues serve as your sources of support in school and out of school. If you can leave your office at a sensible time every day, close the door, and leave the work at work, then you can prevent burnout. It is also important to maintain outside interests and have your personal and professional priorities in proper perspective.

It is important to nurture yourself and do what you love to do, cultivate meaningful friendships, play, exercise, and get excited about trying something new. One can handle the stress in life if one can maintain a positive perspective. Have a sense of humor and laugh at yourself. Don't try to be perfect; we all learn from our mistakes. Sometimes, people will disappoint you; just make sure you don't disappoint yourself. Take care of yourself!

These are words of wisdom from school counselors who have been successful practitioners for a long time. I would add the following suggestions for dealing with the stress of the school counseling roles:

- Forgive yourself when you can't "fix it." Do what you can. Muller-Ackerman (2001) stated, "Although school counselors are trained to help others, one of the most valuable lessons many have learned is when to let go" (p. 21).
- Celebrate small successes. Look for something good that you've done each day.
- If you're feeling discouraged, spend time with the students. This is a good reminder of why you do what you do.

As we consider the future of school counseling, the realities are sometimes overwhelming, but rising to the challenges will only strengthen and unite us as professionals.

Mind How You Go: Your Opportunity and Challenge

Renee, our elementary school veteran, and I typically end our e-mail or phone correspondence with the phrase, "Mind how you go." This was a phrase that we heard at a social outing that we took to mean, "watch out for and take care of yourself." It seems to be an appropriate phrase for the journey you have begun.

It is an exciting time to be in the school counseling profession, and the future of school counseling looks bright and hopeful. The December 2001 issue of *Professional School Counseling* was devoted to the future of school counseling. Articles written by renowned experts in the field offered extensive information, as well as a synopsis of the past, present, and future of the school counseling profession. The emphasis was on the positive accomplishments of the profession, but there was also a challenge to school counselors to meet the needs of a diverse and ever-changing society.

Jones and Granello (2002) identified the common themes that emerged from the articles written for this special issue. These themes were related to role definition, diverse student populations, serving all students, focusing on technology in school counseling, and the continued pursuit of professionalism through professional development (p. 164). Other areas of challenge include outcome-based program evaluation (Green & Keys, 2001), program implementation (Jones & Granello), and the ongoing issues of counseling time in the age of testing and accountability (Baker, 2001). Another primary focus for school counselors is staking their claim in the era of educational reform. School counselors should be included in the planning and implementation of programs that work toward the success of all students. Johnson (2000) made two arguments for school counselor contribution to the educational reform movement.

> First, that in order for the identity of professional school counseling to prosper in this era of educational reform, it must strategically align itself with the chief academic mission of the school; and, second, that in order for the school community at large to come to appreciate this reconceptualized program identity, programs need to pursue a planned professional advocacy campaign that targets all stakeholders, is based on enhanced accountability, and is carried out in progressive phases over a number of years. (p. 39)

The roles and challenges for school counselors offer a tremendous opportunity to contribute to the scholastic experiences of students. The good news is that issues are being addressed by the transformed roles of school counselors and ASCA National Model for School Counseling programs. Further, effective school counseling practices are substantiated and supported by the ASCA National Standards and Ethical Standards. We are confronting the demons head on, which illustrates our movement toward greater action and advocacy.

Professional Perspective

ESTHER (HS)

It is evident that counselors have a dire need and huge responsibility to constantly define and redefine their role in the school setting in order to meet the current, immediate, and changing needs of students and families. If we do not clearly define our role, someone else will do it for us.

As you consider your career in school counseling, let me encourage you to first look at the big picture. We have talked about the many and varied roles and practices of school counselors. In both the traditional roles and the transformed roles, there is an obvious need for leadership and advocacy. Further, we have addressed critical relationships that school counselors should build as they collaborate with school personnel, families, and community members. We have also explored many counseling practices and the perspectives of practitioners and scholars in the field. Finally, and perhaps most importantly, we have considered many of the challenges and opportunities that you may encounter as a school counselor. As mentioned in chapter 1, these are not exhaustive, but they certainly are worth pondering.

School counselors are necessary to the educational mission of schools. Students need the support of a caring individual in the school whose primary responsibility is to advocate for students and help them work toward lifelong goals, including educational and career success. Teachers need supportive colleagues who can focus on the academic performance and career development of students, while addressing the personal and social needs that our youth face in an ever-changing society. Administrators rely on school counselors to supplement and support the academic curriculum, as well as address the unique personal, social, and educational needs of students. Parents need school counselors to serve as resources and guides for helping their children recognize their potential and achieve educational, personal, and career goals. Communities need school counselors to serve as liaisons, referral sources, and partners in programs that benefit the school and community. It is these collaborative alliances that will result in a more tolerant and productive society.

As you begin the journey, I wish you well and welcome you to the profession. Above all else, grasp the opportunities, embrace the challenges, and whatever you do, do it in the best interest of students. While many things in schools change, the priority for school counselors remains the same. Whatever challenges come your way, your school counseling career will be personally and professionally meaningful and significant if your practices and perspectives are focused on the best interests of the students. Mind how you go!

REFLECTION AND CHALLENGE

Consider your reasons for becoming a school counselor and the many roles presented in this book. Choose three professional goals and three personal goals for your journey in school counseling. Display them somewhere where you can see them, and review them frequently. Reevaluate and modify them as needed.

APPENDIX

ASCA's Ethical Standards for School Counselors

Revised June 25, 1998

PREAMBLE

The American School Counselor Association (ASCA) is a professional organization whose members have a unique and distinctive preparation, grounded in the behavioral sciences, with training in clinical skills adapted to the school setting. The school counselor assists in the growth and development of each individual and uses his or her highly specialized skills to protect the interests of the counselee within the structure of the school system. School counselors subscribe to the following basic tenets of the counseling process from which professional responsibilities are derived:

- Each person has the right to respect and dignity as a human being and to counseling services without prejudice as to person, character, belief, or practice regardless of age, color, disability, ethnic group, gender, race, religion, sexual orientation, marital status, or socioeconomic status.
- Each person has the right to self-direction and self-development.
- Each person has the right of choice and the responsibility for goals reached.
- Each person has the right to privacy and thereby the right to expect the counselor-counselee relationship to comply with all laws, policies, and ethical standards pertaining to confidentiality.

In this document, ASCA specifies the principles of ethical behavior necessary to regulate and maintain the high standards of integrity, leadership, and professionalism among its members. The Ethical Standards for School Counselors were developed to clarify the nature of ethical responsibilities held in common by school counseling professionals. The purposes of this document are to:

- Serve as a guide for the ethical practices of all professional school counselors regardless of level, area, population served, or membership in this professional Association;
- Provide benchmarks for both self-appraisal and peer evaluations regarding counselor responsibilities to counselees, parents, colleagues and professional associates, schools, and communities, as well as to one's self and the counseling profession; and
- Inform those served by the school counselor of acceptable counselor practices and expected professional behavior.

A.1. Responsibilities to Students

The professional school counselor:

a. Has a primary obligation to the counselee who is to be treated with respect as a unique individual.

b. Is concerned with the educational, career, emotional, and behavioral needs and encourages the maximum development of each counselee.

c. Refrains from consciously encouraging the counselee's acceptance of values, lifestyles, plans, decisions, and beliefs that represent the counselor's personal orientation.

d. Is responsible for keeping informed of laws, regulations, and policies relating to counselees and strives to ensure that the rights of counselees are adequately provided for and protected.

A.2. Confidentiality

The professional school counselor:

a. Informs the counselee of the purposes, goals, techniques, and rules of procedure under which she/he may receive counseling at or before the time when the counseling relationship is entered. Disclosure notice includes confidentiality issues such as the possible necessity for consulting with other professionals, privileged communication, and legal or authoritative restraints. The meaning and limits of confidentiality are clearly defined to counselees through a written and shared disclosure statement.

b. Keeps information confidential unless disclosure is required to prevent clear and imminent danger to the counselee or others or when legal requirements demand that confidential information be revealed. Counselors will consult with other professionals when in doubt as to the validity of an exception.

c. Discloses information to an identified third party who, by her or his relationship with the counselee, is at a high risk of contracting a disease that is commonly known to be communicable and fatal. Prior to disclosure, the counselor will ascertain that the counselee has not already informed the third party about his or her disease and he/she is not intending to inform the third party in the immediate future.

d. Requests of the court that disclosure not be required when the release of confidential information without a counselee's permission may lead to potential harm to the counselee.

e. Protects the confidentiality of counselee's records and releases personal data only according to prescribed laws and school policies. Student information maintained in computers is treated with the same care as traditional student records.

f. Protects the confidentiality of information received in the counseling relationship as specified by federal and state laws, written policies, and applicable ethical standards. Such information is only to be revealed to others with the informed consent of the counselee, consistent with the counselor's ethical obligation. In a group setting, the counselor sets a high norm of confidentiality and stresses its importance, yet clearly states that confidentiality in group counseling cannot be guaranteed.

A.3. Counseling Plans

The professional school counselor:

works jointly with the counselee in developing integrated and effective counseling plans, consistent with both the abilities and circumstances of the counselee and counselor. Such plans will be regularly reviewed to ensure continued viability and effectiveness, respecting the counselee's freedom of choice.

A.4. Dual Relationships

The professional school counselor:

avoids dual relationships which might impair her or his objectivity and increase the risk of harm to the client (e.g., counseling one's family members, close friends, or associates). If a dual relationship is unavoidable, the counselor is responsible for taking action to eliminate or reduce the potential for harm. Such safeguards might include informed consent, consultation, supervision, and documentation.

A.5. Appropriate Referrals

The professional school counselor:

makes referrals when necessary or appropriate to outside resources. Appropriate referral necessitates knowledge of available resources and making proper plans for transitions with minimal interruption of services. Counselees retain the right to discontinue the counseling relationship at any time.

A.6. Group Work

The professional school counselor:

screens prospective group members and maintains an awareness of participants' needs and goals in relation to the goals of the group. The counselor takes reasonable precautions to protect members from physical and psychological harm resulting from interaction within the group.

A.7. Danger to Self or Others

The professional school counselor:

informs appropriate authorities when the counselee's condition indicates a clear and imminent danger to the counselee or others. This is to be done after careful deliberation and, where possible, after consultation with other counseling professionals. The counselor informs the counselee of actions to be taken so as to minimize his or her confusion and to clarify counselee and counselor expectations.

A.8. Student Records

The professional school counselor:

maintains and secures records necessary for rendering professional services to the counselee as required by laws, regulations, institutional procedures, and confidentiality guidelines.

A.9. Evaluation, Assessment, and Interpretation

The professional school counselor:

a.   Adheres to all professional standards regarding selecting, administering, and interpreting assessment measures. The counselor recognizes that computer-based testing programs require specific training in administration, scoring, and interpretation which may differ from that required in more traditional assessments.

b.   Provides explanations of the nature, purposes, and results of assessment/evaluation measures in language the counselee(s) can understand.

c.   Does not misuse assessment results and interpretations and takes reasonable steps to prevent others from misusing the information.

d.   Uses caution when utilizing assessment techniques, making evaluations, and interpreting the performance of populations not represented in the norm group on which an instrument is standardized.

A.10. Computer Technology

The professional school counselor:

a.   Promotes the benefits of appropriate computer applications and clarifies the limitations of computer technology. The counselor ensures that: (1) computer applications are appropriate for the individual needs of the counselee; (2) the counselee understands how to use the application; and (3) follow-up counseling assistance is provided. Members of under represented groups are assured equal access to computer technologies and are assured the absence of discriminatory information and values in computer applications.

b.   Counselors who communicate with counselees via internet should follow the NBCC Standards for Web Counseling.

A.11. Peer Helper Programs

The professional school counselor:

has unique responsibilities when working with peer helper programs. The school counselor is responsible for the welfare of counselees participating in peer programs under her or his direction. School counselors who function in training and supervisory capacities are referred to the preparation and supervision standards of professional counselor associations.

B. RESPONSIBILITIES TO PARENTS

B.1. Parent Rights and Responsibilities

The professional school counselor:

a.   Respects the inherent rights and responsibilities of parents for their children and endeavors to establish, as appropriate, a collaborative relationship with parents to facilitate the counselee's maximum development.

b.   Adheres to laws and local guidelines when assisting parents experiencing family difficulties that interfere with the counselee's effectiveness and welfare.

c.   Is sensitive to cultural and social diversity among families and recognizes that all parents, custodial and noncustodial, are vested with certain rights and responsibilities for the welfare of their children by virtue of their role and according to law.

B.2. Parents and Confidentiality

The professional school counselor:

a.   Informs parents of the counselor's role with emphasis on the confidential nature of the counseling relationship between the counselor and counselee.

b.   Provides parents with accurate, comprehensive, and relevant information in an objective and caring manner, as is appropriate and consistent with ethical responsibilities to the counselee.

c.   Makes reasonable efforts to honor the wishes of parents and guardians concerning information that he/she may share regarding the counselee.

C. RESPONSIBILITIES TO COLLEAGUES AND PROFESSIONAL ASSOCIATES

C.1. Professional Relationships

The professional school counselor:

a.   Establishes and maintains professional relationships with faculty, staff, and administration to facilitate the provision of optimal counseling services. The relationship is based on the counselor's definition and description of the parameter and levels of his or her professional roles.

b.   Treats colleagues with professional respect, courtesy, and fairness. The qualifications, views, and findings of colleagues are represented to accurately reflect the image of competent professionals.

c.   Is aware of and optimally utilizes related professions and organizations to whom the counselee may be referred.

C.2. Sharing Information with Other Professionals

The professional school counselor:

a.   Promotes awareness and adherence to appropriate guidelines regarding confidentiality; the distinction between public and private information; and staff consultation.

b.   Provides professional personnel with accurate, objective, concise, and meaningful data necessary to adequately evaluate, counsel, and assist the counselee.

c.   If a counselee is receiving services from another counselor or other mental health professional, the counselor, with client consent, will inform the other professional and develop clear agreements to avoid confusion and conflict for the counselee.

D. RESPONSIBILITIES TO THE SCHOOL AND COMMUNITY

D.1. Responsibilities to the School

The professional school counselor:

a.   Supports and protects the educational program against any infringement not in the best interest of counselees.

b.   Informs appropriate officials of conditions that may be potentially disruptive or damaging to the school's mission, personnel, and property while honoring the confidentiality between the counselee and counselor.

c.   Delineates and promotes the counselor's role and function in meeting the needs of those served. The counselor will notify appropriate officials of conditions which may limit or curtail her or his effectiveness in providing programs and services.

d.   Accepts employment only for positions for which he/she is qualified by education, training, supervised experience, state and national professional credentials, and appropriate professional experience. Counselors recommend that administrators hire only qualified and competent individuals for professional counseling positions.

e.   Assists in developing: (1) curricular and environmental conditions appropriate for the school and community; (2) educational procedures and programs to meet the counselee's developmental needs; and (3) a systematic evaluation process for comprehensive school counseling programs, services, and personnel. The counselor is guided by the findings of the evaluation data in planning programs and services.

D.2. Responsibility to the Community

The professional school counselor:

collaborates with agencies, organizations, and individuals in the school and community in the best interest of counselees and without regard to personal reward or remuneration.

E. RESPONSIBILITIES TO SELF

E.1. Professional Competence

The professional school counselor:

a.   Functions within the boundaries of individual professional competence and accepts responsibility for the consequences of his or her actions.

b.   Monitors personal functioning and effectiveness and does not participate in any activity which may lead to inadequate professional services or harm to a client.

c.   Strives through personal initiative to maintain professional competence and to keep abreast of professional information. Professional and personal growth are ongoing throughout the counselor's career.

E.2. Multicultural Skills

The professional school counselor:

understands the diverse cultural backgrounds of the counselees with whom he/she works. This includes, but is not limited to, learning how the school counselor's own cultural/ethnic/racial identity impacts her or his values and beliefs about the counseling process.

F. RESPONSIBILITIES TO THE PROFESSION

F.1. Professionalism

The professional school counselor:

a.   Accepts the policies and processes for handling ethical violations as a result of maintaining membership in the American School Counselor Association.

b.   Conducts herself/himself in such a manner as to advance individual ethical practice and the profession.

c.   Conducts appropriate research and reports findings in a manner consistent with acceptable educational and psychological research practices. When using client data for research or for statistical or program planning purposes, the counselor ensures protection of the individual counselee's identity.

d.   Adheres to ethical standards of the profession, other official policy statements pertaining to counseling, and relevant statutes established by federal, state, and local governments.

e.   Clearly distinguishes between statements and actions made as a private individual and those made as a representative of the school counseling profession.

f.   Does not use his or her professional position to recruit or gain clients, consultees for her or his private practice, seek and receive unjustified personal gains, unfair advantage, sexual favors, or unearned goods or services.

F.2. Contribution to the Profession

The professional school counselor:

a.   Actively participates in local, state, and national associations which foster the development and improvement of school counseling.

b.   Contributes to the development of the profession through sharing skills, ideas, and expertise with colleagues.

G. MAINTENANCE OF STANDARDS

Ethical behavior among professional school counselors, Association members and nonmembers, is expected at all times. When there exists serious doubt as to the ethical behavior of colleagues, or if counselors are forced to work in situations or abide by policies which do not reflect the standards as outlined in these Ethical Standards for School Counselors, the counselor is obligated to take appropriate action to rectify the condition. The following procedure may serve as a guide:

1.   The counselor should consult confidentially with a professional colleague to discuss the nature of a complaint to see if she/he views the situation as an ethical violation.

2.   When feasible, the counselor should directly approach the colleague whose behavior is in question to discuss the complaint and seek resolution.

3.   If resolution is not forthcoming at the personal level, the counselor shall utilize the channels established within the school, school district, the state SCA, and ASCA Ethics Committee.

4.   If the matter still remains unresolved, referral for review and appropriate action should be made to the Ethics Committees in the following sequence:

   - state school counselor association
   - American School Counselor Association

5.   The ASCA Ethics Committee is responsible for educating—and consulting with—the membership regarding ethical standards. The Committee periodically reviews and recommends changes in code. The Committee will also receive and process questions to clarify the application of such standards. Questions must be submitted in writing to the ASCA Ethics Chair. Finally, the Committee will handle complaints of alleged violations of our ethical standards. Therefore, at the national level, complaints should be submitted in writing to the ASCA Ethics Committee, c/o the Executive Director, American School Counselor Association, 801 North Fairfax, Suite 310, Alexandria, VA 22314.

H. RESOURCES

School counselors are responsible for being aware of, and acting in accord with, standards and positions of the counseling profession as represented in official documents such as those listed below:

American Counseling Association. (1995). *Code of ethics and standards of practice.* Alexandria, VA. (5999 Stevenson Ave., Alexandria, VA 22034) 1 800 347 6647 www.counseling.org.

American School Counselor Association. (1997). *The national standards for school counseling programs.* Alexandria, VA. (801 North Fairfax Street, Suite 310, Alexandria, VA 22314) 1 800 306 4722 www.schoolcounselor.org.

American School Counselor Association. (1998). *Position Statements.* Alexandria, VA.

American School Counselor Association. (1998). *Professional liability insurance program.* (Brochure). Alexandria, VA.

Arrendondo, Toperek, Brown, Jones, Locke, Sanchez, and Stadler. (1996). Multicultural counseling competencies and standards. *Journal of Multicultural Counseling and Development.* Vol. 24, No. 1. See American Counseling Association.

Arthur, G.L. and Swanson, C.D. (1993). *Confidentiality and privileged communication.* (1993). See American Counseling Association.

Association for Specialists in Group Work. (1989). *Ethical Guidelines for group counselors.* (1989). Alexandria, VA. See American Counseling Association.

Corey, G., Corey, M.S. and Callanan. (1998). *Issues and Ethics in the Helping Professions.* Pacific Grove, CA: Brooks/Cole. (Brooks/Cole, 511 Forest Lodge Rd., Pacific Grove, CA 93950) www.thomson.com.

Crawford, R. (1994). *Avoiding counselor malpractice.* Alexandria, VA. See American Counseling Association.

Forrester-Miller, H. and Davis, T.E. (1996). *A practitioner's guide to ethical decision making.* Alexandria, VA. See American Counseling Association.

Herlihy, B. and Corey, G. (1996). *ACA ethical standards casebook.* Fifth ed. Alexandria, VA. See American Counseling Association.

Herlihy, B. and Corey, G. (1992). *Dual relationships in counseling.* Alexandria, VA. See American Counseling Association.

Huey, W.C. and Remley, T.P. (1988). *Ethical and legal issues in school counseling.* Alexandria, VA. See American School Counselor Association.

Joint Committee on Testing Practices. (1988). *Code of fair testing practices in education.* Washington, DC: American Psychological Association. (1200 17th Street, NW, Washington, DC 20036) 202 336 5500

Mitchell, R.W. (1991). *Documentation in counseling records.* Alexandria, VA. See American Counseling Association.

National Board for Certified Counselors. (1998). *National board for certified counselors: code of ethics.* Greensboro, NC. (3 Terrace Way, Suite D, Greensboro, NC 27403-3660) 336 547 0607 www.nbcc.org.

National Board for Certified Counselors. (1997). *Standards for the ethical practice of webcounseling.* Greensboro, NC.

National Peer Helpers Association. (1989). *Code of ethics for peer helping professionals.* Greenville, NC. PO Box 2684, Greenville, NC 27836. 919 522 3959. nphaorg@aol.com.

Salo, M. and Schumate, S. (1993). *Counseling minor clients.* Alexandria, VA. See American School Counselor Association.

Stevens-Smith, P. and Hughes, M. (1993). *Legal issues in marriage and family counseling.* Alexandria, VA. See American School Counselor Association.

Wheeler, N. and Bertram, B. (1994). *Legal aspects of counseling: avoiding lawsuits and legal problems.* (Videotape). Alexandria, VA. See American School Counselor Association.

Ethical Standards for School Counselors was adopted by the ASCA Delegate Assembly, March 19, 1984. The first revision was approved by the ASCA Delegate Assembly, March 27, 1992. The second revision was approved by the ASCA Governing Board on March 30, 1998 and adopted on June 25, 1998.

REFERENCES

Allen, J. M. (1992). *Action-oriented research: Promoting school counselor advocacy and accountability.* Washington, D.C.: Office of Educational Research and Improvement. (ERIC Document Reproduction Service No. ED 347477)

American Counseling Association [ACA]. (1995). *Code of ethics and standards of practice.* Alexandria, VA: Author.

American Guidance Service [AGS] Publishing. (2003). *Systematic training for effective parenting [STEP].* Circle Pines, MN: Author.

American Psychiatric Association [APA]. (2000). *Diagnostic and statistical manual of mental disorders (text revision)* (4th ed.). Washington, D.C.: Author.

American School Counselor Association [ASCA]. (1998). *Ethical standards for school counselors.* Alexandria, VA: Author.

American School Counselor Association [ASCA]. (2003a). *The ASCA national model: A framework for school counseling programs.* Alexandria, VA: Author.

American School Counselor Association [ASCA]. (2003b). *Position statement: Child abuse.* Alexandria, VA: Author.

American School Counselor Association [ASCA]. (2002a). *Position statement: Confidentiality.* Alexandria, VA: Author.

American School Counselor Association [ASCA]. (2001). *Position statement: Discipline.* Alexandria, VA: Author.

American School Counselor Association [ASCA]. (2000a). *Position statement: Educational planning.* Alexandria, VA: Author.

American School Counselor Association [ASCA]. (2003c). *Position statement: Evaluation.* Alexandria, VA: Author.

American School Counselor Association [ASCA]. (2002b). *Position statement: Group counseling.* Alexandria, VA: Author.

American School Counselor Association [ASCA]. (2002c). *Position statement: High-stakes testing.* Alexandria, VA: Author.

American School Counselor Association [ASCA]. (2000b). *Position statement: Noncredentialed personnel.* Alexandria, VA: Author.

American School Counselor Association [ASCA]. (1999a). *Position statement: Parent consent.* Alexandria, VA: Author.

American School Counselor Association [ASCA]. (2000c). *Position statement: Sexual orientation.* Alexandria, VA: Author.

American School Counselor Association [ASCA]. (1999b). *Position statement: Special needs students.* Alexandria, VA: Author.

American School Counselor Association [ASCA]. (1999c). *The role of the professional school counselor.* Alexandria, VA: Author.

Anderson, R. S., & Reiter, D. (1995). The indispensable counselor. *The School Counselor, 42*(4), 268–276.

Annie E. Casey Foundation. (2002a). *Kids count 2002 data book online.* Baltimore, MD: Author. Retrieved February 4, 2003 from http://www.aecf.org/kidscount/kc2002/summary.htm.

Annie E. Casey Foundation. (2002b). *2000 census data—Language profile for the United States.* Baltimore, MD: Author. Retrieved February 4, 2003 from http://www.aecf.org/cgi-bin/aeccensus.cgi?action=profileresults&area=1&printerfriendly=0&section=8

Anthony, T. (2002). Reconstructing the Columbine horror. *The Daily Camera.* Retrieved May 9, 2002 from http://www.thedailycamera.com/shooting/reconstruction.html.

Association for Specialists in Group Work (1998). *Best practice guidelines.* Retrieved August 26, 2003 from http://www.asgw.org/best.htm.

Bailey, N. J. (2003). Safety for gay and lesbian students in our schools. *The Education Digest, 68*(6), 46–48.

Bailey, D. F., Getch, Y. Q., & Chen-Hayes, S. (2003). Professional school counselors as social and academic advocates. In B. T. Erford (Ed.), *Transforming the school counseling profession* (pp. 411–434). Upper Saddle River, NJ: Merrill Prentice Hall.

Baker, S. B. (2000). *School counseling for the twenty-first century* (3rd ed.). Upper Saddle River, NJ: Merrill/Prentice Hall.

Baker, S. B. (1994). Mandatory teaching experience for school counselors: An impediment to uniform certification standards for school counselors. *Counselor Education & Supervision, 33*(4), 314–326.

Baker, S. B. (2001). Reflections on forty years in the school counseling profession: Is the glass half full or half empty? *Professional School Counseling, 5*(2), 75–83.

Bauman, S., & Sachs-Kapp, P. (1998). A school takes a stand: Promotion of sexual orientation workshops by counselors. *Professional School Counseling, 1*(3), 42–45.

Beale, A. V., & McCay, E. (2001). Selecting school counselors: What administrators should look for in prospective counselors. *The Clearing House, 74*(5), 257–260.

Bemak, F. (2000). Transforming the role of the counselor to provide leadership in educational reform through collaboration. *Professional School Counseling, 3*(5), 323–331.

Bennis, W., & Nanus, B. (1985). *Leaders: The strategies for taking charge.* New York: Harper & Row.

Birdsall, B. A., & Miller, L. D. (2002). Brief counseling in the schools: A solution-focused approach for school counselors. *Counseling and Human Development, 35*(2), 1–10.

Black, J., & Underwood, J. (1998). Young, female, and gay: Lesbian students and the school environment. *Professional School Counseling, 1*(3), 15–20.

Boes, S. R., VanZile-Tamsen, C., & Jackson, C. M. (2001). Portfolio development for 21st century school counselors. *Professional School Counseling, 4*(3), 229–232.

Borden, W. (1992). Narrative perspectives in psychosocial intervention following adverse life events. *Social Work, 37*(2), 135–141.

Borders, L. D., & Drury, S. M. (1992). Comprehensive school counseling programs: A review for policymakers and practitioners. *Journal of Counseling & Development, 70*(4), 487–498.

Bowen, M. (1978). *Family therapy in clinical practice.* New York: Jason Aronson.

Bowers, J., & Hatch, T. (2002). *ASCA intensive training workshop: The ASCA national model.* Session presented at the annual meeting of the American School Counselor Association, Miami, FL.

Bradley, L., & Lewis, J. (2000). Introduction. In J. Lewis & L. Bradley (Eds.), *Advocacy in counseling: Counselors, clients, & community* (pp. 3–4). Greensboro, NC: ERIC Clearinghouse on Counseling and Student Services.

Brott, P. E., & Myers, J. E. (1999). Development of professional school counselor identity: A grounded theory. *Professional School Counseling, 2*(5), 339–348.

Brown, D. (1999a). *Improving academic achievement: What school counselors can do.* Greensboro, NC: ERIC Clearinghouse on Counseling and Student Services. (ERIC Document Reproduction Service No. ED435895)

Brown, D. (1999b). *Proven strategies for improving learning & achievement.* Greensboro, NC: CAPS Publications.

Brown, D., Pryzwansky, W. B., & Schulte, A. C. (2001). *Psychological consultation: Introduction to theory and practice* (5th ed.). Needham Heights, MA: Allyn & Bacon.

Bruce, M. A. (1995). Brief counseling: An effective model for change. *The School Counselor, 42*(5), 353–363.

Bruce, M. A., & Hopper, G. C. (1997). Brief counseling versus traditional counseling: A comparison of effectiveness. *The School Counselor, 44*(3), 171–184.

Bruce, M. A., Shade, R. A., & Cossairt, A. (1996). Classroom-tested guidance activities for promoting inclusion. *The School Counselor, 43*(3), 224–231.

Burnham, J. J., & Jackson, C. M. (2000). School counselor roles: Discrepancies between actual practice and existing models. *Professional School Counseling, 4*(1), 41–49.

Burns, J. M. (1978). *Leadership.* New York: Harper.

Campbell, C. A., & Dahir, C. A. (1997). *Sharing the vision: The national standards for school counseling programs.* Alexandria, VA: American School Counselor Association.

Capuzzi, D. (2002, May). *The many facets of grief.* Paper used for course entitled *Grief Counseling.* Arlington, VA: Marymount University.

Capuzzi, D., & Gross, D. R. (2003). *Counseling and psychotherapy: Theories and interventions* (3rd ed.). Upper Saddle River, NJ: Merrill Prentice Hall

Carpenter, S. L., King-Sears, M. E., & Keys, S. G. (1998). Counselors + educators + families as a transdisciplinary team = More effective inclusion for students with disabilities. *Professional School Counseling, 2*(1), 1–9.

Cash, J. (1997). What good leaders do. *Thrust for Educational Leadership, 27*(3), 22–25.

Chaves, L. (2000). Responding to public school peer sexual harassment in the face of *Davis v. Monroe County Board of Education. Brigham Young University Education & Law Journal, 2,* 287–306.

Children's Defense Fund. (2002). *The state of children in America's union: A 2002 action guide to Leave No Child Behind®.* Washington, D.C.: Author.

Clark, M. A., & Stone, C. (2000). The developmental school counselor as educational leader. In J. Wittmer (Ed.), *Managing your school counseling program: K–12 developmental strategies* (pp.75–82). Minneapolis, MN: Educational Media Corporation.

Clemente, R., & Collison, B. B. (2000). The relationships among counselors, ESL teachers, and students. *Professional School Counseling, 3*(5), 339–348.

Conroy, E., & Mayer, S. (1994). Strategies for consulting with parents. *Elementary School Guidance & Counseling, 29*(1), 60–66.

Constantine, M. G., & Gainor, K. A. (2001). Emotional intelligence and empathy: Their relation to multicultural counseling knowledge and awareness. *Professional School Counseling, 5*(2), 131–137.

Cooley, J. J. (1998). Gay and lesbian adolescents: Presenting problems and the counselor's role. *Professional School Counseling, 1*(3), 30–34.

Corey, G., Corey, M. S., & Callanan, P. (2002). *Issues and ethics in the helping professions.* Pacific Grove, CA: Brooks/Cole.

Council for Accreditation of Counseling and Related Educational Programs [CACREP]. (2001). *The 2001 standards.* Alexandria, VA: American Counseling Association.

Covey, S. R. (1989). *The seven habits of highly effective people.* New York: Simon & Schuster.

Cromwell, S. (1999). Conflict resolution education: Four approaches. *Education World,* Retrieved October 17, 2001 from http://www.educationworld.com/a_curr/curr171.shtml.

Cuthbert, B. (2002). Involving and responding to parents: Opportunities and challenges. In N. Gysbers & P. Henderson (Eds.),

Implementing comprehensive school guidance programs: Critical leadership issues and successful responses (pp. 79–88). Greensboro, NC: ERIC Clearinghouse on Counseling and Student Services.

Dahir, C. A., & House, R. M. (2002, October). *Connecting pre-service with practice: CACREP-TSCI-National Standards.* Presentation at the biannual conference of the Association for Counselor Education & Supervision, Park City, UT.

Dahir, C. A. (2000). The national standards for school counseling programs: A partnership in preparing students for the new millennium. *NASSP Bulletin, 84*(116), 68–76.

Dahir, C. A., & Tyra, B. (2002, July). *Beyond the National Standards: Building leadership capacity to change paradigms and expectations.* Session presented at the annual conference of the American School Counselor Association, Miami, FL.

Dansby-Giles, G. (2002). Ethics: Handling requests for confidential information is not always as simple as black and white. *ASCA School Counselor, 39*(3), 22–25.

Dansby-Giles, G., Carpenter, J., Howes, J., Hubert, R.M., Huss, S. Norris, Kraus, K., Reed, S., Thomas, R., & Whitledge, J. (1999). *Report of the ASCA Ethics Committee: 1997–1999.* Alexandria, VA: American School Counselor Association. (ERIC Document Reproduction Service No. ED448361)

Daughhetee, C., & Grant, D. (2002). Stress management. *ASCA School Counselor, 39*(6), 16–19.

Davis, J. L. & Mickelson, D. J. (1994). School counselors: Are you aware of ethical and legal aspects of counseling? *The School Counselor, 42*(1), 5–13.

Davis, K. M., & Garrett, M. T. (1998). Bridging the gap between school counselors and teachers: A proactive approach. *Professional School Counseling, 1*(5), 54–55.

Davis, T. E., & Osborn, C. J. (1999). The solution-focused school: An exceptional model. *NASSP Bulletin, 83*(603), 40–46.

Deck, M., Scarborough, J. L., Sferrazza, M. S., & Estill, D. M. (1999). Serving students with disabilities: Perspectives of three school counselors. *Intervention in School & Clinic, 34*(3), 150–155.

de Shazer, S. (1985). *Keys to solution in brief therapy.* New York: W.W. Norton.

de Shazer, S., Berg, I. K., Libchik, E., Nunnally, E., Molnar, A., Gingerich, W., & Weiner-Davis, M. (1986). Brief therapy: Focused solution development. *Family Process, 25,* 207–222.

Dielman, M. B., & Franklin, C. (1998). Brief solution-focused therapy with parents and adolescents with ADHD. *Social Work in Education, 20*(4), 261–268.

Dunn, N. A. W., & Baker, S. B. (2002). Readiness to serve students with disabilities: A survey of elementary school counselors. *Professional School Counseling, 5*(4), 277–284.

Dustin, D., & Ehly, S. (1992). School consultation in the 1990s. *Elementary School Guidance and Counseling, 26*(3), 165–175.

The Education Trust. (2000, July 2). *Summary of proceedings: Transforming School Counseling Initiative.* Session presented at the Education Trust Academy 2000 for Counselors, Fort Worth, TX.

The Education Trust. (2003). *Transforming school counseling initiative.* Retrieved August 19, 2003 from http://www2.edtrust.org/EdTrust/Transforming+School+Counseling.

Edwards, D. L., & Foster, M. A. (1995). Uniting the family and school systems: A process of empowering the school counselor. *The School Counselor, 42*(4), 277–282.

Eliason, M. J. (1996). Identity formation for lesbian, bisexual, and gay persons: Beyond a 'minoritizing' view. *Journal of Homosexuality, 30*(3), 31–58.

The Empower Program. (2001). Washington, D.C.: Author. Retrieved December 11, 2002 from http://www.empowered.org.

Ezell, M. (2001). *Advocacy in the human services.* Belmont, CA: Brooks/Cole.

Federal Interagency Forum on Child and Family Statistics. (2001). *America's children: Key national indicators of well-being.* Washington, D.C.: U.S. Government Printing Office.

Fitch, T., Newby, E., Ballestero, V., & Marshall, J. L. (2001). Future school administrators' perceptions of the school counselor's role. *Counselor Education and Supervision, 41*(2), 89–99.

Florida Department of Education. (2002). "Ride the wave" to success in the classroom: Strategies for classroom management. Office of School Improvement. Retrieved July 1, 2002 from http://osi.fsu.edu/waveseries/wave3.pdf.

Fontaine, J. H. (1998). Evidencing a need: School counselors' experiences with gay and lesbian students. *Professional School Counseling, 1*(3), 8–14.

Gingerich, W. J., & Wabeke, T. (2001). A solution-focused approach to mental health intervention in school settings. *Children & Schools, 23*(1), 33–47.

Gladding, S. T. (2000). *Counseling: A comprehensive profession* (4th ed.). Upper Saddle River, NJ: Merrill Prentice Hall.

Glaser, J. S., & Shoffner, M. F. (2001). Adventure-based counseling in schools. *Professional School Counseling, 5*(1), 42–48.

Glasser, W. (2000). School violence from the perspective of William Glasser. *Professional School Counseling, 4*(2), 77–80.

Glosoff, H. L., & Pate, R. H. (2002). Privacy and confidentiality in school counseling. *Professional School Counseling, 6*(1), 20–27.

Green, A., & Keys, S. (2001). Expanding the developmental school counseling paradigm: Meeting the needs of the 21st century student. *Professional School Counseling, 5*(2), 84–95.

Gysbers, N. C., & Henderson, P. (2000). *Developing & managing your school guidance program* (3rd ed.). Alexandria, VA: American Counseling Association.

Gysbers, N. C., & Henderson, P. (2001). Comprehensive guidance and counseling programs: A rich history and a bright future. *Professional School Counseling, 4*(4), 246–256.

Gysbers, N. C., & Henderson, P. (2002, February). *Steps in developing the yearly guidance program calendar.* Program presented at the Leading & Managing Comprehensive School Guidance Programs Conference, Greensboro, NC: ERIC Counseling and Student Services Clearinghouse.

Hanish, L. D., & Guerra, N. G. (2000). Children who get victimized at school: What is known? What can be done? *Professional School Counseling, 4*(2), 113–119.

Hanke, P. J. (1996). Putting school crime in perspective: Self-reported victimization of high school seniors. *Journal of Criminal Justice, 24*(3), 207–210.

Hart, P. J., & Jacobi, M. (1992). *From gatekeeper to advocate: Transforming the role of the school counselor.* New York: College Entrance Examination Board.

Hatch, T., & Holland, L. (2001). *Moreno Valley Unified school counselor academy handbook.* Moreno Valley, CA: Moreno Valley Unified School District.

Hazler, R. J., & Carney, J. V. (2000). When victims turn aggressors: Factors in the development of deadly school violence. *Professional School Counseling, 4*(2), 105–112.

Henderson, P. (1999). Providing leadership for school counselors to achieve an effective guidance program. *NASSP Bulletin, 83*(603), 77–83.

Hermann, M. A. (2002). A study of legal issues encountered by school counselors and perceptions of their preparedness to respond to legal challenges. *Professional School Counseling, 6*(1), 12–19.

Herring, R. D. (1998). *Career counseling in schools: Multicultural and developmental perspectives.* Alexandria, VA: American Counseling Association.

Herring, R. D., & Furgerson, K. (2000). Counseling issues with sexual minorities: An invisible minority school population. *The Online Journal, 1*(1). Retrieved February 8, 2003 from http://www.aglbic.org/Q/Vol1Num1/Herring.htm.

Hinkle, J. S., & Wells, M. E. (1995). *Family counseling in the schools: Effective strategies and interventions for counselors, psychologists, and therapists.* Greensboro, NC: ERIC/CASS Publications.

Hobbs, B. B., & Collison, B. B. (1995). School-community agency collaboration: Implications for the school counselor. *The School Counselor, 43*(1), 58–65.

House, R. M., & Martin, P. J. (1998). Advocating for better futures for all students: A new vision for school counselors. *Education, 119*(2), 284–291.

Hughey, K. F., & Gysbers, N. C. (1993). Evaluating comprehensive school guidance programs: Assessing the perceptions of students, parents, and teachers. *The School Counselor, 41*(1), 31–35.

Isaacs, M. L., & Stone, C. (1999). School counselors and confidentiality: Factors affecting professional choices. *Professional School Counseling, 2*(4), 258–266.

Jackson, C. M., Snow, B. M., Phillips, P. L., Boes, S. R., & Rolle, G. E. (1999). Professional school counseling: A new vision at State University of West Georgia. *GSCA—Georgia School Counselors Journal, 1*(6), 46–51.

Jackson, C. M., Stanard, R. P., Boes, S. R., Painter, L. C., Wulff, M., & Rolle, G. E. (2001). The school counselor: A key leader in school and community collaboration. *Alabama Counseling Association Journal, 27*(1), 1.

James, S. H., & Greenwalt, B. C. (2001). Documenting success and achievement: Presentation and working portfolios for counselors. *Journal of Counseling & Development, 79*(2), 161–165.

Johnson, L. S. (2000). Promoting professional identity in an era of educational reform. *Professional School Counseling, 4*(1), 31–40.

Jones, S., & Granello, D. H. (2002). School counseling now and in the future: A reaction. *Professional School Counseling, 5*(3), 164–171.

Josephson Institute of Ethics. (2001). *2000 report card: Report #1. The ethics of American youth: Violence and substance abuse: Press release.* Retrieved September 3, 2003 from http://www.josephsoninstitute.org/Survey2000/violence2000-pressrelease.htm.

Jucovy, L. (2000). *Mentoring sexual minority youth. Technical assistance packet #2.* Washington, DC: Office of Juvenile Justice and Delinquency Prevention. (ERIC Document Reproduction Service No. 449434)

Kahn, B. B. (2000). A model of solution-focused consultation for school counselors. *Professional School Counseling, 3*(4), 248–254.

Kelly, F. R., Jr. (1996). "That's not fair!"—Using RET to address the issue of fairness in classroom guidance. *Elementary School Guidance & Counseling, 30*(3), 235–238.

Keys, S., & Lockhart, E. J. (1999). The school counselor's role in facilitating multi-systemic change. *Professional School Counseling, 3*(2), 101–107.

Keys, S. G., & Bemak, F. (1997). School-family-community linked services: A school counseling role for changing times. *The School Counselor, 44*(4), 255–263.

Keys, S. G., Bemak, F., & Lockhart, E. J. (1998). Transforming school counseling to serve the mental health needs of at-risk youth. *Journal of Counseling & Development, 76*(4), 381–388.

Keys, S. G., Bemak, F., Carpenter, S. L., & King-Sears, M. E. (1998). Collaborative consultant: A new role for counselors serving at-risk youth. *Journal of Counseling & Development, 76*(2), 123–133.

Kiselica, M. S., & Robinson, M. (2001). Bringing advocacy counseling to life: The history, issues, and human dramas of social justice work in counseling. *Journal of Counseling & Development, 79*(4), 387–397.

Kopels, S., & Dupper, D. R. (1999). School-based peer sexual harassment. *Child Welfare, 78*(4), 435–460.

Kuranz, M. (2002). Cultivating student potential. *Professional School Counseling, 5*(3), 172–179.

Kurpius, D. J., & Fuqua, D. R. (1993). Fundamental issues in defining consultation. *Journal of Counseling & Development, 71*(6), 598–600.

LaFountain, R. M., & Bartos, R. B. (2002). *Research and statistics made meaningful in counseling and student affairs.* Pacific Grove, CA: Brooks/Cole.

LaFountain, R. M., Garner, N. E., & Eliason, G. T. (1996). Solution-focused counseling groups: A key for school counselors. *The School Counselor, 43*(4), 256–267.

Lankard, B. A. (1991). *Strategies for implementing the National Career Development Guidelines. ERIC Digest No 117.* Columbus, OH: ERIC Clearinghouse on Adult, Career, and Vocational Education. (ERIC Document Reproduction Service No. ED338898).

Lapan, R. T., Gysbers, N. C., & Sun, Y. (1997). The impact of more fully implemented guidance programs on the school experiences of high school students: A statewide evaluation study. *Journal of Counseling & Development, 75*(4), 292–302.

Lee, C. C. (1998). Counselors as agents of social change. In C. C. Lee & G. R. Walz (Eds.), *Social action: A mandate for counselors.* Alexandria, VA: American Counseling Association, 3–16.

Lee, C. C. (2001). Culturally responsive school counselors and programs: Addressing the needs of all students. *Professional School Counseling, 4*(4), 257–261.

Lee, R. S. (1993). Effects of classroom guidance on student achievement. *Elementary School Guidance & Counseling, 27*(3), 163–171.

Lehr, R., & Sumarah, J. (2002). Factors impacting the successful implementation of comprehensive guidance and counseling programs in Nova Scotia. *Professional School Counseling, 5*(4), 292–297.

Leithwood, K., Jantzi, D., & Steinbach, R. (1999). *Changing leadership for changing times.* Philadelphia: Open University Press.

Lewis, J. A., Lewis, M. D., Daniels, J. A., & D'Andrea, M. J. (1998). *Community counseling: Empowerment strategies for a diverse society* (2nd ed.). Pacific Grove, CA: Brooks/Cole.

Littrell, J. M., Malia, J. A., & Vanderwood, M. (1995). Single-session brief counseling in a high school. *Journal of Counseling & Development, 73*(4), 451–458.

Marinoble, R. M (1998). Homosexuality: A blind spot in the school mirror. *Professional School Counseling, 1*(3), 4–7.

McEachern, A. G., & Bornot, J. (2001). Gifted students with learning disabilities: Implications and strategies for school counselors. *Professional School Counseling, 5*(1), 34–41.

McFarland, W. P. (1998). Gay, lesbian, and bisexual student suicide. *Professional School Counseling, 1*(3), 26–29.

Metcalf, L. (1995). *Counseling toward solutions: A practical solution-focused program for working with students, teachers, and parents.* West Nyack, NY: Center for Applied Research in Education.

Miller, J. V. (1992). *The national career development guidelines. Eric Digest.* Washington, D.C.: Office of Educational Research and Improvement. (ERIC Document Reproduction Service No. 347493)

Mostert, D. L., Johnson, E., & Mostert, M. P. (1997). The utility of solution-focused, brief counseling in schools: Potential from an initial study. *Professional School Counseling, 1*(1), 21–24.

Muller, L. E., & Hartman, J. (1998). Group counseling for sexual minority youth. *Professional School Counseling, 1*(3), 38–41.

Muller-Ackerman, B. (2001). What I wish I knew. *ASCA School Counselor, 39*(1), 20–23.

Mullis, F., & Edwards, D. (2001). Consulting with parents: Applying family systems concepts and techniques. *Professional School Counseling, 5*(2), 116–123.

Mulrine, A. (1999, March 3). Once bullied, now bullies—with guns. *U.S. News and World Report,* 24.

Murphy, J. J. (1994). Working with what works: A solution-focused approach to school behavior problems. *The School Counselor, 42*(1), 59–65.

Murphy, J. P., DeEsch, J. B., & Strein, W. O. (1998). School counselors and school psychologists: Partners in student services. *Professional School Counseling, 2*(2), 85–87.

Myers, J. E., Sweeney, T. J., & White, V. E. (2002). Advocacy for counseling and counselors: A professional imperative. *Journal of Counseling and Development, 80*(4), 394–402.

Myrick, R. D. (2003). *Developmental guidance and counseling: A practical approach* (4th ed.). Minneapolis, MN: Educational Media Corporation.

National Center for Student Aspirations. (2001). *Students speak: My education and my future.* Orono, ME: University of Maine, College of Education and Human Development.

National Council for Accreditation of Teacher Education [NCATE]. (2002). *Professional standards for the accreditation of schools, colleges and departments of education.* Washington, D.C.: Author.

National School Safety Center. (2001). *NSSC Review of School Safety Research.* Westlake Village, CA: Author.

Nicoll, W.G. (1994). Developing effective classroom guidance programs: An integrative framework. *The School Counselor, 41*(4), 360–364.

Nicoll, W. G. (1992). A family counseling and consultation model for school counselors. *The School Counselor, 39*(5), 351–361.

Niebuhr, K. E., Niebuhr, R. E., & Cleveland, W. T. (1999). Principal and counselor collaboration. *Education, 119*(4), 674–678.

Nishimura, N. J. (1995). Addressing the needs of biracial children: An issue for counselors in a multicultural school environment. *The School Counselor, 43*(1), 52–57.

Nystul, M. S. (2003). *Introduction to counseling: An art and science perspective* (2nd ed.). Boston: Allyn & Bacon.

Office of Special Education and Rehabilitation Services. (2000). *A guide to the individualized education program: The basic special education process under IDEA.* U.S. Department of Education: Office of Special Education and Rehabilitative Services. Retrieved August 29, 2002 from http://www.ed.gov/parents/needs/speced/iepguide/index.html?exp=0.

O'Hanlon, W. H., & Weiner-Davis, M. (1989). *In search of solutions: A new direction in psychotherapy.* New York: Norton.

Olson, M. J., & Allen, D. N. (1993). Principals' perception of the effectiveness of school counselors with and without teaching experience. *Counselor Education & Supervision, 33*(1), 10–21.

Omizo, M. M., Omizo, S. A., & Okamoto, C. M. (1998). Gay and lesbian adolescents: A phenomenological study. *Professional School Counseling, 1*(3), 35–37.

Otwell, P. S., & Mullis, F. (1997). Academic achievement and counselor accountability. *Elementary School Guidance and Counseling, 31*(4), 343–348.

PACER Center. (1994). *Meeting the needs of all students.* Minneapolis, MN: Parent Advocacy Coalition for Educational Rights. Retrieved August 6, 2002 from http://www.pacer.org/parent/504.html.

Pelsma, D. M. (2000). School counselors' use of solution-focused questioning to improve teacher work life. *Professional School Counseling, 4*(1), 1–5.

Peterson, K. D., & Deal, T. E. (1998). How leaders influence the culture of schools. *Educational Leadership, 56*(1), 28–30.

Peterson, R. L., & Skiba, R. (2001). Creating school climates that prevent school violence. *The Social Studies, 92*(4), 167–175.

Phillips, P. L. (2000). *Leadership development profile.* Unpublished manuscript, State University of West Georgia.

Poland, S., & McCormick, J. S. (1999). *Coping with crisis: Lessons learned (A resource for schools, parents, and communities).* Longmont, CO: Sopris West.

Popkin, M. H. (2003). *Active parenting now for parents of children ages 5–12.* Marietta, GA: Active Parenting Publishers.

Portrait of a young tough. (2000, May). *NEA Today, 18*(8), 23.

Purkey, W. W., & Schmidt, J. J. (1996). *Invitational counseling.* Pacific Grove, CA: Brooks/Cole.

Quarto, C. J. (1999). Teachers' perceptions of school counselors with and without teaching experience. *Professional School Counseling, 2*(5), 378–383.

Quigney, T. A., & Studer, J. R. (1998). Touching strands of the educational web:

The professional school counselor's role in inclusion. *Professional School Counseling,* 2(1), 77–81.

Randolph, D. L, & Masker, T. (1997, Summer). Teacher certification and the counselor: A follow-up survey of school counselor certification requirements. *ACES Spectrum,* 6–8.

Reeder, J., Douzenis, C., & Bergin, J. J. (1997). The effects of small group counseling on the racial attitudes of second grade students. *Professional School Counseling,* 1(2), 15–18.

Remley, T. P., Jr., Hermann, M. A., & Huey, W. C. (Eds.). (2003). *Ethical & legal issues in school counseling* (2nd ed.). Alexandria, VA: American School Counselor Association.

Remley, T. P., Jr., & Herlihy, B. (2001). *Ethical, legal, and professional issues in counseling.* Upper Saddle River, NJ: Merrill Prentice Hall.

Rhyne-Winkler, M. C., & Wooten, H. R. (1996). The school counselor portfolio: Professional development and accountability. *The School Counselor,* 44(2), 146–150.

Rice, G. E., & Smith, W. (1993). Linking effective counseling and teaching skills. *The School Counselor,* 40(3), 201–206.

Richardson, V. (2002, May 13). Zero tolerance takes toll on pupils. *The Washington Times,* pp. A1, A14.

Ripley, V. V., & Goodnough, G. E. (2001). Planning and implementing group counseling in a high school. *Professional School Counseling,* 5(1), 62–65.

Roberts, W. B. Jr., & Morotti, A. A. (2000). The bully as victim: Understanding bully behaviors to increase the effectiveness of interventions in the bully–victim dyad. *Professional School Counseling,* 4(2), 148–155.

Rogers, C. R. (1942). *Counseling and psychotherapy: New concepts in practice.* Boston: Houghton Mifflin

Rogers, C. R. (1961). *On becoming a person: A therapist's view of psychotherapy.* Boston: Houghton Mifflin.

Rowell, L. L, & Hong, E. (2002). The role of school counselors in homework intervention. *Professional School Counseling,* 5(4), 285–291.

Russell, S. T., Driscoll, A. K., & Truong, N. (2002). Adolescent same-sex romantic attractions and relationships:

Implications for substance use and abuse. *American Journal of Public Health,* 92(2), 198–202.

Russell, S. T., & Joyner, K. (2001). Adolescent sexual orientation and suicide risk: Evidence from a national study. *American Journal of Public Health,* 91(8), 1276–1281.

Ryan, C., & Futterman, D. (2001, April/May). Social and developmental challenges for lesbian, gay, and bisexual youth. *SIECUS Report,* 29(4), 5–18.

Safe Communities, Safe Schools. (2001). Bullying Resources Page: Bullying Prevention. Retrieved November 1, 2001 from http://www.colorado.edu/cspv/safeschools/bullying%20resources.htm.

Schmidt, J. J. (2003). *Counseling in schools: Essential services and comprehensive programs* (4th ed.). Needham Heights, MA: Allyn and Bacon.

Schopen, E. A. (1997). Using brief strategic intervention to reduce the school avoidance behavior of seventh graders. *Professional School Counseling,* 1(2), 52–54.

Schwahn, C. J., & Spady, W. G. (1998). *Total Leaders: Applying the best future-focused change strategies to education.* Arlington, VA: American Association of School Administrators.

Sears, S. J. (1999). Transforming school counseling: Making a difference for students. *NASSP Bulletin,* 83(603), 47–53.

Shore, K. (2001). Success for ESL students. *Instructor,* 110(6), 30, 32, 106.

Siebert, A. (2002). Caregiver resiliency. *ASCA School Counselor,* 39(6), 10–13.

Sink, C. A., & MacDonald, G. (1998). The status of comprehensive guidance and counseling in the United States. *Professional School Counseling,* 2(2), 88–94.

Sklare, G. B. (1997). *Brief counseling that works: A solution-focused approach for school counselors.* Thousand Oaks, CA: Corwin Press.

Smith-Heavenrich, S. (2001, May/June). Kids hurting kids: Bullies in the schoolyard. *Mothering,* 106, 70–79.

Smith, S. L., Crutchfield, L. B., & Culbreth, J. R. (2001). Teaching experience for school counselors: Counselor educators' perceptions. *Professional School Counseling,* 4(3), 216–224.

Spruill, D. A., & Benshoff, J. M. (1996). The future is now: Promoting professionalism among counselors-in-training. *Journal of Counseling and Development, 74*(5), 468–471.

Stickel, S. A., Satchwell, K. M., & Meyer, E. C. (1991). The school counselor and discipline: A three-state survey. *The School Counselor, 39*(2), 111–115.

Stone, C. B., & Turba, R. (1999). School counselors using technology for advocacy. *Journal of Technology in Counseling, 1*(1). Retrieved November 18, 2002 from http://jtc.colstate.edu/vol1_1/advocacy.htm.

Studer, J. R., & Sommers, J. A. (2000). The professional school counselor and accountability. *NASSP Bulletin, 84*(615), 93–99.

Studer, J. R., & Allton, J. A. (1996). The professional school counselor: Supporting and understanding the role of the guidance program. *NASSP Bulletin, 80*(581), 53–60.

Tarver-Behring, S., Spagna, M. E., & Sullivan, J. (1998). School counselors and full inclusion for children with special needs. *Professional School Counseling, 1*(3), 51–56.

Taylor, L., & Adelman, H. S. (2000). Connecting schools, families, and communities. *Professional School Counseling, 3*(5), 298–307.

Thompson, R. A. (2002). *School counseling: Best practices for working in the schools* (2nd ed.). New York: Brunner-Routledge.

Thompson, R., & Littrell, J. M. (1998). Brief counseling for students with learning disabilities. *Professional School Counseling, 2*(1), 60–67.

Toporek, R. L. (1999). Developing a common language and framework for understanding advocacy in counseling. Greensboro, NC: ERIC Clearinghouse on Counseling and Student Services. (ERIC Document Reproduction Service No. ED435905).

Trevisan, M. S. (2000). The status of program evaluation expectations in state school counselors' certification requirements. *American Journal of Evaluation, 21*(1), 81–94.

United States Department of Education [DOE]. (1998). *Preventing bullying: A manual for schools and communities* [Brochure]. Washington, D.C.: Author.

United States Department of Education [DOE]. (2002). *No child left behind: A desk reference.* Washington, D.C.: Office of Elementary and Secondary Education.

United States Departments of Education and Justice. (2000, October 26). School violence drops for third straight year: Fewer students carrying weapons to school (Synopsis of the Third Annual Report on School Safety). Retrieved November 28, 2001 from http://www.ed.gov/PressReleases/10-2000/102600.html.

U.S. Census Bureau. (2001a). *United States census 2000.* Washington, D.C.: Government Printing Office.

U.S. Census Bureau (2001b). *Americans with disabilities: 1997,* Table 5: Disability status of children under 15 years old. Retrieved September 14, 2002 from http://www.census.gov/hhes/www/disable/sipp/disab97/ds97t5.html.

Viadero, D. (2000). Lags in minority achievement defy traditional explanation. *Education Week, 19*(28), 1.

Watts, R. E., & Pietrzak, D. (2000). Adlerian "encouragement" and the therapeutic process of solution-focused brief therapy. *Journal of Counseling & Development, 78*(4), 442–447.

Whiston, S. C., & Sexton, T. L. (1998). A review of school counseling outcome research: Implications for practice. *Journal of Counseling & Development, 76*(4), 412–426.

Wittmer, J. (2000). *Managing your school counseling program: K–12 developmental strategies.* Minneapolis, MN: Educational Media Corporation.

Worzbyt, J. C., & Zook, T. (1992). Counselors who make a difference: Small schools and rural settings. *The School Counselor, 39*(5), 344–350.

Wrenn, C. G. (1962). *The counselor in a changing world.* Washington, D.C.: American Personnel and Guidance Association.

Yell, M. L., & Katsiyannis, A. (2000). Student-on-student sexual harassment: What are schools' responsibilities? *Preventing School Failure, 44*(3), 130–132.

Zigarmi, D., Blanchard, K., O'Conner, M., & Edeburn, C. (2000). *Developing leadership & character.* Escondito, CA: The Ken Blanchard Companies.

Zinck, K., & Littrell, J. M. (2000). Action research shows group counseling effective with at-risk adolescent girls. *Professional School Counseling, 4*(1), 50–59.

AUTHOR INDEX

Two indexes are provided for your use. The Subject Index presents all topics discussed in this book; the Author Index lists all authors cited in the text.

SUBJECT INDEX

Two indexes are provided for your use. The Subject Index presents all topics discussed in this book; the Author Index lists all authors cited in the text.

academic development, 107–11, 131
accountability
  action plans, 281–83, *284–85fig*, *286fig*
  evaluation, 276–79, 283–88
  goal setting, 280, 300–302
  reporting results, 288–96
  See also assessment
accreditation standards, 154
ADHD (attention deficit hyperactivity
    disorder), 142
administrators, 82–83, 175–81
  See also schools
advocacy, 227, 232, 259–74
ASCA Ethical Standards for School Counselors,
  31–55
ASCA National Model: A Framework for School
  Counseling Programs (ASCA), 22–24
ASCA National Standards for School Counseling
  (Campbell & Dahir), 20, *21fig*
assessment
  research and, 53, 268
  of student needs, 67, 108–9
  testing, 41–42, 99–103
  See also accountability
attendance officers, 189–90
attention deficit hyperactivity disorder
    (ADHD), 142

behavior contracts, 169–70
Beth (middle school counselor)
  on advocacy, 272
  on collaboration, 155, 166, 170, 176, 181,
    204
  on counseling as a career, 4, 7
  on ethics, 35
  on evaluation, 278, 300
  on leadership, 255
  on professional development, 307, 317
  on roles of counselors, 72, 75–76, 82, 84, 89,
    98, 100
  on student support, 109, 112, 124, 132, 138

Bowers, Judy, 279
Brott, Pamela, 276, 278–97
bullying, 239–45

Career Week coordination plan, 89–95
CD portfolios, 313
changing families/divorce, 113–16
Chart Wizard, 290–93, 294, 295
children
  biracial, 133
  in the 21st century, 106–7
  stress, 111–13
  See also students
Child Study Team, 137–38, 184–86
classroom guidance, 75–79, 140–41, 160–61
  See also counseling services
classroom management, strategies for, 161–
  65
collaboration
  with communities, 85–88, 141–42, 190,
    211–14
  with parents and families, 43–45, 83–85,
    195–211, 213–14
  with school personnel, 141–42, 165–72,
    175–93
colleagues and professionals, 46–50
Columbine High School, 237–39
commitment, 222–23, 225, 230
communication, 226, 231, 288–96
  See also collaboration
communication targets, 293–96
communities
  advocacy action, 262–63, 266
  collaboration with, 85–88, 141–42, 190,
    211–14
  diversity, 133–35
  ethical responsibilities to, 50–51
computers, 42–43, 84, 267–68
conferences
  parent, 170, 203–4
  professional, 54
confidentiality, 33–37, 44–45, 84
  See also sharing information
conflict resolution, 246–52
  See also crisis response teams; intervention;
    violence prevention